Research on Child Language Disorders:

A Decade of Progress

Research on Child Language Disorders:

A Decade of Progress

*A volume marking the Tenth Anniversary
of the Wisconsin Symposium for
Research on Child Language Disorders*

Edited by
Jon F. Miller, Ph.D.
Professor of Communicative Disorder
University of Wisconsin, Madison
and
Associate Director for Development
Waisman Mental Retardation Research Center

8700 Shoal Creek Boulevard
Austin, Texas 78758

Library of Congress Cataloging in Publication Data
Main entry under title:

Research on child language disorders: a decade of progress / Jon F. Miller, editor.
　　　p.　　　cm.
　　　"A volume marking the 10th anniversary of the Wisconsin Symposium for Research on Child Language Disorders.
　　　Includes bibliographical references.
　　　ISBN 0-89079-408-1
　　　1. Language disorders in children. 2. Language disorders in children—Research. I. Miller, Jon F. II. Wisconsin Symposium on Research in Child Language Disorders.
　　　[DNLM: 1. Language Development. 2. Language Disorders–in infancy & childhood. 3. Rsearch. WL 340 R432]
　RJ496.L35R47 1990 ~ 1991
　618.92'855—dc20
　DNLM/DLC
　for Library of Congress   89-25120
                                                                                  CIP

Printed in the United States of America

pro·ed
8700 Shoal Creek Boulevard
Austin, Texas 78758

Contents

Preface

The Wisconsin Symposium for Research on Child Language Disorders has been held at the University of Wisconsin in Madison for the past ten years. The symposium has brought together scholars from the United States and Canada who are conducting research on language disorders in children. Each meeting has featured a keynote speaker, an invited paper or two, and 12 to 15 contributed research papers.

Over the past ten years, we have witnessed an increase in the volume of research on child language disorders, which has improved our understanding of the nature of child language disorders. We have also seen significant advances in the application of technology to research practice, a trend we expect to continue in the future. At the same time, many questions remain unanswered, and there are significant holes in our knowledge about language disorders and the children who experience them. It seems appropriate, therefore, to pause and take stock of our progress and point out the research needs for the next decade.

This volume marks the tenth anniversary of the Wisconsin Symposium on Language Disorders in Children. The keynote speakers for the past nine meetings were invited to submit chapters discussing current theory, development, and disorders, for the first section of this volume; all have contributed papers with the exception of David Crystal. The second section of this volume contains papers from 15 scholars who have made significant contributions to the language disorders research literature. These researchers were invited to write perspective chapters on what they consider to be the primary research needs in their area for the next ten years. The combination of chapters reflects the diversity of the field of language disorders in terms of theory, research methodology, and populations studied.

This research symposium is organized somewhat differently than most meetings because our doctoral students have significant decision and management responsibilities. The symposium committee, formed every year of doctoral students interested in child language disorders, has taken responsibility for selecting keynote and invited speakers, reviewing and selecting contributed papers, organizing all the details of putting on the conference, including the Mildred Berry Distance Classic, a 10-kilometer run along the shore of scenic Lake Mendota.

I would like to thank the many doctoral students who have worked so hard over the past ten years to make the symposium a successful research meeting. I am very grateful to all of these individuals for their contributions to the symposium and to furthering the general goal of improving our understanding of language disorders in children.

The cumulative list of symposium committee members over the past ten years follows. You will recognize many of the names on this list as a result of their productive research efforts since completing their doctoral studies at the University of Wisconsin in Madison. We are very proud of these past and present students and look forward to another decade of progress in research on child language disorders.

Finally, I would like to thank my colleagues in the Department of Communicative Disorders—Robin Chapman, Dee Vetter, Ray Kent, Larry Shriberg, Susan Weismer, Mic McNeil, Peggy Rosin, Gary Gill, Edie Swift, Mary Smith, Karen Carlson, Jamie Murrey-Branch, Linda Hesketh, Koan Kwaitkowski, Mary Lou Vernon, and Anne Heintzelman—for their support of the symposium over the years. In particular, I would like to thank Robin Chapman, who, in addition to giving support and sage advise and counsel, acted as faculty advisor for the 1982 meeting while I was occupied with a university crisis. In addition, those in the University of Wisconsin outreach program in Communicative Disorders directed by Michael Chial are to be commended for their administrative and technical support efforts that go into staging for symposium every year. The success of this meeting is testament to the fact that research on child language disorders has come into its own scientifically.

J.F.M.

Cumulative List
of Symposium
Committee Members

1980–1989

Name	Year(s)
Christine Dollaghan	1980–81, *chair 1980*
Thomas Campbell	1980–83
Rhea Paul	1980
O. T. Kenworthy	1980–83
Kristine Retherford	1980
Sandra Mayfield	1980
Heather MacKenzie	1980–82, *chair 1982*
Thomas Klee	1980–81
Francesca Spinelli	1980–82, *chair 1981*
Jan Bedrosisan	1980–81
Patricia Porter	1980–83
Steve Calculator	1980
Linda Daniel	1980–81
Jeffrey Higgenbotham	1981–84
Linda Milosky	1981–85, *chair 1983*
Susan Ellis Weismer	1981
Marilyn Kertoy	1982–85, *chair 1984*
Barbara MacLachlan	1982–87, *chair 1985*
Pamela Mitchell	1982–83
Elizabeth Crais	1983–86, *chair 1986*
Mark Mizuko	1983–85
Erin Dyer-Smith	1984
Pamela Mathay-Laikko	1984–1988, *chair 1987*
Katherine Odell	1984–89
Sara Pollack	1984–87
Ann Ratcliff	1984–87
Megan Hodge	1986–87
Diane Salmon	1986–87
Edythe Strand	1986
Nancy Streim	1986

Chin-Hsing Tseng	1986–87
Audrey Weston	1986–89, *co-chair 1989*
Christine Caldwell	1987
Roxanne DePaul	1987
Teresa Iacono	1987–88
Elizabeth Kay-Raining Bird	1987–89, *co-chair 1989*
Gordana Miletic	1987
Scott Schwartz	1987–89, *chair 1988*
Kathryn Barrett	1988–89
Marsha Clark	1988
Cynthia Cress	1988–89
Mary J. Graczyk	1988–89
Gregory L. Lof	1988–89
Giuliana Miolo	1988–89
Allison Sedey	1988–89
Ruth Martin	1989
Judith Morrison	1989
Hey-Kyeung Seung	1989
Ying-Chiao Tsao	1989

Contributing Authors

Dorothy M. Aram, Ph.D.
Associate Professor of Pediatrics, Case Western Reserve University
School of Medicine, Cleveland

Elizabeth Bates, Ph.D.
Professor of Psychology and Cognitive Science, University of California,
San Diego

David R. Beukelman, Ph.D.
Professor of Communication Disorders, University of Nebraska, Lincoln

Robin S. Chapman, Ph.D.
Professor of Communicative Disorders, University of Wisconsin,
Madison

Judith A. Cooper, Ph.D.
National Institute on Deafness and Other Communication Disorders,
National Institutes of Health, Rockville, Maryland

Susan Curtiss, Ph.D.
Associate Professor of Linguistics, University of California at Los
Angeles

Peter A. deVilliers, Ph.D.
Professor of Psychology, Smith College, Northampton, Massachusetts

Paul Fletcher, Ph.D.
Reader, Department of Linguistic Science, University of Reading,
England

Kate Franklin, M.S.
Doctoral Student, Department of Special Education and Communication
Disorders, University of Nebraska, Lincoln

Megan Hodge, M.S.
Department of Communication Disorders, Glenrose Rehabilitation
Hospital, Edmonton, Alberta, Canada

David Ingram, Ph.D.
Professor and Head, Department of Linguistics, University of British
Columbia, Vancouver, Canada

Judith R. Johnston, Ph.D.
Professor of Audiology and Speech Sciences, University of British
Columbia, Vancouver, Canada

Ray D. Kent, Ph.D.
Professor of Communicative Disorders, University of Wisconsin,
Madison

Laurence B. Leonard, Ph.D.
Professor of Audiology and Speech Sciences, Purdue University, West
Lafayette, Indiana

Brian MacWhinney, Ph.D.
Professor of Psychology, Carnegie-Mellon University, Pittsburgh

Paula Menyuk, Ph.D.
Professor of Applied Linguistics, Boston University, Boston,
Massachusetts

Jon F. Miller, Ph.D.
Professor of Communicative Disorders, University of Wisconsin,
Madison, and Associate Director for Development, Waisman Mental
Retardation Research Center

Katherine Nelson, Ph.D.
Distinguished Professor of Psychology, City University of New York
Graduate Center, New York, New York

D. Kimbrough Oller, Ph.D.
Professor of Psychology and Pediatrics, University of Miami, Coral
Gables, Florida

Richard G. Schwartz, Ph.D.
Associate Professor of Audiology and Speech Sciences, Purdue
University, West Lafayette, Indiana

Lawrence D. Shriberg, Ph.D.
Professor of Communicative Disorders and Staff Scientist, Waisman
Center on Mental Retardation and Human Development, University of
Wisconsin, Madison

Catherine E. Snow, Ph.D.
Professor of Human Development and Psychology, Harvard Graduate
School of Education, Cambridge, Massachusetts

Carol Stoel-Gammon, Ph.D.
Associate Professor of Speech and Hearing Sciences, University of
Washington, Seattle

Paula Tallal, Ph.D.
Co-Director, Center for Molecular and Behavioral Neuroscience,
Rutgers University, Newark, New Jersey

Donna Thal, Ph.D.
Associate Professor of Communicative Disorders, San Diego University,
San Diego

Dolores Kluppel Vetter, Ph.D.
Professor and Associate Dean of Communicative Disorders, University
of Wisconsin, Madison

Susan Ellis Weismer, Ph.D.
Assistant Professor of Communicative Disorders, University of
Wisconsin, Madison

SECTION I

Introduction

CHAPTER 1

Research on Language Disorders in Children: A Progress Report

JON F. MILLER

INTRODUCTION

Research on child language disorders has made progress in the past ten years in terms of characterizing language disorder and examining causal constructs. The concept of language disorder has expanded to include phonology and a host of language use variables. The study of language development has extended beyond the early school years to now include adolescence and, as a result, the age range of disordered subjects investigated continues to expand. The application of technology, including computer hardware and software, has begun to influence the scope and detail of research, providing opportunity to address questions that could not have been attempted ten years ago. Free speech sample analysis software, for example, provides researchers with the opportunity to study more subjects, in greater detail, more accurately and with greater efficiency than ever before. At the same time there remains a great deal not understood about the nature, cause, and maintenance of language deficits. Fundamental issues, such as the validation of indices of disordered lan-

Preparation of this chapter was supported in part by Research Grants Numbers, RO1-NS2551717, NIDCD, NIH, Judith Johnston and Jon Miller Principle Investigators, and RO1-HD22393, NICHD, NIH, Jon Miller Principle Investigator.

guage performance, have not been addressed consistently in the last decade. This chapter will document the current status of disordered language performance and review the major causal constructs offered as explanations for disordered language performance. Current understanding of language disorders and their causes will be discussed relative to directions for future research.

POPULATION

It is appropriate here to define the population that will be the focus of this chapter. The term *language disorder* will be the label of choice and will be used in place of such terms as *developmentally aphasic, dysphasic, language impaired,* and *language disabled.* The generally accepted definition of *language disorder* follows the one proposed in 1960 by a group of researchers meeting at the Stanford University at the Institute on Childhood Aphasia (PICA, 1962). The Stanford definition assumed maldevelopment or injury to the central nervous system prenatally, perinatally, or postnatally prior to the onset of words. The definition further specified that the language impairment may or may not be associated with other cerebral or neurological pathology. Specifically excluded were language problems associated with mental retardation, hearing impairment, central nervous system damage affecting the peripheral speech mechanism, emotional disturbance, delayed maturation in language development resulting from social and emotional factors, or physical factors not primarily due to central nervous system involvement. The definitions of *language disorder* described in the literature reviewed here generally conform to the definition delineated above, a definition by exclusion of various etiologies and not of a characterization of various inclusion criteria.

SUMMARY OF PAST RESEARCH: LANGUAGE DISORDERS

Despite extensive research over the past ten years focusing on the parsimonious description of language disorder, its characterization remains elusive. Research of this period has often asked the following prototypic question: "Do children with language disorder do 'X' or have/perform 'X'?" The answer has generally been *yes*, at least in the published literature, with disordered children performing less frequently, less accurately, more slowly, or with more errors than their peers on a number of linguistic and nonlinguistic tasks. In general, language-disordered children show a later onset of language skills, their rate of acquisition is slower, and they may never have the language skills of their peers, even as adults (Aram, Ekelman & Nation, 1984; Schery, 1985; Weiner, 1985).

Language disorder was considered a unitary construct in the late 1970s and early 1980s with notable exceptions (Johnston & Kamhi, 1984). In most studies of this period, single aspects of language performance (e.g., vocabulary, syntax, pragmatics) were studied. Recent review papers have argued that research focusing on the identification of individual variables as parsimonious characterizations of disordered performance is inadequate (Johnston, 1988; Van Kleeck, 1988). Rarely do children exhibit unique deficits at a single level; rather, children usually exhibit deficits at several levels of language performance simultaneously. Recent research, which has investigated how deficits at one level of language performance impact other levels of performance, appears to support this view. For example, Leonard, Camarata, Schwartz, Chapman and Messick (1985) and Camarata and Schwartz (1985) have explored the effects of phonological limitations on lexical acquisition. Similarly, syntactic deficits will alter performance on a variety of pragmatic tasks (Miller, 1978, 1981; Johnston & Kamhi, 1984; Johnston, 1988). Johnston (1988) argues that language-disordered children are communicatively impaired precisely because they lack command of language form. "Without sufficient grammatical resources, they have difficulty constructing cohesive texts, repairing conversational breakdowns, and varying their speech to fit social situations" (p. 693). Clearly we need to understand not only the interrelationships between linguistic levels but also the asynchronies within linguistic levels.

Developmental asynchronies have been observed within linguistic levels, (i.e., syntax) and between processes (i.e., comprehension and production). Example of within-level asynchrony can be found in studies that have documented simple sentence patterns developing in advance of grammatical functors and propositional embedding (Johnston & Kamhi, 1984; Liles & Watt, 1984). Asynchronies between language comprehension and production have been observed for some time in normal children (Chapman & Miller, 1975) and in various disordered populations, children with language disorders and mental retardation (Miller, 1987b, 1988; Miller, Chapman & MacKensie, 1981). Over the next ten years it will be important to investigate the proposition that asynchronies observed in the language profiles of language-disordered children may continue to change throughout the developmental period. Disordered language performance may look different at different points in time as a result of continued development, adaptation, or intervention. The concept of changing profiles of language disorder complicates the problem of characterizing disordered language performance.

Despite the extended number of variables investigated and the extended age range of the subjects studied, the general picture of the language disordered child remains the same (i.e., delays exist in the rate of acquisition of specific linguistic devices). Johnston (1988) summarizes the research to date that compares language-matched normal and disordered populations as follows. At the lexical level, lexical organization and phonological limitations on lexical acquisition were the same for normal and disordered speakers (Camarata & Schwartz, 1985), suggesting similar skills at the same language levels. At the sentence level, language-matched disordered speakers acquire the major grammatical categories and the rules for combination in the same order as normal children. Grammatical morphology appears to be the slowest among grammatical skills to develop, but does follow the same sequence as normal children. Text-level grammars are clearly delayed, but the developmental sequence of these skills requires more study. Children with language disorders evidence strengths in conversation skills. They are purposeful and responsive; however, communication is limited by their mastery of grammatical form. This summary of language performance is not much different than our conclusions ten years ago, though the range of language variables has clearly expanded and the developmental period required to reach adult language competence has been extended through adolescence. The characterization of language disorder and proposed causal constructs are closely linked, if for no other reason than the general definition of language disorder first used. The circular relationship between the definition of what constitutes language disorder and causal constructs put forth as explanations should be considered seriously. The next section reviews the causal constructs put forth to explain language disorder, with consideration of the circularity of the cause-consequence argument in language disorder.

STUDIES OF CAUSAL CONSTRUCTS

GENERAL SYMBOLIC DEFICIT

Studies of causal explanations for language disorders have focused primarily on cognitive constructs using Piaget's developmental model. This work has centered around symbolic function since Morehead (1972) first proposed that language disorders were but one manifestation of a general symbolic deficit. Children with language disorders were predicted to have deficits in all areas of representational thought. Early research by Inhelder (1966) and de Ajuriaguerra (1966) supports this view and three recent studies examining visual imagery (Johnston & Weismer, 1983), anticipatory imagery (Savich, 1984), and analogic reasoning (Nippold, Erskine & Freed, 1988) provide further detail about this causal construct. In general, as the imagery demands increased, the performance of the language-disordered subjects on these three different imagery tasks decreased significantly compared to the control subjects. The extent to which cognition can be shown to govern language acquisition (Johnston, 1985) influences the extent to which cognitive constructs will be investigated as possible causal constructs for language disorder. The link between cognitive deficit and neurological impairment in children is too compelling not to explore given the extensive work on the brain-language relationship in adults with aphasia. Are these deficits in symbolic function indications of neurological impairment or simply less general linguistic ability?

General symbolic functioning has also been investigated in younger children using tasks designed to tap representational or symbolic play. Terrell, Schwartz, Prelock and Messick (1984) found higher symbolic play scores for language-matched disordered children than normals at the one-word stage of development. The scores were below Chronological Age (CA) expectations for the language-disordered group. Roth and Clark (1987) studied older subjects using individual and dyadic play tasks. They found significant deficits in the play of the language-disordered subjects compared with language-matched normals. Terrell and Schwartz (1988) argued that play must involve object transformation to be considered representational or symbolic. They studied disordered children with age- and language-matched control groups on three play tasks: concrete, representational and symbolic. All three types of play were exhibited by the disordered and normal groups. The disordered children performed fewer high-level representational/symbolic play activities compared with concrete play activities. These studies support the work documenting a general representational deficit in children with language disorders. An extension of the work on the representational aspects of cognition is a series of studies on hypothesis testing, thought to be essential for language learning.

DEFICITS IN HYPOTHESIS TESTING

Hypothesis testing has been considered a central component of theories of language acquisition, particularly syntax, since the 1960s (Brown & Fraser, 1964; Miller & Ervin, 1964). According to these views, language acquisition involves actively analyzing language input, formulating hypotheses about linguistic structure, and then testing these hypotheses with new data. Several investigators have proposed that hypothesis-testing deficits are responsible for the limited language learning skills of language-disordered children (Kamhi, Catts, Koening & Lewis, 1984; Kamhi, Nelson, Lee & Gholson, 1985; Nelson, Kamhi & Apel, 1987). The results of these studies are inconsistent. Kamhi et al. (1984, 1985), report no group differences for normal and language-disordered children on verbal and nonverbal hypothesis testing tasks, but noted some language-disordered subjects did experience difficulty on the verbal tasks. The Nelson et al. (1987) study found that the language-disordered subjects solved fewer problems and needed more trials to find solutions than MA-mental age and CA-matched normal subjects. They explain their findings, however, as caused by less capacity and efficiency in verbal processing as well as nonverbal information processing. Further, they argue that language-disordered children have particular difficulty encoding information into short-term memory (STM) as opposed to storing and retrieving it. The performances noted in these studies may be related to STM deficits with the variability between study results accounted for by the STM load of the experimental tasks.

In a more specific investigation of short-term memory abilities of language-disordered children, Kirchner and Klatzky (1985) found STM rehearsal strategy deficits in language-disordered children when compared to control subjects. They suggest a general deficit in the verbal ability to actively maintain and regenerate items in STM. They also noted that coding in memory was different for the two groups when they evaluated their errors. The disordered children coded words semantically for recall and the normal children coded them phonetically. This view is somewhat supported by a "fast mapping" study reported by Dollaghan (1987). She found that both language-disordered and language-matched normal children exhibited similar comprehension skills for a single presentation of a novel word, but the disordered children differed significantly in their ability to produce the word. All children seemed to process the same information about the novel words in associating the word with its referent but the disordered children appeared to have difficulty producing the appropriate phonological sequence. This suggests the information storage requirements do not demand the same phonological mapping for comprehension as is required for production.

AUDITORY PROCESSING DEFICITS

The other major area of research into causal constructs has been in the area of auditory processing. Research through the 1970s produced improved research methods that allowed the identification of specific auditory processing in language-disordered children (Tallal & Piercy, 1973a, 1973b, 1974, 1975; Tallal, 1976). These studies identified the processing of rapid acoustic events as the primary deficit in children with language disorders. Research has continued in this area, exploring temporal processing skills in both visual and auditory modes and with linguistic and nonlinguistic stimuli. The results of this work indicate that children with language disorders have difficulty with temporal processing of brief, rapidly sequenced events regardless of mode or stimuli (Stark & Tallal, 1981; Tallal, Stark, Kallman & Mellits, 1981). While these deficits have received a great deal of attention as explanations for disordered-language performance, the causal link between perceptual deficits and language performance has not been made. Work in the past ten years has pointed out the complexity of auditory processing relative to the constructs of discrimination, attention, and higher cognitive processes. Auditory processing deficits can be viewed equally as causes or outcomes of disordered-language performance and at present researchers are unlikely to explain language disorders by simple appeal to perceptual deficits (Johnston, 1982, 1988).

OBSERVATIONS

LANGUAGE OUTCOMES PREDICTED BY VARIOUS CAUSAL CONSTRUCTS

Miller (1983) discussed the language outcomes associated with a variety of causal factors broadly classified as neuropsychologic factors, structural and physiological factors, and environmental factors. Language outcomes were categorized as deficits in comprehension, production, and use of language for communication for a number of general causal conditions. It is quite clear that a wide variety of conditions is associated with language disorder. There have been no studies, however, of the specific language-performance outcomes of the causal constructs reviewed in this chapter, with the exception of Curtiss and Tallal (see chapter 9) in this volume. The authors brings a fresh perspective to validating causal constructs proposed as explanations for language disorder. The analysis of productive language aimed at documenting performance deficits associated with temporal processing problems is an example of how future research will have to pursue the problem of linking cause and consequence in language disorder.

DESCRIPTIVE DATA CHARACTERIZING DISORDERED-LANGUAGE PERFORMANCE

One of the basic problems in this field is the lack of broad-based descriptive data on populations of children with language disorders. Careful description of the language, perceptual, cognitive, and neurological status of language-disordered populations is needed. This detailed description of disordered performance would lead to testable hypothesis about causal constructs that one day might explain the range of performance deficits evidenced by these children. The description of disordered language performance, however, will need to be expanded. The primary view of language disorders, at present, is developmental. Arguments claiming that disorders could only be defined relative to developmental status, as first proposed by Morehead and Ingram (1973), have dominated research. This view has been very productive in distinguishing developmental "errors" from deviant performance, but at the same time it may have discouraged investigators from pursuing performance "errors" lest they be viewed as developmentally ignorant. It is now time to consider the description of language disorder from two perspectives—development and error patterns. The clinical error categories proposed by Miller (1987) may serve as a beginning (see also Fletcher, chapter 8). Careful developmental and error pattern descriptions of language disorder would be useful in developing and testing hypotheses about potential causal constructs as well as individual adaptations to linguistic or cognitive deficits. The evidence for different patterns of language disorder will be taken up in a subsequent section of this chapter.

POPULATION CHARACTERISTICS

The variability of performance of language-disordered children on experimental tasks can be attributed in part to very general subject inclusion criteria within studies and a lack of consistent population definition among studies. Several population characteristics that are consistently documented in research populations warrant comment.

Neurological Status

Advancing technology makes statements frequently found in subject descriptions such as "no known neurological impairment" uninterpretable. Ten years ago, this statement reflected the state of the art of clinical neurological assessment. Today the statement simply means that the child's neurological status using the new sophisticated scanning devices available has not been explored (see Courchesne, Yeung-Courchesne, Press, Hesselink and Jernigan, 1988; Courchesne, in press) for recent neuroanatomical data on autistic children. Advancing technology has brought many new tools for documenting neurological status. Investigators must begin to use them on experimental populations in order to document neurological similarities and differences among subjects, rather than defining groups by exclusion. There may be a variety of causal conditions that minimally affect the nervous system that are not explored when constituting experimental groups. Advances in medical technology may help in defining a population of language-disordered children that truly has no "known cause." Developments in describing neurological status will be instrumental in linking models of child language disorders with models of adult language disorders. A life-span view of language performance would be important for the advance of theories of disordered-language performance.

Genetic Status

Advances in cytogenetic and amino acid analysis technology have allowed the identification of new disease processes for previously undiagnosed conditions. Such documentation is important for characterizing the biological status of potential research subjects. A recent case in the Madison (Wisconsin) public schools, involving a child with an IQ of 85 with language learning and behavioral problems, serves as an example. A cytogenetic evaluation revealed this child had fragile-X syndrome. It should be noted that mental retardation was not evident, though it is usually associated with this condition. Inclusion of such children in research populations of "language-disordered children" would certainly contribute to the heterogeneity of the results.

Mental Age/IQ

Characterizing the IQ or mental age of language-disordered and control subjects frequently ignores the research documenting the role of cognition in language development (Johnston, 1985). Investigators limit the IQ/mental age of their subjects on the lower end to avoid the classification of mental retardation. However, frequently IQ/mental age are left free to vary at the upper end, going as high as IQ 145 in more than half of the published research. This can only be interpreted as an indication that these investigators believe that advanced cognitive status will not accelerate language learning in the same way low IQ will dampen it, which is a curious interpretation of the literature. This practice certainly adds to the variability of experimental data.

Hearing Status

The impact of otitis media on language development is becoming more clearly documented (Hasenstab, 1987; Wallace, Gravel, McCarton & Rubin, 1988). Research involving young children should provide careful description of otitis history. Hearing status should be documented for middle ear integrity as well as acuity at the time the experimental measures are administered.

Socioeconomic Status

SES has been shown to affect language development negatively in almost all areas of language performance (McCarthy, 1954). Yet fewer than 35% of the published research studies on language disorders document SES status. Measures of SES using the 1980 census data are available (Stevens & Cho, 1985) updating the widely accepted Duncan (1961) occupational classification system for determining social status. For documenting SES as a variable associated with developmental progress, a combination of parent education level and occupation should be used. This information is readily available and should be routinely reported. If SES were routinely reported, it might be easier to generalize the results of research conducted in different parts of the country, in urban versus rural settings.

Intelligibility

The majority of studies reviewed have not reported the speech intelligibility status of the subjects. The high frequency of intelligibility deficits among this population suggests a significant difficulty. The practice of including only intelligible subjects may underrepresent the population and may limit the opportunity of documenting relationships that may exist between intelligibility and word- or utterance-formulation deficits in children. This aspect of productive performance is critical to understanding the relationship between speech and language at both the linguistic and motor levels.

CONTROL GROUPS

The use of control groups has become standard practice when investigating language disorders. Usually two types are used, a chronological- or mental-age matched group and a language-age matched group. The language measures used to match subjects are quite variable, ranging from comprehension test scores to Mean Length of Utterance (MLU). A number of recent studies of older children have not used language matches at all. The rationale for constituting control groups must come from the hypothesis tested in each study; therefore uniformity in control group description should not necessarily be expected. It is surprising, however, that less than 50% of the studies published in the past ten years have employed language-matched control groups. Without such controls, generalization across studies is difficult, if not impossible, because the general language ability of the experimental group cannot be measured accurately. However, several conditions have posed limitations on investigators wishing to employ language-matched control groups, most notably the lack of measures of general language performance. Investigators matching on language comprehension must choose between vocabulary measures, like the PPVT or syntactic measures like the M-Y or the TACL. MLU has been the most frequently used measure of language production for quantifying stage of productive performance for defining language-matched control groups. MLU is a valuable measure for the following reasons: (1) the high correlation with age; (2) it is stable; (3) the almost linear change across age; and (4) it allows investigators to predict an age range of normal children to sample (Miller & Chapman, 1981; Klee, Schaffer, May, Membrino & Mougey, 1989). MLU has limited functional utility in predicting age. It is applicable only to the first five years of life prior to when complex syntax is infrequently used. However, MLU has been criticized as a general measure of production because asynchronies have been noted in semantic and syntactic variables in disordered children at the same MLU level (Johnston & Kamhi, 1984). There are no general measures of language production that can be used either to identify disordered performance or to quantify general language development to define language-matched control groups for subjects older than 4–5 years of age. Such measures will be critical for the development of future experimental work on language disorders. See Miller (chapter 10 in this volume) for a detailed discussion of general measures of language production.

SUMMARY

Research on language disorders in children has addressed two major issues: (1) the linguistic skills and abilities that may characterize language disorder; and (2) the causal constructs that may explain deficits in language learning relative to other nonverbal cognitive skills. The general characterization of language disorder appears to be developmental. The data overwhelmingly support a view of disorder as delayed acquisition with grammatical features central to the disorder construct. Relative to causal constructs, the literature suggests that children with language disorders evidence deficits in nonverbal cognition, particularly in representational skills. The link between these cognitive deficits and language performance is weak and no causal direction can be proposed from the research to date. Other cognitive deficits noted in the literature on short-term memory for ordered stimuli and temporal aspects of auditory processing suggest a more molecular level of explanation. Future research into causal constructs will be helped by a more complete description of disordered-language performance.

The problem of language disorder has only been seriously examined from a developmental perspective (Miller, 1987a). The only substantive differences in acquisition between disordered and normal speakers are differences in rate of acquisition of various grammatical and semantic features compared to normal children. Johnston (1988) interprets these asynchronies as developmental differences because they deal with rate of learning, not deviant language form or meaning. The literature currently portrays language disorder as a delay in the acquisition of language, involving comprehension and production together or language production alone. This characterization suggests a performance deficit model where the language learned is not impaired but the acquisition rate is slow, which may be a reflection of various performance deficits.

Even with the extensive work to date, the description of language disorder remains incomplete. Investigators frequently comment in the discussion section of research papers that disordered subjects "make more frequent errors," respond with "much less facility," and produce the same complex utterance types but "less frequently." None of these terms is usually quantified or included as part of the experiment. However, these comments may provide important clues to descriptive categories overlooked since Menyuk first used them in 1964 (Menyuk, 1964). If the language production of a group of five-year-old language-disordered children was examined from a developmental as well as an "error" point of view, the results would find them delayed on developmental measures of form, with remaining differences among the children's language that can be described as errors of omission, formulation, rate, and fluency (Miller, 1987a). This view is supported by clinical data (Miller, 1987a) and suggests the existence with two different but related levels of description, one developmental, and one of the errors produced. This view can be tested empirically by asking if there are unique patterns of language disorder defined by analysis of productive language performance.

EVIDENCE FOR UNIQUE TYPES OF LANGUAGE DISORDER

General types of language disorder, generated by clinicians (Miller, 1987a) are included in Table 1-1. Documenting unique patterns of productive language performance requires validating the measures defining each type. Each potential measurement category listed in Table 1-1 must be evaluated to determine if it is measuring what researchers claim it is measuring (i.e., word finding, sentence formulation etc.). Validity is one of the most difficult constricts to deal with because of the private-event nature of much of language performance. Language production is directly observable and measurable. Recent advances in computer analysis of language production (SALT, Miller & Chapman, 1982–87; CHILDES, MacWhinney & Snow, 1986) provide the tools to examine the issues of validity of measurement categories and unique disorder types. An example of what will be required to document disorder types follows.

The set of measures examined here appear to be indications of formulation difficulty, false starts, repetition and reformulations and were called "mazes" by Loban (1976). The private-event nature of message

Table 1-1. A clinical typology of language disorders

Clinical Types	Measurement Level	Measurement Category
Sentence Formulation		A. Errors
		1. Overgeneralization
		2. Incomplete Utterance
		3. Word Choice
Word Finding	Word/Morpheme	4. Word Order
		5. NP-VP Symmetry
		6. Redundancy
Rate/Hyper and Hypo-Verbal		B. Substitutions
	Utterance	Omissions
Discourse/Pragmatic		C. Rate
		1. Words Per Minute
		2. Utterances Per Minute
	Discourse	
Semantic/Reference		D. Fluency
		1. False Starts
		2. Repetition
Delay		3. Reformulation
		4. Pause; Within and Between Utterances
		E. Development (Syntax)
		1. NP
		2. VP
		3. Negatives
		4. Questions
		5. Complex Sentences

Adapted from Miller (1987). Based on an ongoing project with the speed-language clinicians of the Madison Metropolitan School District.

formulation requires developing inferential measures based on utterances produced in various speaking conditions. Through controlling the speaking context, utterances can be analyzed, using measurement categories assumed to provide insight into the message formulation process. Miller (1987a) examined mazes to determine if they were valid indicators of utterance-formulation load. The study argued that the frequency of mazes was directly attributable to the message-formulation load placed on the speaker either internally or externally. Two hypotheses were examined. First, the frequency of mazes would be significantly higher in the narrative speaking condition as the result of increased formulation load over conversational speech. Narratives require the speaker to determine the form, content, and organization of messages, as well as monitor the listener's understanding of the message sequence. The second hypothesis asserted that speakers choosing to present messages in longer utterances would produce more mazes than speakers producing shorter utterances. Longer utterances are more likely to be multipropositional, requiring complex syntax with each proposition increasing the formulation load on the speaker, though self-induced.

The data set consisted of conversation and narrative samples from 162 normal children, 3–13 years of age. There were 27 children in each of six age groups at 3, 5, 7, 9, 11, and 13 years of age. False starts, repetitions, and reformulations (mazes) were coded in two 100 complete and intelligible utterance transcripts, one conversation and one narration, for each child. Mazes were coded together as one set of behaviors to determine their overall validity in documenting formulation load. SALT was used to analyze the frequency of mazes produced for each speaking condition and at each age. Table 1-2 contains the mean frequency of mazes for the 100 complete and intelligible utterance versions of the transcripts. The subjects produced significantly more mazes in the narrative condition than in conversation at each age. A striking feature of these data is the high frequency of false starts, repetitions and reformulations found in these transcripts. It has been generally assumed that normal speakers are fluent, producing relatively few formulation errors.

The contribution of utterance length to message formulation was examined by calculating the proportion of utterances containing mazes at each utterance length for each speaker. The analysis of these data reveal that speakers produce more mazes as utterances get longer in both speaking conditions, and this trend continues with increasing age. As speakers attempt utterances of longer length, they are more likely to produce a false start, repetition, or reformulation.

These data support the hypothesis that increasing internal and external demands on formulation will result in increased maze production. Mazes are therefore confirmed as valid indicators of utterance formulation complexity. Given these data we are now in position to examine the utterance formulation characteristics of language-disordered children.

Table 1-2. Mean percent of utterances with mazes in 100 complete and intelligible utterance samples for each age group. (n = 162, 27 at each age)

	Age					
	3	5	7	9	11	13
Conversation	.15	.19	.23	.23	.22	.23
Narration	.18	.25	.28	.30	.38	.33

Data from Miller (1986) SALT Reference Data Base Project, Language Analysis Laboratory, Waisman Center, University of Wisconsin–Madison.

Two different conditions associated with language disorders, each identified by mazes, have been discussed in the literature. Word-finding problems have been identified at least in part by maze behaviors (German, 1987). Utterance-formulation problems have been documented by MacLachlan and Chapman (1988). Both studies used normal control groups and found that children with language disorders produced more mazes than control subjects in narrative samples. The two studies confirm that mazes are produced more frequently by groups of language-disordered children. It is not possible to determine if these behaviors reflect a difficulty in accessing or recalling lexical items or in organizing them to formulate coherent messages. Several studies of word retrieval have found, however, that language-disordered children have word-storage deficits. They are less likely to store a word and less consistent in retrieval (Leonard, Nippold, Kail & Hale, 1983; Kail, Hale, Leonard, & Nippold, 1984). Studies attempting to document word-finding problems using free speech sample data have used the following behaviors: incomplete statements, grammatical errors, pauses, repetitions, reformulations, starters, time fillers, empty words, and word substitutions (German, 1987; Schwartz & Solot, 1980). This is a very diverse set of characteristics and the frequency and distribution of these behaviors in normal children is largely unknown, except for mazes. It is compelling that word-finding problems are expected in some children with language disorders (McGregor & Leonard, 1989), though it is doubtful that researchers would agree on the defining properties of this problem.

It is likely that both formulation and word-finding problems have unique patterns of productive language performance, but they remain to be described and explained. At present, clinicians recognize these as distinct categories, but there is considerable overlap in the dependent measures that have been used to describe each. Experience to date has shown some language-disordered children with high frequencies of mazes, more than one standard deviation above the mean for their age group, with longer mazes and more mazes per utterance than normal children. Other children combine long pauses with "ums" and "ers" prior to verb phrases, as well as frequently correcting word choices. The next step is to examine the length, content, and position of mazes to determine if clusters of characteristics are evident. References to individual variation in language patterns in language-disordered children are increasing, implying not that we are dealing with a single group, but perhaps several groups of disorders, each independent in character and perhaps independent in causal mechanisms.

Language production is the most often affected among language-disordered children. Production seems to be affected at a number of linguistic levels, as well as the frequency of utterances per unit time. Frequency is the most often used measure of disordered performance, from less frequent use of specific forms to less talking in general. Researchers are often heard to complain about how long it will take to gather language samples of comparable length from disordered as compared to normal children. A general measure of language performance should tap as many linguistic levels as possible without focusing on any single characteristic. Such a measure should capture rate, as well as form and content aspects of the language system. Several candidates have emerged from an ongoing project of productive language development in normal children (see Miller, chapter 10 in this volume).

SUGGESTIONS FOR FUTURE RESEARCH

1. Language disorder has been studied from a developmental perspective. There is ample evidence to suggest that it is time to study the errors, omissions, substitutions, and formulation problems of these children as well. The developmental perspective is necessary but not sufficient to document the range of communication problems evidenced by this population. The "error" perspective will be necessary to document different types of language impairment, should they exist.

2. Experimental groups of language-disordered children should be defined by the experimenter and not the child's service system. Differences both within and between service systems relative to criteria, as to who can receive services, testing methods, data, and interpretation create variability among subject groups and reduce the generalizability of the results. At present, it cannot be said with any confidence that a language-disordered child in Madison is the same as one in Los Angeles or Omaha.

3. Language-control groups need to be uniformly employed, which is more easily said than done. New measures will be needed to define age-matched groups on language variables that predict age through the developmental period. Some work has begun on this problem (see chapter 10). A great deal more work needs to be done to document predictive variables and how they function individually and collectively.

4. We can expect technology to continue to open new avenues of research. The computerized free speech sample analysis programs now available (Miller & Chapman, 1986; MacWhinney & Snow, 1986) and new approaches to comprehension testing (Cauley, Golinkoff, Hirsh-Pasek, & Gorden, 1989; Miller & Chapman, 1983) offer new opportunities for creative experimental work.

5. More descriptive work must be done using multidimensional models of language performance. The course of language development in disordered populations is subject to a variety of environmental stresses not experienced by normal children, including adaptation and intervention. Future research must address the relationship among variables through

the developmental period, the impact of lexical deficits on syntax, of syntactic deficits on discourse, and affect of unintelligible speech on message form and frequency for example. Characterizing developmental change and "error" patterns in language-disordered children should be the primary objective of the next ten years.

REFERENCES

Aram, D. M., Ekelman, B. L., & Nation, J. E. (1984). Preschoolers with language disorders: Ten years later. *Journal of Speech and Hearing Research, 27,* 232–244.

Brown, R., & Fraser, C. (1964). The acquisition of syntax. In U. Bellugi & R. Brown (Eds.), *The acquisition of language.* Monograph of the Society for Research in Child Development, No. 92. 29, 43–78.

Camarata, S. M., & Schwartz, R. G. (1985). Production of object words and action words. *Journal of Speech and Hearing Research, 28,* 323–330.

Cauley, K., Golinkoff, R., Hirsh-Pasek, K. & Gordon, L. (1989) Revealing Hidden Competencies: A New Method for Studying Language Comprehension in Children with Motor Impairments. *American Journal of Mental Retardation, 94,* (1), 53–63.

Chapman, R., & Miller, J. (1975) Word order in early two and three word utterances: Does production precede comprehension? *Journal of Speech and Hearing Research, 18,* 355–371.

Courchesne, E. (In Press) Comparison of Neurophysiological and Neuroanatomical Indices of Human Postnatal Brain Development. In K. Gibson, M. Konner & A. C. Peterson (Eds.) *Brain and Behavioral Development: Biosocial Dimensions* Hawthorne, New York: Aldine Press.

Courchesne, E., Yeung-Courchesne, B., Press, G., Hesselink, J., & Jernigan, T. (1988). Hypoplasia of cerebellar vermal lobules VI and VII in autism. *New England Journal of Medicine 318,* 1349–1354.

de Ajuriaguerra, J. (1966). Speech disorders in childhood. In E. Carterette (Ed.), *Brain function: Speech, language and communication* (Forum on Medical Sciences No. 4). Berkeley: University of California.

Dollaghan, C. A. (1987). Fast mapping in normal and language-disordered children. *Journal of Speech and Hearing Disorders, 52,* 218–222.

Duncan, O. (1961). A socioeconomic index for all occupations. In A. Reiss (Ed.), *Occupations and social status* (pp. 109–138). New York: Macmillan.

German, D. J. (1987). Spontaneous language profiles of children with word-finding problems. *Language, Speech and Hearing Services in the Schools, 18,* 217–230.

Hasenstab, M. S. (1987). *Language learning and otitis media.* Boston: College Hill.

Inhelder, B. (1966). Cognitive development and its contribution to the diagnosis of some phenomena of mental deficiency. *Merrill-Palmer Quarterly, 12,* 299–316.

Johnston, J. (1982). Interpreting the Leiter IQ: Performance profiles of young normal and language-disordered children. *Journal of Speech and Hearing Research, 25,* 291–296.

Johnston, J. (1985). Cognitive prerequisites: Evidence from children learning English. In D. Slobin (Ed.), *The cross-linguistic study of language acquisition* (Vol. 2). Hillsdale, NJ: Erlbaum.

Johnston, J. (1988). Specific language disorders in the child. In N. Lass, L. McReynolds, J. Northern, & D. Yoder (Eds.), *The handbook of speech pathology.* Philadelphia: W. B. Saunders.

Johnston, J., & Kamhi, A. (1984). The same can be less: Syntactic and semantic aspects of the utterances of language-impaired children. *Merrill-Palmer Quarterly, 30,* 65–86.

Johnston, J. R., & Weismer, S. E. (1983). Mental rotation abilities in language-disordered children. *Journal of Speech and Hearing Research, 26,* 397–403.

Kail, R., Hale, C. A., Leonard, L. B., & Nippold, M. A. (1984). Lexical storage and retrieval in language-impaired children. *Applied Psycholinguistics, 5,* 37–49.

Kamhi, A. G., Catts, H. W., Koenig, L. A., & Lewis, B. A. (1984). Hypothesis-testing and nonlinguistic symbolic abilities in language-impaired children. *Journal of Speech and Hearing Disorders, 49,* 169–176.

Kamhi, A. G., Nelson, L. K., Lee, R. F., & Gholson, B. (1985). The ability of language-disordered children to use and modify hypotheses in discrimination learning. *Applied Psycholinguistics, 6,* 435–452.

Kirchner, D. M., & Klatzky, R. L. (1985). Verbal rehearsal and memory in language-disordered children. *Journal of Speech and Hearing Research, 28,* 556–565.

Klee, T., Schaffer, M., May, S., Membrino, I., & Mougey, K. (1989). A comparison of the age-MLU relation in normal and specifically language impaired preschool children. *Journal of Speech and Hearing Disorders, 54,* 226–233.

Leonard, L. B., Camarata, S., Schwartz, R. G., Chapman, K., & Messick, C. (1985). Homonymy and the voiced-voiceless distinction in the speech of children with specific language impairment. *Journal of Speech and Hearing Research, 28,* 215–224.

Leonard, L. B., Nippold, L., Kail, R., & Hale, C. A. (1983). Picture naming in language-impaired children. *Journal of Speech and Hearing Research, 26,* 609–615.

Liles, B., & Watt, J. (1984). On the meaning of "language delay." *Folia Phoniatr, 36,* 40–48.

Loban, W. (1976). *Language development: Kindergarten through grade twelve* (Research Rep. No. 18). Urbana, IL: National Council of Teachers of English.

MacLachlan, B. G., & Chapman, R. S. (1988). Communication breakdowns in normal and language learning–disabled childrens' conversation and narration. *Journal of Speech and Hearing Disorders, 53,* 2–7.

MacWhinney, B., & Snow, C. (1986). CHILDES: Child Language Data Exchange System. Pittsburgh: Carnegie-Mellon University, Dept. of Psychology.

McCarthy, D. (1954). Language development in children. In L. Carmichael (Ed.), *The manual of child psychology* (pp. 492–630). New York: Wiley.

McGregor, K., & Leonard, L. (1989). Facilitating word finding skills of language impaired children. *Journal of Speech and Hearing Research, 54,* 141–147.

Menyuk, P. (1964). Comparison of grammar of children with functionally deviant and normal speech. *Journal of Speech and Hearing Research, 37,* 427–446.

Miller, J. (1978). Assessing children's language behavior: A developmental process approach. In R. Schiefelbusch (Ed.), *The basis of language intervention.* Baltimore: University Park Press.

Miller, J. (1981). *Assessing language production in children.* Baltimore: University Park Press.

Miller, J. (1983). Identifying children with language disorders and describing their language performance. In J. Miller, D. Yoder, & R. Schiefelbusch (Eds.), *Contemporary issues in language intervention* (Asha Rep. No. 12). Rockville, MD.

Miller, J. (1987a). A grammatical characterization of language disorder. In A. Martin, P. Fletcher, P. Grunewell, & D. Hall (Eds.), *First international symposium: Specific speech and language disorders in children* (pp. 100–114). London: AFASIC.

Miller, J. (1988). The developmental asynchrony of language development in children with Down syndrome. In L. Nadel (Ed.), *The psychobiology of down syndrome.* New York: Academic.

Miller, J., & Chapman, R. (1981). The relation between age and mean length of utterance in morphemes. *Journal of Speech and Hearing Research, 24,* 154–161.

Miller, J., & Chapman, R. (1982–87). *SALT: Systematic Analysis of Language Transcripts*: A computer program designed to analyze free speech samples—Apple II Version. Madison: University of Wisconsin, Language Analysis Laboratory, Waisman Center.

Miller, J., & Chapman, R. (1983). Using microcomputers to advance research in language disorders. *Theory into Practice 12,* 301–307.

Miller, J., Chapman, R., & MacKenzie, H. (1981). Individual differences in the language acquisition patterns of mentally retarded children. *Proceedings of the Second Wisconsin Symposium on Research in Child Language Disorders,* 130–146. University of Wisconsin-Madison, Madison, Wisconsin.

Miller, J. F. (1987b). Language and communication characteristics of children with Down syndrome. In S. Paschel, C. Tingey, J. Rynders, A. Crocker, & D. Crutcher (Eds.), *New perspectives on Down syndrome* (pp. 233–262). Baltimore: Brooks.

Miller, W., & Ervin, S. (1964). The development of grammar in child language. In U. Bellugi & R. Brown (Eds.), *The acquisition of language.* Monographs of the Society for Research in Child Development, 29(92) 9–34.

Morehead, D. (1972). Early grammatical and semantic relations: Some implications for a general representational deficit in linguistically deviant children. *Papers and Reports in Child Language Development,* no. 4. Stanford: Stanford University, Committee on Linguistics.

Morehead, D., & Ingram, D. (1973). The development of base syntax in normal and linguistically deviant children. *Journal of Speech and Hearing Research, 16,* 330–352.

Nelson, L. K., Kamhi, A. G., & Apel, K. (1987). Cognitive strengths and weaknesses in language-impaired children: One more look. *Journal of Speech and Hearing Disorders, 52,* 36–43.

Nippold, M. A., Erskine, B. J., & Freed, D. B. (1988). Proportional and functional analogical reasoning in normal and language-impaired children. *Journal of Speech and Hearing Disorders, 53,* 440–448.

PICA. (1962). *Proceedings of the Institute on Childhood Aphasia.* San Francisco: National Society for Crippled Children and Adults.

Roth, F. P., & Clark, C. M. (1987). Symbolic play and social participation abilities of language-impaired and normally developing children. *Journal of Speech and Hearing Disorders, 52,* 17–29.

Savich, P. A. (1984). Anticipatory imagery in normal and language-disabled children. *Journal of Speech and Hearing Research, 27,* 494–501.

Schery, T. K. (1985). Correlates of language development in language-disordered children. *Journal of Speech and Hearing Disorders, 50,* 73–83.

Schwartz, R., & Solot, L. (1980). Response patterns characteristic of verbal expressive disorders. *Language, Speech and Hearing Services in Schools 11,* 139–144.

Stark, R., & Tallal, P. (1981). Perceptual and motor deficits in language impaired children. In R. Keith (Ed.), *Central auditory and language disorders in children* (p. 121). Austin, TX: PRO-ED.

Stevens, G., & Cho, J. (1985). Socioeconomic indexes and the new 1980 census occupational classification scheme. *Social Science Research 14,* 142–168.

Tallal, P. (1976). Rapid auditory processing in normal and disordered language development. *Journal of Speech and Hearing Research, 19,* 561–571.

Tallal, P., & Piercy, M. (1973a). Developmental aphasia: Impaired rate of non-verbal processing as a function of sensory modality. *Neuropsychologia, 11,* 389–398.

Tallal, P., & Piercy, M. (1973b). Defects of non-verbal auditory perception in children with developmental aphasia. *Nature, 241,* 468–469.

Tallal, P., & Piercy, M. (1974). Developmental aphasia: Rate of auditory processing and selective impairment of consonant perception. *Neuropsychologia, 12,* 83–93.

Tallal, P., & Piercy, M. (1975). Developmental aphasia: The perception of brief vowels and extended stop consonants. *Neuropsychologia, 13,* 69–74.

Tallal, P., Stark, R., Kallman, C., & Mellits, D. (1981). A re-examination of some nonverbal perceptual abilities of language-impaired and normal children as a function of age and sensory modality. *Journal of Speech and Hearing Research, 24,* 351–357.

Terrell, B. Y., & Schwartz, R. G. (1988). Object transformations in the play of language-impaired children. *Journal of Speech and Hearing Disorders, 53,* 459–466.

Terrell, B. Y., Schwartz, R. G., Prelock, P. A., & Messick, C. K. (1984). Symbolic play in normal and language-impaired children. *Journal of Speech and Hearing Research, 27,* 424–429.

Van Kleek, A. (1988) Language delay in the child. In N. Lass, L. McReynolds, J. Northern, & D. Yoder (Eds.), *The handbook of speech pathology.* Philadelphia: W. B. Saunders.

Wallace, I., Gravel, C., McCarton, C., & Rubin, R. (1988). Otitis media and language development at one year of age. *Journal of Speech and Hearing Disorders 53,* 245–251.

Weiner, P. (1985). The value of follow-up studies. *Topics in Language Disorders* (June), *5,* 78–92.

SECTION II

Language Development:
Theory and Models

CHAPTER 2

The Biogenesis of Speech: Continuity and Process in Early Speech and Language Development

RAY D. KENT AND MEGAN HODGE

THE CONTINUITY HYPOTHESIS AND A BIOLOGICAL PERSPECTIVE

The bulk of recent evidence in several areas of human development favors the continuity hypothesis, namely, that during infancy and childhood, behavioral development unfolds in a smooth or continuous fashion with age rather than exhibiting sharp discontinuities (Bornstein & Sigman, 1986; Kent & Bauer, 1985; Vihman, Macken, Miller, Simmons & Miller, 1985). Developmental changes under the continuity hypothesis may be regarded as behavioral organizations and reorganizations that, correlated with remodeling of the nervous and musculoskeletal systems, maintain a substantial degree of underlying order. This view is consistent with three general developmental principles founded in biology. First, despite significant individual differences in quantitative aspects, the sequence in which major behavioral developments follow one another in a given species is remarkably consistent when typical conditions prevail. The second and third principles involve the notions of differentiation and hierarchical integration. Gottlieb (1983) points out that the behavior of nearly every developing organism evolves toward greater versatility and differentiation. These changes can be seen in more detailed perceptual representations, more refined motor activities, greater achievements in the cognitive sphere, and increasing individualization of style or personality. As one level of differentiation builds on a preceding one, identifiable integrated hierarchies form.

The theoretical challenge of this view is to identify aspects of organization that link various points of development, so as to maintain continuity, while also showing how this organization accommodates changes in the child's behavioral repertoire, so as to account for the maturation of behavior. From a clinical perspective, the continuity hypothesis has an important corollary: The continuity of development implies that (1) one can predict behavior at a later point in development from an appropriate behavioral organization at an earlier time, or (2) in some instances, later behavior is in some way dependent on an earlier appropriate behavioral organization. Of course, the word *appropriate* is key to the enterprise.

The continuity hypothesis holds not only across molar aspects of behavior, such as cognition, but also across the relatively molecular aspects, such as the perceptual representation of a class of speech sounds and the control of the speech apparatus to perform movements with particular acoustic consequences. Development, then, is viewed as an interacting confluence of several domains of behavior. Although this chapter emphasizes the development of sensorimotor systems that support language development, the authors recognize the inevitable and necessary interaction of sensorimotor development with other developmental domains, including language, perception, cognition, voluntary movement and socialization. Focus here will be primarily on the infant. The word *infant* means, literally, "without speech," but that is not to say that the infant is without capacities that significantly preconfigure spoken language. The continuity hypothesis and various lines of evidence argue that certain aspects of the organization of oral-verbal behavior should be identifiable during infancy. This chapter will suggest what some of these precursors are in the perceptual and motor domains and describe how they link with the form of spoken language behaviors.

The infant is viewed as a biological system whose development of oral-verbal behavior, and potential disruption of this development, are best understood using the theories, concepts, and principles of biology. Following Albert, Munson and Resnick (1988), the following primary principles should apply: (1) biological organisms are goal-directed; (2) these organisms require information (whether direct, indirect, or both) for their operation; and (3) they are programmed systems in the sense that processes at various levels of biological organization are under the control of collectives of information that become operative under specific and identifiable sets of conditions.

Biological systems are physical systems of a special kind because processes of the system are controlled by programs that are acquired and developed during evolution. In a given period of time, a population of organisms will possess a characteristic genetic program. Individual variations of this species-specific genetic program interact with internal and external environmental factors to direct the development of individual organisms at all levels of organization. The programs that regulate activities within cells or within physiologic or behavior sequences are ones that impart a goal-directed character to the systems and subsystems of the organism. These programs may be *closed*, that is, entirely the result of the decoding of information contained in the genome and its expression through internal biological systems such as the central nervous system or the cardiovascular system. Other biological phenomena require an interaction between the programmed system and the external environment for their operation. For these *open* programs, learning or conditioning is necessary. Some programs begin as open but become closed after required conditions are satisfied. Clinically, a biologic perspective has an important corollary: an oral-verbal disorder implies a failure or disruption in the operation of biological programs of information. Such disorders exist apart from social norms and values and apart from a society's ability to identify a condition or disorder, although the extent to which a handicap exists will depend on the particular individual and environment. In this view, research aimed at understanding both the information stored and acted upon in biological programs and the modes by which they operate to serve the function of spoken language is necessary to understand how such disruptions can occur and how they can be prevented or their effects on the developing child ameliorated.

STRUCTURAL AND MOTOR FACTORS IN EARLY VOCALIZATIONS

This biological perspective will be applied here to infant behaviors that the authors believe are linked to the eventual acquisition of language. A starting point for this inquiry is to consider the contemporary understanding of vocal behaviors during the first two years of life. Describing these behaviors is commonly approached in terms of a stage model. Stage models can be misleading in their inherently discontinuous portrayal of development (Kent, 1982) and because they capture only the nomothetic aspects of observable behavior rather than the range of normal individual differences necessary to apply the information to a particular case (Rutter, 1981). However, they are a convenient form of summary, used here for exactly this purpose and not to endorse them as the preferred means of understanding developmental processes. Stage descriptions will be taken as a point of departure.

Several stage models of vocal development in the first year of life are given in Table 2-1. It is immediately evident that the models differ in several respects, although they presumably are intended to represent a common developmental pattern (assuming that the infant subjects on whom these models are based did in fact behave as a homogeneous population). Significantly, the models differ not only in the stage labels but also in the number and duration of the stages. This outcome may mean that the behaviors lack sufficient discontinuity in their patterns to permit independent investigators to identify reliably equivalent categorical stages in vocal development. However, certain common features run through the various stage models, and it is these features, rather than the discrete stages themselves, that will be focused on in this chapter.

One general feature is an early (birth to one or two months) dominance of phonations that generally lack articulatory components other than vocalic elements. Holmgren, Lindblom, Aurelius, Jalling, and Zetterstrom (1986) observed that these vocalizations may develop in two phases, a first phase of continuous phonations and a later phase of interrupted phonations. Following this period is an interval in which the infant produces an increased number of consonants, most of which appear as single articulations accompanying a continuous or interrupted phonation. Oller (1978) termed this interval the expansion stage, because during this time the infant's phonetic repertoire increases substantially. Kent offered an anatomic interpretation of this stage, noting that it corresponds closely to the age at which the infant's vocal tract anatomy undergoes a major change (Figure 2-1). At about this time, the larynx descends within the neck, so that the pharynx lengthens and the larynx and velopharynx disengage. This anatomical remodeling of the vocal tract may permit a reliable distinction of nasal versus nonnasal sounds, a fundamental contrast that lays the groundwork for further increases in phonetic repertoire.

At this same time, or somewhat later, important changes occur in normal phonetic behaviors. Koopmans-van Beinum and van der Stelt (1986) presented data showing that during the period of about 2–5 months, there is a marked increase in sound productions associated with a single articulatory movement per breath unit. This behavior is essentially a consonantal articulation. The data of Holmgren et al. (1986) indicate that at about 5–6 months, a significant change occurs in the proportion of utterances that contain glottal/phonatory modulation versus the proportion of utterances that contain a supraglottal articulation. This

Table 2-1. Comparison of stage descriptions of vocal development during the first year of life.

Age, weeks

| 0 2 4 6 8 10 12 14 16 18 20 22 24 26 28 30 32 34 36 38 40 42 44 46 48 50 52 |

STARK (1979)
- Reflexive crying and vegetative sounds
- Cooing and laughter
- Vocal play
- Reduplicated babble
- Nonreduplicated babble and expressive jargon →

OLLER (1978)
- Phonation | GOOing | Expansion | Canonical babble | Variegated babble →

HOLMGREN ET AL. (1986)
- Cont. Phon. -Artic. | Int. Phon. -Artic. | Cont. or Int. Phon. + one Artic. | Phonatory variants ± Artic. | Cont. or Int. Phon. + Reduplicated articulatory movements →

ELBERS (1982)
- ← Vocalizing → | Repetitive → | Concatenating (manner — Place) | Mixing →

KENT
- Phonation I | Phonation II | Simple articulation with phonatory variants | Multisyllabic babbling (Reduplicated and variegated babbling developing in parallel) →

Selected stage systems are shown against age in weeks. The systems are from the sources given in the table. Abbreviations used in the table are as follows: Cont. Phon. = continuous phonation; Artic. = articulation; Int. Phon. = interrupted phonation.

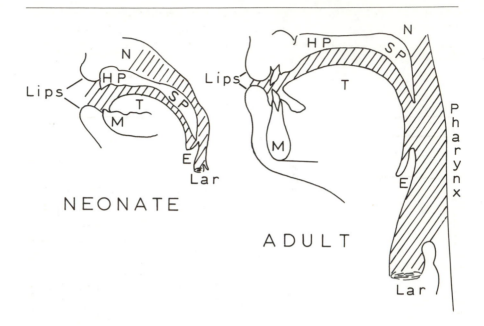

Fig. 2-1. Sketches of the vocal tracts (midsagittal sections) of an infant and an adult. Note differences in oropharyngeal channel (more right-angled in adult), laryngeal-velopharyngeal separation (greater in adult), larynx height (lower in adult), and relative tongue size (more fully occupying the oral cavity in the infant). Abbreviations: E = epiglottis; HP = hard palate; Lar = larynx; M = mandible; N = nasal cavity; SP = soft palate; T = tongue.

glottal/supraglottal shift may be a major phonetic milestone in that it points to increasing supraglottal articulation.

The various stage models agree in recognizing a major developmental advance at about 6 months, at which time an infant's vocalizations increase in complexity to include productions of multisyllabic trains. Until recently, this period of multisyllabic babbling commonly was thought to consist of two subphases, a stage of reduplicated babbling (in which phonetic elements are essentially repeated in a syllable train), and a stage of variegated babbling (in which alteration of phonetic elements occurs in a syllable train). However, recent studies do not confirm this pattern (Mitchell & Kent, submitted; Smith, Brown-Sweeney, & Stoel-Gammon, 1988). They point to a pattern in which reduplicated and variegated babbling develop concurrently rather than sequentially. Kent's stage model recognizes a consolidated stage of reduplicated-variegated babbling beginning at about 6 months. (The distinction between reduplicated and variegated babbling may reflect categorical effects in adult perception as much as it reflects genuine differences in the infant's vocal tract function. The infant may produce rhythmical opening and closing gestures with slight variations in velocity and positioning of the oral, pharyngeal, and laryngeal structures. The temporal and spectral consequences of this variability in sequential movements would then be subjected to differential categorization by the adult listener's phonetic decision space.)

There is an interesting congruence between repetitive babbling and repetitive body movements (Kent, 1982, 1984). Thelen (1981) observed that the peak occurrence of rhythmic stereotypies (repetitive movements) in the limbs, fingers, neck, and trunk is at about 9 months of postnatal life, corresponding to the age at which reduplicated babbling is typically observed. The question arises, is the repetitive organization of babbling an expression of a general tendency toward rhythmic and repetitive organization of movement, that is, a developmental proclivity across motor systems? Some support for this idea comes from the observation that reduplication is one of the few phonological processes not characteristic of both L1 and L2 acquisition. The peculiar association of reduplication with L1 is consistent with the view that reduplication reflects maturational processes and not a language learning process per se.

From the point of view of voluntary motor control, multisyllabic babbling represents a chaining or sequencing of motor responses. The multisyllabic pattern may be a useful preconfiguration of more complex multisyllabic patterns in adult speech. But, at the least, these utterances would seem to provide the infant with sensorimotor experience pertaining to articulatory movements and their auditory consequences. The enjoinment of auditory product with articulatory activity is strongly indicated by research on vocalizations in hearing-impaired infants. Contrary to some early reports, deaf children do indeed babble. However, the babbling is not the same as that in hearing children. One particular difference between hearing and hearing-impaired infants is that the former have an earlier onset of multisyllabic babbling constituted of CV (consonant-vowel) structures (Oller, Eilers, Bull & Carney, 1985; Kent, Osberger, Netsell & Hustedde, 1987; Stoel-Gammon & Otomo, 1986). The fact that hearing-impaired infants babble differently from hearing infants indicates that this early vocalization behavior is conditioned by auditory awareness. Support for this conclusion also comes from studies showing that some aspects of babbling are influenced by the language of the caregivers; that is, babbling is to some degree language-sensitive (De Boysson-Bardies, Sagart & Durand, 1984).

Hodge (1989) obtained acoustic measures of relative speech timing in reduplicated CV ([d ae]) chains (three syllables) spoken by eight infants between 7–9 months and compared these to similar chains produced by older children and adults. Despite rather large differences in the absolute durations of the segments and in the relative contribution of tongue and jaw movements, the mean ratio of the duration of the opening and closing gestures in the first syllable to the duration of the total cycle (opening to opening gesture) in the second to third syllables was strikingly similar for 3-year-olds, 5-year-olds, 9-year-olds, and adults (ratio of 0.75) and not statistically different (df 4, 35; $p = 0.70$) from that for the infants (ratio of 0.67). This result perhaps indicates that the relative timing of stop-vowel sequences is a stable property of vocal behavior, despite wide variations in the absolute durations of the sequence and of the articulatory actions used to produce the sequence. Temporal properties of this kind may characterize what some authors have termed *canonical babbling* (Oller, 1986).

In learning to produce speech, the infant ultimately needs to acquire the capability to produce a set of motor behaviors that realize linguistic intentions for the parent language. Each member of the behavioral set is itself a set of muscle contractions, a pattern of activity. Speech is typically described as one of many motor acts performed with a multilinked or multiarticulate system. In such a system, several muscle subsystems are mechanically joined to form a larger assembly. For example, the fingers, hand, wrist, lower arm, upper arm, and shoulder are part of a larger system, the *arm*. To control such a system effectively, we need to know the properties of the component systems and the ways in which the smaller systems cooperate for multilink movements. The developmental emergence of such a motor capability is partly a matter of what Thelen and Cooke (1987) termed *individuation*. They described this phenomenon with reference to the development of walking. The stepping responses of newborns are highly synchronous flexions and extensions of the hip, knee, and ankle joint. The transition from this infantile pattern to mature walking involves "the individuation of joint action from the obligatory synergy of the newborn period" (p. 392).

Individuation of muscle actions in speech may involve special, if not unique, phenomena. Consider that what is called the speech apparatus consists of systems with quite different structures and functions. Vocalization requires coordination of the relatively massive respiratory system consisting of bones, muscles, cartilages, and elastic lung tissue, with control of the vocal folds housed in the muscular and ligamentous structure of the larynx. The vocal tract itself is constituted of different types of muscle systems: the basically sphincteric systems of the velopharynx and the lips, the muscle and bone tissues of the jaw, and the muscular fluid-filled bag we know as the tongue.

The tongue deserves special note, both because of its primary role in vowel and consonant formation and because it remains the least understood component of the vocal tract. It has been termed a *muscular hydrostat* (Kier & Smith, 1985; Smith & Kier, 1989) in recognition of its essential structure—a fluid-filled bag, incompressible at physiologic pressures, that relies on muscle fibers not only for motion but also for skeletal shaping and support. The tongue is a muscular organ that achieves movement and shaping without the benefit of joints. It can be likened to a bag of jelly: a change in any one dimension causes a compensatory change in at least one other dimension. Thus, protrusion of the tongue is accompanied by a narrowing of its body. Flattening of its surface is accompanied by a widening of the body. To understand how the infant comes to articulate most consonants and all vowels, we need to understand how the infant learns to regulate a muscular bag of fluid.

In the infant, the tongue can be likened to a relatively broad and flat fluid-filled bag lying in the gradually sloping oropharyngeal channel (Figure 2-2). Local extensions and contractions of the muscular hydrostat would seem to be most effective in accomplishing a reciprocating or back-and-forth motion of the tongue, as is required for sucking and swallowing. Early vowel sounds in the first year of life are predominantly low vowels or mid vowels. The articulation of these vowels is somewhat akin to resting the fluid-filled bag—the tongue—on the floor of the mouth. Low and mid vowels can be produced by varying the amount of jaw lowering. Deformation of the tongue is minimal. The high vowels represent a more demanding articulation. For these vowels, the tongue must be significantly extended in some regions, and this extension is accompanied by a narrowing in its lateral dimension. High vowels like /i/ and /u/, rather infrequently observed in infant vocalizations, represent a significant modification of the muscular hydrostat from that appropriate for low or mid vowels. Although /i/ and /u/ tend to be infrequently produced by infants younger than about one year, these high vowels emerge as accurately produced vowels in at least some contexts during the second year (Hodge, in preparation; Otomo, 1988). In Otomo's data, the vowels /I/ and /e/ tended to be raised toward /i/, which result he interpreted to mean that /i/ functioned as a "motoric anchor." The differentiation of /I/ and /e/ from /i/ may require intermediate adjustments of the tongue hydrostat between its maximal extension for /i/ and its minimal extension for /ae/. Vowel /i/ may serve as a motoric anchor because it represents the pattern of muscle activity that accomplishes the maximum elevation of the tongue mass in the anterior oral cavity. In addition, vowel /i/ is a perceptual anchor. It marks the endpoint of a vowel axis that runs diagonally in the Bark F2-F1 by Bark F1 plane in the progression /a/ to /ae/ to /E/ to /e/ to /I/ to /i/ (Figure 2-3) and is typically characterized by high intelligiblity scores in identification tasks (Peterson & Barney, 1952).

During the course of consonant mastery, the hydrostat is put through additional maneuvers. Of particular relevance is bending. As Smith & Kier (1989) point out, bending of a muscular hydrostat requires two simultaneous adjustments: a decrease in length on one side and a resistance to change in diameter. If resistance to diameter change is not present, the

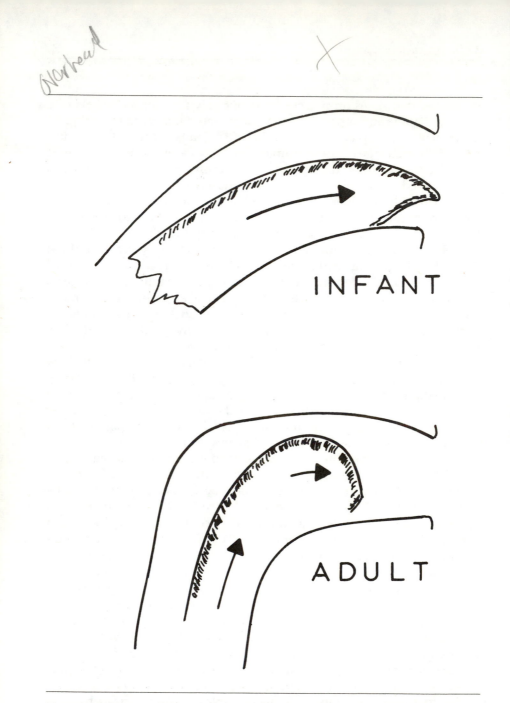

INFANT

ADULT

Fig. 2-2. Diagrammatic representation of the tongue as a muscular hydrostat in the adult and the infant. The infantile tongue is oriented more horizontally when head is in upright position, and regional extension is primarily in the area indicated by the arrow. Adult tongue has regional expansion-contraction possibilities in the areas indicated by arrows.

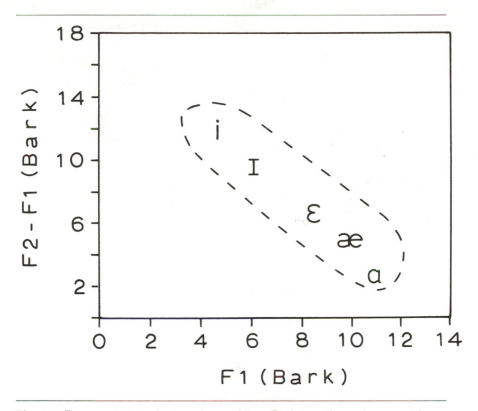

Fig. 2-3. Representation of selected vowels in a Bark-transformed space with Bark F1 and Bark F2-F1 as its axes. Note linear arrangement in this transformed space.

hydrostat will shorten on one aspect but not bend. The liquids /l/ and /r/ generally are produced with an articulation that requires bending. This adjustment of the muscular hydrostat may be a difficult skill for the young child, and it is relevant that gliding of liquids is a frequently noted phonologic process in early speech development (Figure 2-4). As is also shown in Figure 2-4, the earliest consonants to be mastered (/p m h n w g k d f j/) involve little or no bending of the tongue. Sounds that require bending tend to be acquired later. The achievement of motor control over the hydrostat may be a limiting factor on phonologic development.

Three general factors that may control important advances in speech sound capability, Velopharyngeal valving, motor sequencing of syllabic elements into trains, and control of the tongue contour, may condition later

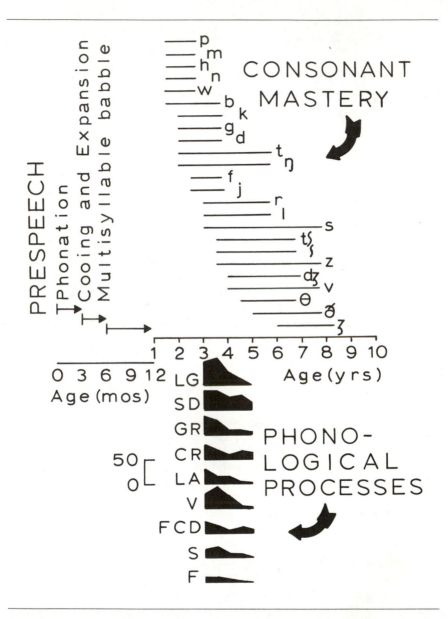

Fig. 2-4. Composite graph of the development of consonant articulation in children, showing: prespeech stages; consonant mastery, or age span for mastery by 90% of children (after Sander, 1972); phonological processes, or frequency of occurrence of phonological process errors (after Haelsig and Madison, 1986). For consonant mastery, consonants are identified by phonetic symbol: for phonological processes, the abbreviations are as follows: LG = liquid gliding; SD = syllable deletion; GR = glottal replacement; CR = cluster reduction; LA = labial assimilation; V = vowelizing; FCD = final consonant deletion; S = stopping; and F = fronting. Data are for American English.

prominent events in phonologic development. Certainly, these are not the only factors to be considered but they are sufficient to make the case that structural and motoric constraints are relevant to the operations of early vocalization.

THE DEVELOPMENTAL ORGANIZATION OF AUDITORY PERCEPTION

Recent work on speech discrimination by infants has been interpreted to support the hypothesis that perceptual capability is subject to either maintenance or loss, depending on experience. In the strong form of this hypothesis, the infant is born with the capacity to make the auditory discriminations required for the phonetic categories of language (Kuhl, 1988; Mehler et al., 1988; Werker, 1989). Some potential discriminations are lost because they are not supported by suitable auditory experience. Others are maintained through environmental interaction. A brief summary of research on this issue was given by Werker (1989), who also reported that recovery of a nonnative sensitivity is possible with considerable experience. Olsho's (1986) work indicates that infants' psychoacoustic abilities may have been underestimated in some earlier investigations. Taken together, these studies show that the human infant possesses a considerable ability to process the acoustic patterns of speech.

An interpretation of these results is that the infant is not a *tabula rasa*, on which the records of sensory experience are written, but rather a genetically programmed multipotential system. The capability for phonetic discriminations is lost without appropriate auditory exposure but they do not seem to be completely unrecoverable. In other words, the system does not completely lose its plasticity. At the same time, it would be misleading to assert that exposure to sound plays no role whatever in the perceptual discriminations required for speech. According to Edelman (1987), perceptual categorization is a prior ability that is seen as centrally important but is not in itself sufficient to generate adaptive behavior. In his view, nervous systems evolved to generate individual behavior that is adaptive within a species econiche in relatively short periods of time. Such behavior in an individual requires initial categorization of salient aspects of the environment so that adaptation can occur on the basis of resultant categories.

Neither a stringently stable nor a persistently plastic system would serve well the purposes of establishing recognition codes for speech. Rather, recognition codes would be most robust while permitting necessary modification in a system that has both stable and plastic modes. Such a system has been described by Carpenter and Grossberg (1987) in their account of stable self-organizing neural recognition codes. They point out in discussing the stability-plasticity dilemma that a system must be plastic to cope with new events but stable in the presence of irrelevant or frequently repeated events. The infant (and indeed the human throughout life) faces this dilemma. The irrelevant auditory experiences to which humans are continuously exposed would lead to a degradation of learned codes unless the organism is prepared to deal with these stimuli. Carpenter and Grossberg proposed that this degradation can be prevented if the system is sensitive to novelty so that it can distinguish between familiar and unfamiliar events, between expected and unexpected events. This requirement is met by the interaction of two subsystems, an attentional subsystem and an orienting subsystem. The attentional subsystem processes familiar events and, in so doing, maintains stable representations of these events and also establishes learned expectations (top-down processing) to stabilize processing. The orienting subsystem can reset the attentional subsystem upon the occurrence of an unfamiliar event. This subsystem determines if an event is familiar and adequately represented by an existing recognition code, or unfamiliar and therefore requiring a new code.

Seen in this way, the infant's recognition code for speech sounds (and therefore language) reflects an interplay of the attentional and orienting subsystems. A highly important question is when and how this recognition code influences the child's own vocal behaviors. As mentioned earlier, evidence points to a strong perceptual influence on babbling at least in the second half-year of life, and possibly earlier. The general scheme of the interactions among language environment, auditory perception of speech, and vocal (motor) behavior is sketched in Figure 2-5. Both perceptual and motor functions are controlled in part by genetic programs. For perception, this means that the infant possesses signal processing programs with normalized multicategory potential for phonetic discriminations. For motor functions of the vocal apparatus, this means that early sound production will exhibit universal (language-independent) phonetic proclivities (Locke, 1983). Underlying these phonetic proclivities for vocalizations are species-specific spectral and temporal patterns in their corresponding acoustic signals. Through exposure to the spoken expression of language, the infant develops a recognition code that increasingly matches the recognition code of the adult users of the language. Eventually, this recognition code will influence the child's own productions as he or she discovers the capability to replicate self-produced and other-produced auditory events. To some degree, this process may involve the incremental acquisition of individual phonetic elements in the

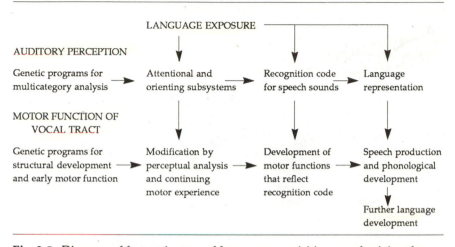

Fig. 2-5. Diagram of factors in normal language acquisition, emphasizing the interaction of genetic programs with experience.

perception and production systems. Alternatively, a more powerful process that enables rapid acquisition would be based on parameter fixation (Chomsky, 1981; Halle, 1988). Halle proposed that all human languages can be characterized with abstract and universal principles of parameter fixation. Perceptual-productive experience with speech sounds in the infant may be the expression of such a fixation.

Of course, this treatment of the subject leaves much that is unknown about children's recognition codes for language. A particularly interesting question is whether these codes come about through the development of perceptual algorithms (Bernstein, 1982) or through nonalgorithmic means. One possibility for the latter is an annealing process (Hastings & Waner, 1984, 1987). An annealing system consists of a state space, a potential energy function mapped on the state space, and a stochastic noise. Stable regions in the state space are local energy minima, or "potential wells." Figure 2-6 is a simple sketch of such wells. To give this meaning for speech recognition, think of each well on the surface as an emerging phonetic category, that is, an attractor of speech inputs. As a well deepens and broadens, it becomes a broader attractor. This system can achieve an evolutionary learning if its states are modes of information and its state transitions depend on environmental inputs combined with ergodic searching.

This kind of system seems consistent with two powerful features of auditory perception that are present even in the infant: phonetic equivalence and prototypicality (Greiser & Kuhl, in press). Phonetic equivalence is observed when stimuli that differ in their acoustic properties are treated as the same stimulus category, for example, the same phoneme.

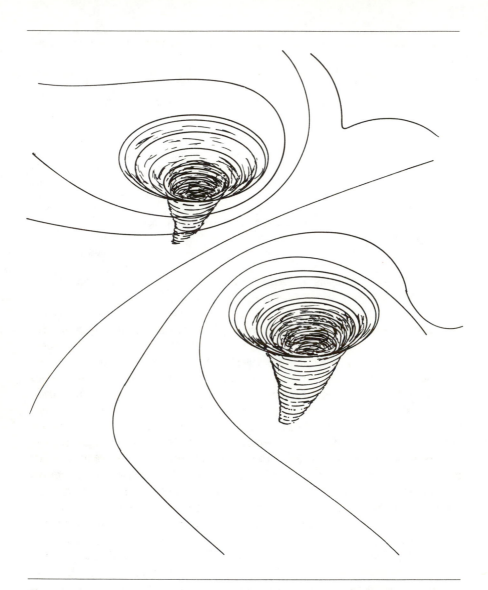

Fig. 2-6. Artistic impression of "potential wells" that serve as attractors in an energy space. Wells are analogous to phonetic categories in auditory perception and may be one aspect of the genetic program for signal processing.

Prototypicality means that despite this categorical bundling of different stimuli, they are not equally effective as category exemplars. A prototypical stimulus is a "best" stimulus, one that most effectively or reliably evokes the category in question. It seems reasonable that a prototypical stimulus would be at the center of an energy well whereas other stimuli within the category would be within the well but not necessarily at its center.

THE BIOLOGY OF CHANGE

It should be emphasized that a biological perspective does not assume or necessarily predict a high degree of uniformity in normally developing behaviors. The logical outcome of complex interactions of both stable and changing genetic and environmental influences over time must be individual differences in behavior, therefore predicting pluralism in behavioral developments such as speech. In their study of ten children aged 9 to 16 months, Vihman, Ferguson and Elbert (1986) observed substantial individual differences even in the earliest developmental period for phonetic tendencies, consonant use in babbling and early words, and phonological word-selection patterns. Vihman et al. concluded from their data that "the origins of phonology must be traced to the prelinguistic period" (p. 36), and that the general pattern of phonological development is toward greater uniformity as language knowledge grows. These two conclusions are complementary. The first points to the essential continuity of the developmental process. The second points to the constraining influence of the ambient language, which under normal circumstances inevitably must shape the vocal behaviors of the child.

Studies of the development of other motor skills also show that infants can reach a comparable behavioral capability through quite different developmental routes. This conclusion was reached for locomotor strategies by Bottos et al. (1989). Their study included a control (normal) group of 154 infants. These infants as well as an index group of infants from a neonatal intensive care unit were observed to determine the locomotor strategies that preceded independent walking. As shown in Figure 2-7, four major patterns were observed: crawling on hands and knees (70% of the control group), stomach creeping (5%), bottom shuffling (9%), and no distinct locomotor pattern before erect walking (16%). Figure 2-7 illustrates the range of onset age and mean age for crawling, creeping, and shuffling. The mean age of unaided walking for each subgroup is shown by the diamond symbol. The mean age for unaided walking is in the range of 12–14 months for the four subgroups. Apparently, the timely occurrence of walking does not depend on a specific pattern of preceding locomotory experience although some experiences are more common than others and at-risk infants may show different locomotor patterns (Bottos et al., 1989).

The development of walking is relevant here for another reason. Zelazo (1983) has argued for a behavioral-cognitive perspective on the development of walking, hypothesizing that an improving access to memory permits the integrative capacity for balance and coordination.

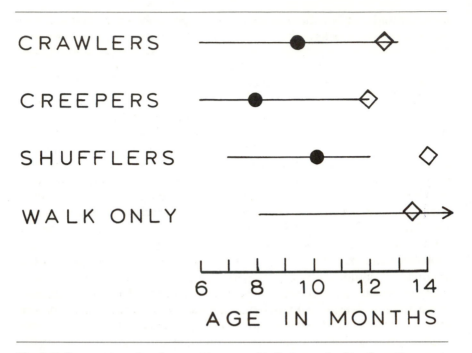

Fig. 2-7. Locomotory development in normal infants graphed to show the onset of the earliest form of locomotion (crawling, creeping, shuffling, or "just standing up and walking") and the onset of unaided walking. Drawn from data reported by Bottos et al. (1989).

Thelen (1983), on the other hand, rejected the cognitive explanation and proposed that the development of walking is readily accounted for by considerations of motivation, central nervous system development, and physical changes in body proportions and bone and muscle strength. The same kind of disagreement between cognitive and physical factors is implicitly, if not explicitly, present in many discussions of babbling. If cognitive development is critical to babbling, as Elbers (1982) concluded, then what the cognitive developments are and how they relate to patterns in babbling and early language productions must be defined.

AUDITORY-PERCEPTUAL AND MOTORIC FOUNDATIONS OF LANGUAGE

Speech as an environmental stimulus consists of time-varying long- and short-term patterns of acoustic energy. Because speech is the acoustic representation of language, it is a physical event (externally verifiable) that links two or more human nervous systems via shared information regarding encoding and decoding processes and cognitive representation. The infant's goal in learning speech is to identify the acoustically definable contrasts in the ambient language, to organize these contrasts into repertoires or categories that support representation, and to learn how to control the vocal tract to produce the acoustic contrasts so determined. The developmental process was roughly sketched in Figure 2-5 as a progressive interaction of genetic programs with environmental influences.

Language is a serially ordered behavior in which competence demands the capability to recognize and produce sequences of some kind. Language expressed as speech is a temporal pattern of sounds. Multisyllabic babbling perhaps preconfigures the serial properties of adult speech, and it is possible that infant babbling of the multisyllabic variety shares with language a competent serial structure. In babbling, the competence rests in the capacity to assemble consonants and vowels into syllable strings uttered in one breath group. Babbling has paradigmatic and syntagmatic components of at least a simple sort. The paradigmatic accomplishments are in the repertoire of sounds, especially consonants, which give syllabic shaping to utterances and comprise the elements from which complex sequences are formed. The syntagmatic aspects of babbling reside both in the formation and concatentation of syllables (and hence the discovery of syllabic and intersyllabic phonologic regularities) and in the prosodic envelopes expressed over sequences of syllables. The serial competence of spoken language is in more demanding capacities (e.g., to recognize and generate specified phonologic strings, to parse and produce syntactic groupings of words, and to maintain coherence in heard or self-uttered discourse). Tallal and associates (Tallal, 1988) reported that factors of temporal processing were sufficient to distinguish language-impaired children from normal children in their sample. We are not suggesting that temporal factors are the whole story; rather, temporal factors are an important early chapter in language acquisition.

The developmental importance of some aspects of infant vocalizations is demonstrated in studies of speech and language development in children developing normally and in children who present with communication delays or disorders. Murphy, Menyuk, Liebergott and Schultz (1983) reported that the articulation of CV syllables ("structured vocalizations") was a significant predictor of the age at which children would produce 50 different words. Menyuk, Liebergott and Shultz (1986) interpreted this result to point to a developmental linkage among early CV production, early word production, and the production of word-final consonants. Vihman et al. (1986) reached a similar conclusion from their study of phonological development in 10 children. Their data indicated that the frequency of usage of consonants in babbling and words at 1 year predicts relative phonological advance at 3 years.

In an investigation of perinatal risk factors and vocalizations in the first year, Jensen, Boggild-Andersen, Schmidt, Ankerhus and Hansen (1988) compared the development of 9 children in a risk group and 20 normally developing controls. Compared with the control infants, the infants with neonatal risk factors had significantly reduced numbers of reduplicated syllables and consonants in their first-year spontaneous vocalizations. Moreover, all of the risk infants who later had abnormal scores on a preschool language test showed significant reductions in different reduplications and consonants in the first-year vocalizations. The authors concluded that prelinguistic sound production may be useful in the identification of infants at risk for developmental language disorders. Camp, Burgess, Morgan and Zerbe (1987) related scores on the Verbalization factor of the Bayley Scales of Infant Development at 11–15 months with earlier monthly measures of infant vocalization. They reported an overall trend of increasing vocalization with the most reliable individual differences at 4, 5, and 6 months. The 4–6 month interval was therefore recommended as the best time to assess vocalization with a minimal set of observations. Interestingly, this period corresponds roughly to Oller's Expansion Stage, that is, a point in development at which the infants' sound repertoire increases and vocal tract anatomy is being remodeled.

Another behavior that is pertinent to spoken language and appears to be appropriately sampled at 4 months, is pause or silence in vocalization. Pausing takes two forms that have been most commonly investigated, the first being the intrapersonal pause or silence between vocalizations of the same speaker. The second form is the switching pause, or silence between the vocalizations of two different speakers. The regulation of these two kinds of pauses proceeds differently in development. Beebe, Alson, Jaffe, Feldstein and Crown (1988) concluded that mothers and their 4-month-olds matched switching pauses, but not intrapersonal pauses. These pausing patterns may be a precursor of dialogue. Beebe et al. also reported that although the group data did not show a significant matching of intrapersonal pause durations, the level of infant engagement within a dyad was correlated with intrapersonal pause matching. Thus, affective engagement is a potent factor in the regulation of intrapersonal pause congruence.

Table 2-2 gives an overview of the relationships among Piaget's (1955) stages of cognitive development, Stark and Heinz's (1988) levels of vocal communication, and major developmental milestones. What eventually will need to be known is whether causality patterns can be drawn among the three columns of the table. But lacking secure knowledge of causality relationships, increasingly refined descriptions of the behaviors related to each entry in the table can be worked toward. In doing so, a profile of potentials and processes pertinent to speech and language development may eventually be generated.

Table 2-2. Descriptions of developmental patterns based on Piaget (1953) and Stark and Heinz (1988)

Month	Piaget's Stages	Stark-Heinz Levels	Milestones
0	1: Use of reflexes	Reflexive	Cries
1	2: Primary circular reactions		Coos, smiles
2		Reactive	Orients to voice
3			Vocalizes, laughs
4		Activity	Ah-goo, razz turn taking
5	3: Secondary circular reactions		Rolls from prone to supine
6			Reduplicated babble
7		Personal	
8	4: Coordination of secondary schemes		Gestures
9		Intentional communication: instrumental, regulatory, interactional, heuristic/ imaginative	Crawls, sits
10			Imitates speech
11			First word
12			Walks

One facet of this enterprise is to model the biological program and its operational processes for oral-verbal behavior. Such a model should enhance the ability to evaluate environmental interactions as they relate to communicative behavior and the development of spoken language. It might also provide an early organizational framework for the development of nomothetic principles that apply to ideographic circumstances of child-situation, vocal-verbal interactions (cf. Rutter, 1981). It is beyond the scope of this chapter to discuss the vital role of nervous system development in the acquisition of spoken language. Speech is a behavior, unique to humans, that depends on many differentiated and integrated functions of the central and peripheral nervous systems. Any condition that disrupts or limits development of the nervous system has the potential to disrupt or limit oral-verbal behavior. For review of neural mechanisms, see several sources (Eggermont, 1989; Elbers, 1981; Goodman, 1987; & Parmalee & Sigman, 1983).

A theoretical convergence between biology and language has appeared in Piatelli-Palmarini's (1989) writings on selectivity and parameter setting.

The crux of Piatelli-Palmarini's conception is schematized in Figure 2-8. The CNS in the neonate and infant is assumed to be profligate in its neuronal capacity. Through massive cell death and synaptic degeneration, certain potentials for neuronal organization are lost while others are preserved. The selectivity comes about in part through exposure to stimuli in the environment. Especially for language, environmental stimuli underdetermine the structures to be acquired because the stimuli are poor, variable and underconstrained. However, even occasional exposure to poor language stimuli is sufficient to fix the parameters for a particular language or dialect. Basically, the parameters are preassigned combinatorial options. Parameter fixation enables the child to accomplish a projective reconstruction of language (Chomsky, 1981). Piatelli-Palmarini takes as support for this view the ability of children who are congenitally deaf (or who become deaf before acquiring language) to develop verbal faculties. Although Piatelli-Palmarini perhaps understates the difficulty of spoken language acquisition in such circumstances, the basic point remains: auditory exposure to the ambient language is not absolutely critical to acquiring some level of spoken language competence.

Piatelli-Palmarini's arguments go far beyond the relatively modest claims of this chapter, so far, in fact, as to deny that language is *learned* in the usual sense of the word. An innatist-selectivist explanation is proposed

Fig. 2-8. A schematic representation of Piatelli-Palmarini's innatist-selectivist conception of language acquisition. See text for description.

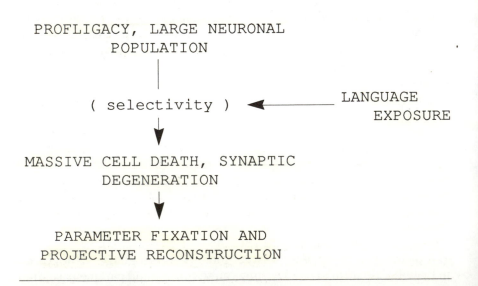

as the alternative to instructivism. What is held in common with Piatelli-Palmarini is the assertion that the genetic potential for spoken language is considerable. This chapter suggests that genetic programs underlie the biology of speech perception and speech production. If parameter fixation applies to the phonological level, as Halle (1988) maintains, then the genetic program coupled with an exposure to the sound patterns in a language can fix the parameters of the phonological system. Halle suggests a dual richness in this parameter fixation in that the abstract parameters pertain to *both* the mental representations of words and to the neural patterns of their spoken productions. An hypothesis that follows is that babbling incorporates some aspects of parameter fixation. These aspects may include rhythmic patterns, syllable structures, stress patterns and vowel preferences. Indeed, properties very similar to these begin to emerge well before the age of 1 year (De Boysson-Bardies et al., 1984; De Boysson-Bardies et al., 1989).

The particular innatist assumptions of parameter theory need not be made if one takes an alternative view that has been termed *epigenetic selection* (Sachs, 1988). Sachs addresses problems in biology that are conceptually similar to those confronting students of language development. Sachs's thinking was that development is basically selection from an excess of genetically equivalent possibilities. Considering evidence from such diverse sources as synaptic formation of nerve fibers, the differentiation of plant stomata, and the development of insects and rodents, Sachs noted common biologic facts such as the following. First, with respect to individual cells or groups of cells, some developmental events are discontinued or the developmental course may even be reversed. Second, there is large variability at the cellular level and in the course of maturation of individual structures. Third, for any given structure, there is a typical excess capacity or potential for development. These features accord in a striking way with features of language development. Sachs' conception of epigenetic selection stressed a developmental process in which the final state, rather than individual events, is strictly specified and which allows for the correction of developmental mistakes.

Some of the proposed mechanisms or rules of epigenetic selection in biology would seem to apply to language. One rule of interest is a negative correlation among the development of similar events. In biology, Hydra "heads" inhibit, though not necessarily prevent, the formation of similar structures. Likewise, in language, the formation of one phoneme or one syntactic structure would inhibit, but not always prevent, the formation of similar ones.

Another rule is a positive correlation for events that are different or complementary. In biology, one tissue can induce differentiation of another tissue. In language, one development might induce others, such as the case of certain semantic distinctions (negation) requiring a syntactic expression.

A related rule is that, during development, there is an increasing positive feedback between complementary processes. An example in plant growth is that rapidly growing buds induce vascular differentiation and root initiation. It is easy to imagine analogous effects in language, such as an expanding lexicon inducing phonological differentiation on the one hand and semantic growth on the other. Increasing positive feedback enables continued development with even a weaker stimulus or governing signal. In botany, this means that plant cells that began to differentiate in response to a particular signal could continue differentiation even if the signal diminishes. In language, this means that a differentiation of syntactic devices, once underway, may proceed even if the pertinent language phenomena that support this differentiation become more subtle or less frequent.

Finally, Sachs proposes that internal controls limit developmental processes as cells (or, by analogy, language components) reach *determinate* states. That is, the process is self-limiting. When the developmental structure is complex, the internal controls could have a different function, one of promoting a transition from one set of interactions to another. For example, reaching a certain vocabulary size (such as 50 words) may force a phonological reorganization through the introduction of new sets of interactions.

SUMMARY AND IMPLICATIONS

In conclusion, a four-part response will answer the challenge that was posed at the outset; namely, to identify aspects of oral-verbal behavioral organization, observable in infancy, that link with later points in speech development.

1. Evidence points to at least two major aspects of vocal organization observed in infants that have adult-like characteristics. The first is temporal congruence in between-speaker switching pauses (turn-taking) and the second is the relative timing of certain acoustic events corresponding to opening and closing gestures in stop-vowel syllable chains. These aspects reflect an early stable temporal organization, both within and between speakers, that is basic to spoken communication. Other types of potential organization relate to rhythmic pattern, syllable structure or vowel preference (De Boysson-Bardies et al., 1984, 1989). As these patterns are identified, they define the envelope of vocalization pertinent to a particular language. Conceivably, some of these patterns are complementary and

therefore may be mutually inductive or reinforcing (through positive feedback).

2. Both direct and indirect evidence point to several aspects that, although not stable across development, maintain continuity by conditioning oral-verbal behavior at a later point in time. These include the following:

a.   The descent of the larynx, at around 2–4 months, with a consequent lengthening of the pharynx and disengagement of the larynx and velopharynx. This change permits the production of nasal versus nonnasal phonetic elements, and the emergence of the component structures of the velopharyngeal valving mechanism required for the production of high-pressure consonants.

b.   The control of tongue position, contour, and movement within a growing vocal tract. The tongue is a unique and versatile articulator that is fundamental to the child's increasing ability to generate vocal tract shapes and transitions necessary for vowel and consonant mastery.

c.   The quantity and quality of vocalizations at certain points during the first year of life. The frequency of vocalizations between 4–6 months and the number of different consonant sounds and multisyllabic sequences in the second half of the first year have been reported to be predictive of later oral-verbal abilities.

d.   Sufficient auditory awareness and exposure to the parent spoken language(s) of the infant's sociolinguistic environment. This appears necessary to shape the infant's recognition code which is the basis for the correspondence between acoustic cues and meaning and for the encoding and decoding operations of language. In addition to awareness and exposure to spoken language, the infant needs attentional and orienting systems that enable the processing of both familiar and novel acoustic stimuli.

3. The significant change that occurs during the latter part of the first year is the infant's goal for vocal communication. With increasing synaptic density and neuronal connectivity linking the increasingly differentiated areas of the cerebral cortex with each other and with subcortical structures, it is assumed that the infant grows in the capacity to process incoming sensory information and to associate and integrate thought with action to gain control over the environment. Confronted with the task of generating sound-meaning relationships to exercise some degree of control over the environment, the child shifts from producing speech-like but linguistically unspecified "social babbling" to the goal of producing acoustic signals that convey linguistic information to an audience. The process may not be one of simple incremental learning of phonetic elements but rather one of parameter fixation or epigenetic selection. Consistent with general developmental principles, the strategies and length of time used to achieve

the goal of spoken language will exhibit pluralism across individuals. Oral-verbal behavior will demonstrate increasing differentiation and integration with time, barring disruptions in the biological program and/or the information and conditions required for its operation.

4. Based on the previous discussion, the following conditions have the potential to disrupt the emergence and development of oral-verbal behavior in the first year:

a. Alterations in the anatomy or interference with the normal processes of anatomical remodeling of the vocal tract in the first year will restrict the potential diversity of the infant's phonetic repertoire.

b. Generalized or specific CNS damage may disrupt oral-verbal development in many aspects. For example, it may reduce control over the vocal tract muscular components, especially the tongue and velum. It may interfere with the generation of sequences of movements to produce rhythmical action patterns or to perceive the sensory components of these. It may limit, distort, or mask the infant's auditory awareness of the spectral-temporal patterns of the ambient language or the ability to orient and attend to these patterns. It may slow and constrain the differentiation and integration of the cortical and subcortical areas.

c. Departures from typical environmental conditions such that the child does not have adequate exposure to the parent language in age-appropriate interactions or is not motivated to use verbal behavior to gain control over the environment also may relate to abnormalities in oral-verbal development.

REFERENCES

Albert, D., Munson, R., & Resnick, M. (1988). *Reasoning in medicine: An introduction to clinical inference.* Baltimore: Johns Hopkins University Press.

Beebe, B., Alson, D., Jaffe, J., Feldstein, S., & Crown, C. (1988). Vocal congruence in mother-infant play. *Journal of Psycholinguistic Research, 17*, 245–259.

Bernstein, L. E. (1982). Ontogenetic changes in children's speech-sound perception. In N. J. Lass (Ed.), *Speech and language: Advances in basic research and practice, Vol. 8* (pp. 191–220). New York: Academic.

Bornstein, M. H., & Sigman, M. D. (1986). Continuity in mental development from infancy. *Child Development, 57*, 251–274.

Bottos, M., Barba, B. D., Stefani, D., Pettena, G., Tonin, C., & D'Este, A. (1989). Locomotor strategies preceding independent walking: Prospective study of neurological and language development in 424 cases. *Developmental Medicine and Child Neurology, 31*, 25–34.

Camp, B., Burgess, D., Morgan, L., & Zerbe, G. (1987). A longitudinal study of infant vocalization in the first year. *Journal of Pediatric Psychology, 12*, 321–331.

Carpenter, G. A., & Grossberg, S. (1987). Discovering order in chaos: Stable self-organization of neural recognition codes. In S. H. Koslow, A. J. Mandell, & M. F.

Shlesinger (Eds.), *Perspectives in biological dynamics and theoretical medicine* (pp. 33–50). *Annals of the New York Academy of Sciences, 504.*

Chomsky, N. (1981). *Lectures on government and binding (the Pisa Lectures).* Dordrecht, Netherlands: Foris.

De Boysson-Bardies, B., Halle, P., & Durand, C. (1989). A crosslinguistic investigation of vowel formants in babbling. *Journal of Child Language, 16*, 1–17.

De Boysson-Bardies, B., Sagart, L., & Durand, C. (1984). Discernible differences in the babbling of infants according to target language. *Journal of Child Language, 11*, 1–15.

Edelman, G. (1987). *Neural Darwinism: The theory of neuronal group selection.* New York: Basic Books.

Eggermont, J. (1989). The onset and development of auditory function: Contributions of evoked potentials. *Journal of Speech-Language Pathology and Audiology, 13*, 5–16. [Also see accompanying peer commentary.]

Elbers, E. (1981). Maturation of the central nervous system. In M. Rutter (Ed.), *Scientific Foundations of Developmental Psychiatry* (pp. 25–39). Baltimore: University Park Press.

Elbers, L. (1982). Operating principles in repetitive babbling: A cognitive continuity approach. *Cognition, 12*, 45–63.

Goodman, R. (1987). The developmental neurobiology of language. In W. Yule and M. Rutter (Eds.), *Language Development and Disorders. Clinics in Developmental Medicine*, No. 101/102, pp. 129–145. Oxford: Blackwell Scientific.

Gottlieb, G. (1983). The psychobiological approach to developmental issues. In M. Haith & J. Campos (Eds.), *Mussen's Handbook of Child Psychology (4th ed.). Vol. II. Infancy and Developmental Psychobiology* (pp. 1–26) New York: Wiley.

Greiser, D., and Kuhl, P. K. (in press). The categorization of speech by infants: Support for speech-sound prototypes. *Developmental Psychology.*

Haelsig, P. C., and Madison, C. L. (1986). A study of phonological processes exhibited by 3-, 4-, and 5-year-old children. *Language, Speech and Hearing Services in Schools, 17*, 107–114.

Halle, M. (1988). The immanent form of phonemes. In W. Hirst (Ed.), *The making of cognitive science: Essays in honor of George A. Miller.* Cambridge: Cambridge University Press.

Hastings, H. M., & Waner, S. (1984). Low dissipation computing in biologic systems. *Biosystems, 17*, 241–244.

Hastings, H. M., & Waner, S. (1987). Evolutionary learning in simulated neural networks. In S. H. Koslow, A. J. Mandell, & M. F. Shlesinger (Eds.), *Perspectives in biological dynamics and theoretical medicine* (pp. 289–290). *Annals of the New York Academy of Sciences, Vol. 504.*

Hodge, M. (1989). *A comparison of measurements across speaker age: Implications for an acoustic characterization of speech maturation.* Ph.D. dissertation, University of Wisconsin–Madison.

Holmgren, K., Lindblom, B., Aurelius, G., Jalling, B., & Zetterstrom, R. (1986). On the phonetics of infant vocalization. In B. Lindblom and R. Zetterstrom (Eds.), *Precursors of early speech* (pp. 51–63). New York: Stockton.

Jensen, T. S., Boggild-Andersen, B., Schmidt, J., Ankerhus, J., & Hansen, E. (1988). Perinatal risk factors and first-year vocalizations: Influence on preschool language and motor performance. *Developmental Medicine and Child Neurology, 30*, 153–161.

Kent, R. D. (1982). Structure and function times three. Paper presented at the Symposium on Research on Children's Language Disorders, University of Wisconsin–Madison, June 1982.

Kent, R. D. (1984). The psychobiology of speech development: Co-emergence of language and a movement system. *American Journal of Physiology, 246,* R888–R894.

Kent, R. D., & Bauer, H. R. (1985). Vocalizations of one year olds. *Journal of Child Language, 12,* 491–526.

Kent, R. D., Osberger, M. J., Netsell, R., & Hustedde, C. G. (1986). Phonetic development in identical twins differing in auditory function. *Journal of Speech and Hearing Disorders, 52,* 64–75.

Kier, W. M., & Smith, K. K. (1985). Tongues, tentacles, and trunks: The biomechanics of movement in muscular-hydrostats. *Zoological Journal of the Linneas Society, 83,* 307–324.

Koopmans-van Beinum, F. J., and van der Stelt, J. M. (1986). Early stages in the developments of speech movements. In B. Lindblom & R. Zetterstrom (Eds.), *Precursors of early speech* (pp. 37–50). New York: Stockton.

Kuhl, P. K. (1988). Auditory perception and the evolution of speech. *Human Evolution, 3,* 19–43.

Locke, J. L. (1983). *Phonological acquisition and change.* New York: Academic.

Mehler, J., Jusczyk, P., Lambertz, G., Halsted, N., Bertoncini, J., & Amiel-Tison, C. (1988). A precursor of language acquisition in young infants. *Cognition, 29,* 143–178.

Menyuk, P., Liebergott, J., & Schultz, M. (1986). Predicting phonological development. In B. Lindblom and R. Zetterstrom (Eds.), *Precursors of early speech* (pp. 79–93). New York: Stockton.

Mitchell, P. R., and Kent, R. D. (submitted). Phonetic variation in multisyllabic babbling.

Murphy, R., Menyuk, P., Liebergott, J., & Schultz, M. (1983). Predicting rate of lexical acquisition. Paper presented at the Biennial Meeting of the Society for Research in Child Development, Detroit.

Oller, D. K. (1978). Infant vocalizations and the development of speech. *Allied Health and Behavioral Science, 1,* 523–549.

Oller, D. K. (1986). Metaphonology and infant vocalizations. In B. Lindblom and R. Zetterstrom (Eds.), *Early precursors of speech* (pp. 21–35). Basingstoke: Macmillan.

Oller, D. K., Eilers, R. E., Bull, D. H., and Carney, A. E. (1985). Prespeech vocalizations of a deaf infant: A comparison with normal metaphonological development. *Journal of Speech and Hearing Research, 28,* 47–62.

Olsho, L. W. (1986). Early development of human frequency resolution. In R. W. Rubels et al. (Eds.), *The biology of change in otolaryngology* (pp. 71–90). Amsterdam: Elsevier.

Otomo, K. (1988). Development of vowel articulation from 22 to 30 months of age: Preliminary analyses. Paper presented at 1988 Child Phonology Conference, University of Illinois, Urbana-Champaign.

Parmalee, A. H., and Sigman, M. D. (1983). Perinatal brain development and behavior. In M. Haith & J. Campos (Eds.), *Mussen's Handbook of Child Psychology (4th ed.). Vol. IV. Infancy and Developmental Psychobiology* (pp. 95–155). New York: Wiley.

Peterson, G., and Barney, H. (1952). Control methods used in a study of the vowels. *Journal of the Acoustical Society of America, 24,* 175–184.

Piaget, J. (1955). *The language and thought of the child.* (M. Gabain, Trans.) Cleveland: Meridian Books.

Piatelli-Palmarini, M. (1989). Evolution, selection and cognition: From "learning" to parameter setting in biology and in the study of language. *Cognition, 31,* 1–44.

Rutter, M. (1981). Introduction. In M. Rutter (Ed.), *Scientific Foundations of Developmental Psychiatry* (pp. 1–7). Baltimore: University Park Press.

Sachs, T. (1988). Epigenetic selection: An alternative mechanism of pattern formation. *Journal of Theoretical Biology, 134,* 547–559.

Sander, E. (1972). When are speech sounds learned? *Journal of Speech and Hearing Disorders, 37,* 55–63.

Smith, B., Brown-Sweeney, S., & Stoel-Gammon, C. (1988). A quantitative analysis of reduplicated and variegated babbling. Paper presented at the Child Phonology Conference, University of Illinois, Urbana-Champaign, May 6–7, 1988.

Smith, K. K., & Kier, W. M. (1989). Trunks, tongues, and tentacles: Moving with skeletons of muscle. *American Scientist, 77,* 29–35.

Stark, R. (1979). Prespeech segmental feature development. In P. Fletcher & M. Garman (Eds.), *Language acquisition* (pp. 15–32). New York: Cambridge University Press.

Stark, R. E., & Heinz, J. M. (1988). Learning to talk. The first two years. Paper presented at the 1988 Convention of American Speech-Language-Hearing Association, Boston, November 1988.

Stoel-Gammon, C., & Otomo, K. (1986). Babbling development of hearing-impaired and normally hearing subjects. *Journal of Speech and Hearing Disorders, 51,* 33–41.

Tallal, P. (1988). Developmental language disorders. In J. F. Kavanagh & T. J. Truss, Jr. (Eds.), *Learning disabilities: Proceedings of a national conference* (pp. 181–272). Parkton, MD: York.

Thelen, E. (1981). Rhythmical behavior in infancy: An ethological perspective. *Developmental Psychology, 17,* 237–257.

Thelen, E. (1983). Learning to walk is still an "old" problem: A reply to Zelazo (1983). *Journal of Motor Behavior, 15,* 139–161.

Thelen, E., & Cooke, W. D. (1987). Relationships between newborn stepping and later walking: A new interpretation. *Developmental Medicine and Child Neurology, 29,* 380–393.

Vihman, M. M., Ferguson, C. A., & Elbert, M. (1986). Phonological development from babbling to speech: Common tendencies and individual differences. *Applied Psycholinguistics, 7,* 3–40.

Vihman, M. M., Macken, M. A., Miller, R., Simmons, H., & Miller, J. (1985). From babbling to speech: A reassessment of the continuity issue. *Language, 61,* 397–445.

Werker, J. F. (1989). Becoming a native listener. *American Scientist, 77,* 54–59.

Zelazo, P. R. (1983). The development of walking: New findings and old assumptions. *Journal of Motor Behavior, 15,* 99–137.

CHAPTER 3

Toward a Theory of Phonological Acquisition

DAVID INGRAM

INTRODUCTION

When theories of phonological acquisition are discussed today, three proposals usually come to mind. First, there is the seminal work by Jakobson (1968), which introduced the notion of the universal development of a set of distinctive features. Next, there is natural phonology as developed by Stampe (1969), where the concept of natural phonological process was introduced to account for the systematic nature of children's errors. Lastly, much attention has been paid of late to the so-called cognitive theory of Macken and Ferguson (1983), which focuses on the problem-solving capacity of children as well as their individual variation.

Each of these theories has captured an important aspect of development, but has come up shorthanded in others. For Jakobson's theory, there is the difficulty of handling the individual variation that has been found in data-oriented studies. Further, as stressed in Ingram (1988a), the theory suffers

This chapter contains material that was originally part of a longer paper entitled, "Language Acquisition, Learnability, and Phonological Acquisition," which was divided into this and another, entitled "Underspecification Theory and Phonological Acquisition," which was presented at the annual meeting of the Linguistic Society of America, December 1988.

from methodological difficulties in actually applying the theory. Natural phonology has provided mechanisms to determine the course of acquisition, but has not come up with a universal set of phonological processes or means to limit the extent of possible variation that it allows. Lastly, the cognitive theory has had difficulties in even being identifiable as a theory at all. It is based on no adult theory of the phonological system and has emphasized individual variation to the virtual exclusion of any general patterns.

In the development of my own ideas on this topic, I have duly spent time exploring each of these theories as well as others (e.g., Waterson, 1971), in an effort to understand better the nature of phonological acquisition. During the last few years in particular, I have come to a set of beliefs about this process which has the form of an emerging theory. Since so much work in this field is really an extension of Jakobson's original ideas, I refer to this view as a neo-Jakobsonian theory. It attempts to combine the gains of all of the three theories above with current research into nonlinear phonology (c.f. van der Hulst & Smith, 1985, for a review).

In examining the current state of the field, it has been my impression that the work of both Jakobson and Stampe is perceived by many to be primarily of historical interest. At least for the more traditional field of child language, the most discussed theory currently appears to be the cognitive theory of Macken and Ferguson. Since I have some difficulties with their use of the term 'cognitive' in this context, I refer to this growing literature as the Stanford theory, in recognition of the institution where much of this line of research has been developed. This theory has all of the following properties: (1) emphasis on individual variation among children; (2) the claim that the first unit of organization used by children is the syllable (Macken, 1979); and (3) few noticeable general patterns of acquisition across children.

The theory that I will be discussing takes virtually the opposite position to the Stanford theory on each of these points. Like both Jakobson and Stampe, it recognizes individual variation, but attempts to constrain it through universal principles. Second, it argues that children begin acquisition with the same phonological units as adults, this being the distinctive feature. Lastly, it proposes that we will find general patterns of acquisition, and that these patterns will show consistent cross-linguistic variation. For example, both English and French children will show general patterns of acquisition, but they will not be the same for both groups of children.

Here, I will present an overview of the neo-Jakobson theory which underlies my current views on this topic. I will do this by outlining twelve important findings on phonological acquisition, with each followed by a discussion of its theoretical implications.

ASPECTS OF PHONOLOGICAL ACQUISITION

Accounts of phonological acquisition have by and large been what Wasow (1983) recently referred to as "local theories."

[F]irst it [Child Language :DI] tends to be inductive, in the sense that the hypotheses are generated from patterns observed in corpora, and second, the hypotheses are typically "local," i.e., they posit strategies for dealing with particular phenomena at a specific stage of development, rarely attempting to relate to general issues in linguistic theory. (Wasow, 1984, p. 191)

Another way to describe this orientation is to say that the focus has been for much of this work on the basic facts and assumptions that need to be part of the theory of acquisition.

The discussion will summarize some observations and hypotheses from both the field at large, and some recent studies of my own which have approached phonological acquisition from this perspective (e.g., Goad & Ingram 1987, Ingram 1988a, 1988b, Tse & Ingram 1987, Pye, Ingram & List 1987). These studies are part of a rich literature in child phonology, which has discussed these issues from different perspectives and with different degrees of controversy. While data-oriented, however, the hypotheses drawn attempt to go beyond the kind of local theory commented upon by Wasow.

1. *Phonetic perceptual development.* In the first year of life, infants show the ability to perceive a broad range (and possibly all) of the acoustic characteristics of speech sounds in at least simple syllables. This research, initiated by the early findings of Eimas, Siqueland, Jusczyk and Vigorito (1971), has blossomed into an extensive literature demonstrating the excellent perceptual ability of infants. Indeed, researchers have had difficulty even finding discriminations that infants can't perceive, and those ones that are claimed to be such are met with controversy.

Given this ability, I propose the following initial hypothesis about the child's representation of his first words:

Acoustic Representation Hypothesis: Children first represent their early vocabulary in the form of fully specified phonetic feature matrices.

This, of course, makes no claims about the child's later phonological organization. Rather it makes the proposal that the child has the acoustic information he needs for eventual phonological analysis. A word like *pig*, for example, will be phonetically represented as [phI:g], with the child having acoustic awareness of the aspiration of the initial stop as well as the length of the vowel.

2. *The development of the receptive vocabulary.* There is an important issue of how long an acoustic representation might exist before phonological analysis begins. One possibility is that children will store several words before any analysis is initiated. A clue into this process can be obtained, then, by looking at vocabulary growth in both the child's understanding and production.

The assumption has always been made that receptive vocabulary precedes the productive one. Only recently, however, has this relationship been made more precise. The most important study in this regard is Benedict (1979), where Benedict studied the vocabulary development of eight children from their first words in comprehension up to their fiftieth word in production. Some startling results came from this study, which showed that receptive vocabulary is much in advance of the spoken vocabulary. Some of these results are summarized in (1). One striking finding is that the children on the average acquired nearly 100 words receptively before their first words were produced.

1. Ages when first and fiftieth words appear in comprehension and production, based on Benedict (1979)

    Comprehension: 0 words   0 ; 10(14)
                      50 words   1 ; 1(5)
    Production: 0 words   1 ; 1(21)
                      50 words   1 ; 6(15)

Further, when children acquire their fiftieth word in production around 1;6, they have a much larger receptive vocabulary—around 250 words.

Given this situation, it seems unlikely that all of these words are simply acoustically stored without any phonological analysis whatsoever. Instead, I suggest the following hypothesis:

The Onset Hypothesis: The size of the child's receptive vocabulary in this period, combined with his or her perceptual ability, is sufficient for the child to begin phonological organization at the time of the first words in production.

This hypothesis also leads to the prediction that the child's early words should show such organization, which in fact will be argued for below.

3. *The development of the spoken vocabulary.* We have known for some time that the first words in production are acquired quite slowly from around 1;0 to 1;6, with a word spurt around 1;6. The following data from Smith (1926) documented this observation several years ago.

2. Age	Number of Words
0 ; 8	0
0 ; 10	1
1 ; 0	3
1 ; 3	19
1 ; 6	22
1 ; 9	118

At the same time, the bulk of the literature on phonological acquisition is based on the acquisition of the first 50 words in production (e.g., Menn, 1971; Ferguson & Farwell, 1975; Waterson, 1971). Given the previous finding on receptive vocabulary, it should be obvious that the productive vocabulary will be behind the receptive one. This leads to the following caution about claims about the child's phonology based only on production data:

> *Caution*: Given the discrepancy between spoken and receptive vocabularies just mentioned, spoken vocabulary should be considered a conservative estimate of the child's phonology.

In other words, the child's phonological knowledge of the receptive vocabulary may be well in advance of what is demonstrated in the spoken language.

4. *The word spurt*. As just mentioned, children show a word spurt in their spoken language around 1;6. An unresolved issue is the cause of this change. One possibility is that it is the result of the child's attainment of the symbolic function, in the sense of Piaget (1948). On the surface, this seems a reasonable possibility, since the symbolic function will be needed for extensive vocabulary development to take place. There are at least two problems, however, with this account of the word spurt. One is the fact that children undergo a similar word spurt several months earlier in their receptive vocabulary development (Gibson & Ingram, 1983). That milestone is a more likely candidate for evidence for the development of the symbolic function. Second, if the symbolic function were the cause of the word spurt in production, one would expect a semantic difference in the nature of the child's words before and after. One such difference would be in the use of overextensions. Research by Rescorla (1980), among others, however, has found no such change in overextensions (see review in Ingram, 1989a).

An alternative explanation is to argue that the word spurt results from a change in the child's phonological system. Some evidence for the nature of this difference can be found in Velten (1943). Before the word spurt, Joan Velten acquired a small set of basic phonological distinctions with severe co-occurrence restrictions. Then, at 22 months, Joan acquired over 100 new words in a matter of weeks. Velten comments that this new vocabulary did not show much expansion of the phonological distinctions that Joan had already acquired, but instead an expansion of their combinatorial possibilities.

Such data support a range of other research since Jakobson (1968), which claims that the child, during the first months of phonological development, concentrates on the development of a basic set of phonological distinctions, followed by the exploration of their co-occurrence. This suggests then, that the word spurt in production may be a significant milestone in the child's phonological development. If true, then the theory of phonological acquisition will need to contain a mechanism to account for this. I can only offer a suggestion of what this might be at this time, which is that the spurt may be linked to a significant development in the child's phonological analysis of the receptive vocabulary in terms of phonotactics.

5. *The first units of organization.* As mentioned in the introduction to this chapter, researchers differ concerning the nature of the child's first phonological units. There are two possible views on this, which I will refer to as the *developmental* and *universal* views respectively. The developmental view, most forcefully expressed in Macken (1979), proposes that the child goes through several stages, beginning with the "word" as the unit of organization, proceeding to the "syllable," and eventually to the "feature." Development is seen, then, as a series of reorganizations. The universal view, on the other hand, argues that the child's phonological formalism is essentially adult-like at the onset of acquisition. This is, whatever the units are of the theory of the adult system, these will be the ones with which the child begins development.

In Ingram (1986a), I give five arguments against the developmental view. First, there is the problem already mentioned of the child's large receptive vocabulary. If the child's first words in production are stored as wholes with no internal organization, then presumably so are the words in understanding. It seems unlikely, however, that so many words could be acquired with no internal phonological organization. Second, the claim that the word is the first unit of organization at least indirectly predicts that there should be no evidence in babbling of awareness of individual segments. Reports on babbling, however, indicate that such as the case. For example, a babbling sequence of [bi], [ba], [bu] is much more likely to be found than one of [bi], [mu], [ta]. Also, the early vocabulary is more apt to look like the former rather than the latter. Third, while the "word" is an important unit within this approach, it is not defined within any phonological theory. Is there a total discontinuity in development, or is word retained and built upon with additional units? Fourth, the child will need to shift eventually from the word to features, yet there is no mechanism provided to account for this shift in organization. Fifth, there is no real testing of this hypothesis because there is no methodology provided that will determine the existence of features as a unit of organization. That is, we can't claim the child does or does not use features until we have method to show when they exist.

In several recent reports, I have been developing such a method and applying it to data. *This* methodology was first introduced in Ingram (1981) and expanded in Ingram (1988a, 1988b, 1989), and Goad and Ingram (1987). It makes use of a criterion of frequency before claims about the child having particular sounds and phonemes can be made. It uses the criterion to divide the child's sounds into marginal, used, and frequent sounds. The analyses that this method yields consistently show the preference for certain segments over others. This type of pattern is given for one child in Table 3-1. Most important, the preferred sounds are not random, but tend to fall into natural oppositions that can be separated from one another by a single distinctive feature. The next observation concentrates on the nature of these first contrasts.

Somewhat less controversial is the observation that these first words also are usually restricted to a small set of syllable shapes. I combine this fact with the above hypothesis to make the following claim about acquisition:

Assumption about feature acquisition: The child first establishes one or two basic, or "canonical" syllable shapes to start with, and uses these for the initiation of distinctive feature acquisition.

6. *The development of contrasts*. Phonological contrasts often first enter the child's system in a very restricted way. For example, a child who has the consonants /p/, /b/, /t/, and /k/ has only acquired the voicing contrast for the labial position. This gradual development of contrasts can be seen by looking at the data presented in Table 3-1. This figure presents data taken from Ferguson and Farwell (1975) on the acquisition of the first 50 words by a girl referred to as "T." Applying the methodology just referred to results in the following order of acquisition of word initial consonants:

3. T's acquisition of word initial consonants

1.	l d l		2.	l b l	l d l	3.	l b l	l d l
							l s l	
4.	l b l	l d l	5.	l b l	l d l	6.	l b l	l d l
	l p l			l p l	l t l		l p l	l t l	l k l
		l s l			l s l			l s l

We can see that T is acquiring distinctive features in a gradual but consistent fashion. T first acquires a place distinction, and then [voice] for each. The pattern predicts that she should next acquire a [g]. Individual analyses of children such as these will enable us to determine the extents

Table 3-1. T's acquisition of English word initial consonants

Session	Phonetic Inventory										
	[m	n	b	d	p	t	k	s	S	h	w]
1				d							
2				d			(k)			(h)	
3	(m)			*d						h	
4	(m)		b	*d		(t)			(S)	(h)	
5	(m)		b	*d		(t)		s	(S)		(w)
6	(m)	(n)	*b	d	*p	t		s	S	(h)	(w)
7	m	(n)	*b	d	*p	*t	(k)		(S)	(h)	w
8	(m)	(n)	*b	d	p	*t	(k)		S	(h)	w
9	(m)	(n)	*b	d	*p	*t	k	s	(S)	(h)	w

Session	Matches and Substitutions													
	/m	n	b	d	p	t	k	s	S	c	h	w	j	r/
1				d			(h)							
2				d			(h)				(?)			
3	(m)		(d)	d	(t)		(h)	(g)			(h)			
4	(m)		b	d			(S)	(S)			(h)			
5	(m)		b	d			s	(S)			(?)			(w)
6	(m)	(n)	b	d	p	(t)		s	(S)		(h)		(j)	(w)
7	m	(n)	b	d	p	t	(k)	(S)	(S)	(t)	(h)	(w)	(j)	(w)
8	(m)	(n)	b	d	p	t	(T)	S	(S)	(t)	(h)	(w)	(j)	(w)
9	(m)	(n)	b	d	p	t	k	s	(S)	(t)	(h)	(w)	(j)	(b)

Source: Based on the adaptation in Ingram (1989a) of data from Ferguson and Farwell (1975). S indicates a voiceless alveopalatal fricative. Bold indicates acquired sounds.

and limits in variation between children, and thus the general patterns that emerge. For example, the above data suggest that children initially restrict a new feature to a previously acquired one.

To capture such changes, this developmental theory will need a phonological theory of universal phonological features. Fortunately, recent research in phonological theory has returned to the question of the nature of phonological features. In particular, researchers are examining the possibility that there is an internal geometry to features, much as was originally suggested in Jakobson and Halle (1956). While this work has yet to reach a consensus (see review in den Dikken and van der Hulst, in press), it holds promise for the investigation of language acquisition in that the developmental data may help to provide evidence for certain proposals and against others.

7. *The occurrence of selection and avoidance.* Recent research by Schwartz

and Leonard (1982) has shown that children select certain sounds of adult words to attempt and avoid others. They established this through a very clear research design in which they taught nonsense words to children in the second year of life. One set of words were IN words, meaning that they were created with phonetic characteristics that were present in the child's spontaneous language. These were contrasted with OUT words, which contained features outside of the child's language. The results indicated that the children acquired the IN words much more quickly than the OUT ones.

This finding indicates that the diary samples collected from children in this age range may be more reliable samples than has been thought to be the case. If children do indeed select and avoid words on the basis of their current phonological abilities, then the gaps that we find in reasonably careful diaries should represent *systematic gaps* in the data. This observation does not add to the theory of acquisition, but it allows stronger conclusions from the analyses of diary data than it might otherwise.

It also shows that children do not begin acquisition by attempting to express all of the phonemes in the adult language. Instead, they only attempt a restricted set of these. For example, an English child's attempts at words with initial stop consonants may be restricted to those beginning with voiced consonants. This suggests that the distinctive features used in children's first spoken words reflect, from the onset, their phonological organization of the much larger receptive vocabulary.

8. *The appearance of substitutions.* Children's first substitutions are at first restricted in the same way as contrasts are, as stated in paragraph 6. For example, a child might first use [b] for adult words beginning with /b/, and then spread its use to words beginning with /p/ and /f/. We can see this kind of spread in operation in the hypothetical data presented below, which are typical of how substitutions develop:

4. Stage	/b/	/p/	/d/	/t/	/k/
1			d		
2	d		d		
3	b		d		
4	b	b	d	d	d

Our hypothetical child has acquired [d] for /d/, and then spreads its use to /b/. We can actually see this same pattern in Figure 3-1 for T in session 3. Next [b] appears for /b/, and later spreads to /p/. Meanwhile [d] has spread even farther now to /t/ and /d/.

The importance of such patterns is not just in the generalizing of a substitution, but in examining the nature of the adult phonemes that it spreads to. I would like to argue that such patterns are restricted by the nature of the child's phonological system. Stated somewhat differently, the determination of the child's distinctive features must not just consider the child's spoken forms, but also the target phonemes of the language. The child at stage 3 above has the same sounds as stage 4, but the system is more developed. This is because the child at stage 4 has identified a distinctive feature beyond those adult phonemes that are absolute matches with the child form.

A distinctive feature analysis of the data in (4) is provided in (5). Two features are being acquired and spreading, [cont(inuant)], and [labial]. (Nothing crucial is being implied by the selection of these particular features, which is only for demonstration purposes.) The place feature develops in stage 3, and spreads in stage 4.

5. Stage	Features	/b/	/p/	/d/	/t/	/k/
1	cont			−		
2	cont	−		−		
3	cont	−		−		
	labial	+		−		
4	cont	−	−	−	−	−
	labial	+	+	−	−	−

The subsequent pronunciation of these forms is by natural phonological processes much like those proposed by Stampe. I formulate these, however, as default feature rules as developed by Archangeli and Pulleybank (1986). A possible set of default rules for this example could be the following:

6. Default rules: [−labial]   →   [+coronal]
                        [Uvoice]   →   [+voice]

The first rule states that sounds that are nonlabial are most naturally produced as coronals. In the second rule, the "U" stands for "unmarked for." It states that any sound not indicated for [voice] will be naturally voiced. Such rules will fill in values for features that have not yet become distinctive for the child. Representing phonological processes this way allows them to be related to the current distinctive features in the child's system. It differs from natural phonology, however, in placing more prominence in the formal system to the representation of distinctive features. Ingram (1988c) provides a more detailed discussion of the use of this particular formalism.

It should be pointed out that an analysis along these lines is very much as originally suggest in Jakobson (1968). As mentioned in Ingram (1988a), there has been some misunderstanding of Jakobson in thinking he claims that the child develops a system independent from the adult system. The truth, however, is that he constantly makes reference to the adult target sounds that the child is attempting.

9. *Patterns of sound development.* I have argued thus far that children begin to acquire distinctive features at the onset of their acquisition of a production vocabulary. A further issue concerns when it can be concluded that such oppositions exist. Research suggests that there are three patterns of emergence of contrasts over the first six months of acquisition. First, there is a *lexical pattern* in which a contrast exists only between individuals words. In Table 3-1, for example, T has a distinction between initial [m] and [n] for several sessions. This distinction, however, was only evident in the words for "mama" and "no." Second, there is a *gradual pattern* in which the contrast spreads slowly from one word eventually to several. This appears to be the most common situation, as one might expect. Last, there is an *abrupt pattern* where a contrast suddenly appears in several words over a very short period. T shows this for the acquisition of [p]. At this point, I am not sure if the difference between the abrupt and gradual patterns reflects a sampling effect, or a psychological difference between the two. This will only be determined through careful analyses of individual children.

The fact that such patterns exist is clear evidence that the child's words do not all equally reflect the underlying phonological system. I have argued that we should not make claims about the child's system on the basis of lexical contrasts (Ingram, 1988a), but only on those contrasts that are used and frequent. Following a child's development of contrasts through identifying these patterns should allow more confident decisions about the nature of the child's phonological system.

10. *Cross-linguistic regularities.* Previous work by Jakobson proposed that all children would follow initially the same course of acquisition. This, he argued, was the result of restrictions imposed by his model of universal grammar on the acquisition process. As mentioned in Ingram (1989a), this universal sequence was only true for the very earliest vocalic and conso-nantal oppositions. Soon after, the influence of the specific system being acquired would be manifested.

A stronger version of this position has recently been put forth in Locke (1983). Locke differs from Jakobson by suggesting that the universally shared aspects of early phonological acquisition result from biological restrictions on the child's speech apparatus. Also, he is more explicit about when he believes children will show language specific processing. He states, "I will suggest that no genuine accommodations to the adult system will be evident until the child reaches the systemic stage of phonological acquisition, which probably occurs at some time after the first fifty words are in use" (p. 84). In other words, linguistic processing and language specific effects should not be found until after the word spurt in language acquisition.

In a series of research reports, my colleagues have found these predictions not to be true. Instead, we have consistently found cross-linguistic differences in the early phonologies of children acquiring different languages. It has led us to the conclusion that the child's perceptual and articulatory ability at the onset of speech production is adequate for them to attempt most of the more prominent sounds in a language.

This finding was first reported in Pye, Ingram and List (1987), where we compared the early phonetic inventories of English and Quiché children (Quiché is a Mayan language spoken in Guatemala). We found that children in each language tended, with some individual variation, to acquire a "basic" set of sounds for that language. The basic set of initial consonants we observed for English and Quiché are presented below:

7. English   Quiché
    m   n   m   n
    b   d   g
    p   t   k   p   t   č   k   ?
    f   s   h   x
    w   w
                                          l

An important aspect about these two sets of basic sounds is that there were sounds that the two languages shared that appeared in one set but not in the other. For example, Quiché has an /s/, but it was not an early acquisition in Quiché. On the other hand, both /l/ and /c/ were among the first sounds acquired in Quiché, but are not early in English.

Results like these for other languages have also been reported in Ingram (1988b). There I observed diary studies on three children acquiring Estonian, Swedish, and Bulgarian respectively. In all three cases, the children showed early use of [v], a notoriously late acquisition in English. Here, for example, are the early initial consonants for a Swedish girl reported in Rasmussen (1931) who, at 1 ; 9, had only 34 words. Those sounds with asterisks are those which were particularly frequent.

8.   *m   *n
      *b   *d   g
       p   t   *k
      *v   *s
               r

We can see that [v] is both early and frequent. A similar kind of finding has recently been found for French where the mid vowels [e] and [o] are acquired before the high ones [i] and [u] (Ingram, in prep. a).

The explanation for these results, as initially presented in Pye, Ingram and List (1987) is that these early inventories reflect the phonological prominence of these sounds in the language. In Swedish, for example, there are several words that are common in the vocabulary of young children which begin with a [v]. Swedish children, therefore, will be presented with several words showing the phonological importance of this sound in Swedish. Importantly, it is the linguistic prominence of the sound which is crucial. The voiced dental fricative [ð] in English is frequently heard, but not an early acquisition. Our account is because it nonetheless only occurs in a restricted set of words.

This aspect of phonological acquisition contributes to the earlier evidence for the claim that children are doing linguistic organization of their language early on. It provides a fruitful hypothesis that can be tested by future cross-linguistic research. Interestingly, a recent report by De Boysson-Bardies, Halle, Sagart and Durand (1989) even suggests that these features may begin to emerge in the later stages of babbling.

11. *The nature of phonotactic constraints and early syllable structure.* It has been known for some time that the child's first words are subject to severe phonotactic constraints. As mentioned earlier, these appear to be relaxed after the first fifty words or so when the basic set of phonemes has been acquired. That is, development after the word spurt appears to be primarily the spreading of the "basic" sounds into new combinations, rather than the addition of new sounds. The documentation of these changes for a Spanish child can be found in detail in Macken (1978).

Eventually, analyses of their development will allow us to know more about how such restrictions get loosened. Also, the data may shed some light on how we may want to represent ultimately the skeletal structure of phonological representations. Let me give just one example of how this may be pursued. A current issue under discussion in phonological theory is whether we wish to represent the timing of phonological structure as sequences of Cs and Vs (CV theory), or as morae. One argument for mora theory (Hayes, 1988) is that it captures the facts of compensatory lengthening. For example, a language that has heavy syllables (i.e., two morae) will show lengthening of the vowel if the final consonant is deleted (see 9a and b, below [where m stands for a mora]). The vowel can be said to be lengthened to maintain the empty mora which is left behind.

```
9.   a.   m   m          b.   m   m
          /|  |               /|  /
          d a  t              d   a:
```

Mora theory predicts that there will never be compensatory lengthening into the onset position if a consonant deletes, because onsets cannot have morae of their own.

Given certain assumptions, we can propose that mora theory makes certain predictions about children's productions. One would be that we should see compensatory lengthening when children delete final consonants, but not when they delete initial ones. If such patterns prove to be true, they can be used as evidence in favor of the existence of morae.

12. *The representation of distinctive features.* Last, there is the issue of what features children actually acquire, and how they are represented. As stated earlier, I propose that they acquire distinctive features from the onset of acquisition. Goad and Ingram (1987) suggests as a hypothesis that the first features are only specified for minimal contrasts. So, the child with /b/, /p/, and /t/ only has the [voice] feature for /b/ and /p/. Such a hypothesis restricts both the nature of the feature proposed to be acquired as well as its specification for specific phonemes.

Despite this hypothesis, there will still be a number of instances where the nature of a minimal contrast is not obvious. For example, take a hypothetical child with the system /m/, /p/, and /b/ → [m]. We have a choice here between the features [nasal] and [voice], as shown in 10.

10. *a.*   /m/ /p/ /b/   *b.*   /m/ /p/ /b/
           nasal +   −   +   voice +   −   −

In fact, the feature systems available are sufficiently rich that there will be many such choices found. Ingram (1988c), I propose the following hypothesis to restrict the features that we may assign to the child's words:

> *Distinctive Feature Hypothesis*: Children phonologically analyze and represent their first words in distinctive features selected from the set of available phonetic features in the fully specified phonetic representation. Further, any phonological feature assigned to an element underlying rule must be available within the fully specified phonetic representation.

The beauty of this hypothesis is that it restricts dramatically what can be specified underlyingly. In the case of the example in 10, it rules out 10*a* since the sound /b/ does not have the feature nasal in its phonetic representation.

THE NATURE OF PHONOLOGICAL DISABILITY

So far, I have outlined a general view of phonological acquisition with reference only to data from normal children. What, then, is the relation between these observations and phonological acquisition in children with phonological dysfunction?

Ingram (1987a, 1987b) argues that a theory of phonological disorders will only be possible in reference to a theory of phonological acquisition in general. Further, it is proposed that unique patterns of phonological delay will only be identifiable once there is a theory of the extent and limits of normal children.

Unfortunately, there is no theory of normal variation at this time. As pointed out in Ingram (1987b), cases of so-called normal children can be found which show patterning every bit as strange as those of disordered children. It is somewhat ironic, in fact, that we tend to view variation among normal children as evidence for linguistic creativity, yet variation among disordered children as instances of "deviance."

My proposal was that for the time being we should continue to assume the conclusion that patterns of delayed acquisition are similar to those for normal children. We can, however, begin inquiries into what might lead children in either group toward more unusual acquisition patterns. Ingram (1989b) also proposed what I refer to as a hypothesis about phonological deviance that applies to all children as follows:

> *Hypothesis about Phonological Deviance*: "The extent of a child's phonological deviance is the consequence of an inverse relation between his stage of phonological acquisition and the size of his vocabulary" (p. 163).

This hypothesis argues that children who show unusual acquisition patterns will be those who are at an early stage of phonological acquisition yet have an extensive vocabulary.

One such child who looked deviant in this sense is the famous Hildegard Leopold (Leopold, 1947). As shown in Ingram (1985), Hildegard maintained an extremely small consonantal inventory over the first year of phonological acquisition, as shown in 11.

11. Hildegard's consonants at 1;11

word initial	m-	n-	word final	-t		-k
	b-	d-				
	w-	h-			S	

While her consonantal inventory remained constant, Hildegard continued to expand her vocabulary, resulting in a remarkable increase in homonymy within her system. This is atypical in the sense that the use of homonymy for most children tends to decrease rather than increase.

I should emphasize that this position just outlined does not assume that the search for differences between normal and disordered children should cease. It simply states that the current data are inclusive thus far, and require a more developed theory of normal acquisition. Each of the observations in the previous section, in fact, are possible candidates to explore for potential differences.

Indeed, in research just completed, Ingram (in prep. b) has identified what may be a significant difference between at least some disordered children and normal children. In this study, 35 normal children were compared with 35 disordered ones on one narrow aspect of acquisition—

the acquisition of English stop consonants (i.e., /b/, /d/, /g/, /p/, /t/, /k/). The typical pattern for the normal children is to acquire the entire voiced series /b/, /d/, /g/, before the voiceless ones. The disordered children, however, showed a marked preference to acquire voicing before or simultaneously with place. In particular, voice tended to be acquired before two place distinctions within the lingual stops. So, for example, systems such as (1) b,p,t ; (2) b,p,t,d and even (3) t,d in some extreme cases might be found.

This finding can be interpreted by recognizing the independence of the larynx from the developing control of the tongue. The children who show this pattern are having difficulty enacting the tongue movements necessary to make both alveolar and velar place distinctions. This problem, however, does not impede them from continuing their development by acquiring [voice] as a distinctive feature. This early difficulty in lingual control for disordered children is more obviously seen in later development with their notorious problem with fricatives. Once again, the children's ability to cope with an articulatory problem with alternative linguistic development is seen.

A theory of normal phonological acquisition is not only prerequisite for research such as the above, but also for the development of programs of phonological remediation. Ingram (1986b) has attempted to show how findings on cross-linguistic normal acquisition lead to significant gains in the understanding of remediation. In particular, several aspects of normal acquisition, such as those presented earlier, are outlined, which can be used in several of the remedial procedures suggested in Hodson and Paden (1983). For example, the simple observation that children show receptive knowledge of linguistic aspects 3 to 4 months before productive use should be sufficient to doom traditional speech therapy from the onset. As findings on normal development expand, they should lead to new and interesting attempts to explore them through phonological intervention.

SUMMARY

As the title of this paper indicates, I have outlined some ideas that are moving toward a theory of phonological acquisition. The overall picture is something like the following: The child acquires an accurate acoustic representation of an initial receptive vocabulary. As he or she begins to speak, these words begin to be represented phonologically. This phonological representation will consist of some form of skeletal structure representing syllable structure (Cs and Vs, or morae). Feature acquisition will also begin by the child selecting these from UG, combined with the prominence of specific features in the language. As each feature is acquired, a parameter of phonological acquisition is set. Pronunciation consists of the interaction of those features acquired with a universal set of redundancy rules (or markedness statements) as found in natural phonology.

As can be seen, this model adapts the strong points of Jakobson's theory and natural phonology within the basic structure of currently discussed nonlinear phonology. Also, the method for analysis develops explicit analytic procedures, as argued for in Ferguson and Farwell (1975). Details about its nature will emerge as more phonological analyses of children acquiring a range of languages are done, as well as those of children with marked phonological delay.

REFERENCES

Archangeli, D., & Pulleyblank, D. (1986). The content and structure of phonological representations. Manuscript, University of Arizona and University of Southern California.

Benedict, H. (1979). Early lexical development: Comprehension and production. *Journal of Child Language, 6*, 183–200.

De Boysson-Bardies, B., Halle, P., Sagart, L., & Durand, C. (1989). A crosslinguistic investigation of vowel formants in babbling. *Journal of Child Language, 16*, 1–17.

Dikken, M. den, & Hulst, H. van der. (in press). Segmental heirarchitecture. In H. van der Hulst & N. H. S. Smith (Eds.), *Features, segmental structure and harmony processes.* Dordrecht: Foris.

Eimas, P., Sigueland, E., Jusczyk, P., & Vigorito, J. (1971). Speech perception in infants. *Science, 171*, 303–318.

Ferguson, C. A., & Farwell, C. B. (1975). Words and sounds in early language acquisition. *Language, 51*, 419–439.

Gibson, D., & Ingram, D. (1983). The onset of comprehension and production in a language delayed child. *Applied Psycholinguistics, 4*, 359–375.

Goad, H., & Ingram, D. (1987). Individual variation and its relevance to a theory of phonological acquisition. *Journal of Child Language, 14*, 419–432.

Hayes, B. (1988). Compensatory lengthening in moraic phonology. Manuscript, University of California, Los Angeles.

Hodson, B., & Paden, E. (1983). *Targeting intelligible speech: a phonological approach to remediation.* San Diego: College Hill.

Hulst, van der, H., & Smith, N. (1985). The framework of nonlinear generative phonology. In *Advances in nonlinear phonology* (pp. 1–55). Dordrecht: Foris.

Ingram, D. (1981). *Procedures for the phonological analysis of children's language.* Baltimore: University Park Press.

Ingram, D. (1985). On children's homonyms. *Journal of Child Language, 12*, 671–680.

Ingram, D. (1986a). In defense of the segment in phonological acquisition. Paper presented at the annual meeting of the Linguistic Society of America, New York.

Ingram, D. (1986b). Explanation and phonological remediation. *Child Language Teaching and Remediation, 2*, 1–29.

Ingram, D. (1987a). Categories of phonological disorder. *Proceedings of the First International Symposium on Specific Speech and Language Disorders in Children* (pp. 88–99). Surrey: Association for All Speech Impaired Children.

Ingram, D. (1987b). Phonological impairment in children. Paper presented at the International Symposium entitled Language Acquisition and Language Impairment, Parma, Italy, June 4–6, 1987.

Ingram, D. (1988a). Jakobson revisited: Some evidence from the acquisition of Polish phonology. *Lingua, 75,* 55–82.

Ingram, D. (1988b). The acquisition of word-initial [v]. *Language and Speech, 31,* 77–85.

Ingram, D. (1988c). Underspecification theory and phonological acquisition. Paper presented to the annual meeting of the Linguistic Society of America, New Orleans, December 1988.

Ingram, D. (1989a). *First language acquisition: Method, description, and explanation.* Cambridge: Cambridge University Press.

Ingram, D. (1989b). *Phonological disability in children, 2nd ed.* London: Cole & Whurr.

Ingram, D. (in prep.a). The acquisition of French vowels.

Ingram, D. (in prep.b). The acquisition of the feature [voice] in normal and phonologically delayed children.

Jakobson, R. (1968). *Child language, aphasia, and phonological universals.* (R. Keiler, Trans.). The Hague: Mouton. (Original German version published in 1941.)

Jakobson, R., & Halle, M. (1956). *Fundamentals of language.* The Hague: Mouton.

Leopold, W. (1947). *Speech development of a bilingual child: a linguist's record: Vol. 2, Sound learning in the first two years.* Evanston, IL: Northwestern University Press.

Locke, J. (1983). *Phonological acquisition and change.* New York: Academic.

Macken, M. A. (1978). Permitted complexity in phonological development: One child's acquisition of Spanish consonants. *Lingua, 44,* 219–253.

Macken, M. A. (1979). Developmental reorganization of phonology: A hierarchy of basic units of acquisition. *Lingua, 49,* 11–49.

Macken, M. A., & Ferguson, C. (1983). Cognitive aspects of phonological development: Model, evidence, and issues. In K. E. Nelson (Ed.), *Children's language, Vol. 4* (pp. 256–282). Hillsdale, NJ: Erlbaum.

Menn, L. (1971). Phonotactic rules in beginning speech. *Lingua, 26,* 225–251.

Piaget, J. (1948). *Play, dreams and imitation in childhood.* New York: Norton.

Pye, C., Ingram, D., & List, H. (1987). A comparison of initial consonant acquisition in English and Quiche. In K. E. Nelson & A. Van Kleeck (Eds.), *Children's Language, Vol. 6* (pp. 175–190). Hillsdale, NJ: Erlbaum.

Rasmussen, V. (1931). *Diary of a child's life from birth to the fifteenth year.* London: Gylendal. (Original Swedish edition published in 1922.)

Rescorla, L. (1980). Overextensions in early language development. *Journal of Child Language, 7,* 321–335.

Schwartz, R., & Leonard, L. (1982). Do children pick and choose? An examination of phonological selection and avoidance in early acquisition. *Journal of Child Language, 9,* 319–336.

Smith, M. (1926). An investigation of the development of the sentence and the extent of vocabulary in young children. *University of Iowa Studies in Child Welfare* 3.5

Stampe, D. (1969). The acquisition of phonemic representation. *Proceedings of the Fifth Regional Meeting of the Chicago Linguistic Society,* 433–444.

Tse, S., & Ingram, D. (1987). The influence of dialectal variation on phonological acquisition: A case study on the acquisition of Cantonese. *Journal of Child Language, 14,* 281–294.

Velten, H. (1943). The growth of phonemic and lexical patterns in infant speech. *Language, 19,* 281–292.

Wasow, T. (1983). Some remarks on developmental psycholinguistics. In Y. Otsu, H. van Riemsdijk, K. Inoue, A. Kamio, & N. Kawasaki (Eds.), *Studies in generative grammar and language acquisition,* Editorial Committee, Division of Languages, International Christian University. (pp. 191–196). Tokyo.

Waterson, N. (1971). Child phonology: A prosodic view. *Journal of Linguistics, 7,* 179–211.

CHAPTER 4

Connectionism as a Framework for Language Acquisition Theory

BRIAN MACWHINNEY

Connectionism is "in." Not since the Dark Ages of the pre-Chomskyan era have we seen so much interest in associationist models of human thinking. Streaming forth from their banishment in the Skinnerian dungeons are dozens of detailed computational models based on the new language of networks, nodes, and connections. At the crest of this wave are the Parallel Distributed Processing (PDP) models of Rumelhart, McClelland, and their colleagues (1986). Proponents of these new models present them as a major challenge to the *ancien régime*—a definitive revolution in the way in which we understand the human mind. Yet revolutions in academia are seldom bloodless. Inevitably, the proponents of the new paradigm tend to over-state their case and, inevitably, the Old Guard tries to form a unified front to challenge the contributions of the newcomers. The ensuing confusion infuriates some, galvanizes others, and perplexes everyone. All of these things are happening now in the Great Debate that is taking place between the New Connectionism and the Classical Model.

From the viewpoint of the onlooker to this controversy, what most characterizes this debate is the amount of heat being generated and the uniform avoidance of compromise positions or mixed models. From the general viewpoint of the human sciences, both the connectionists and their opponents seem to agree on many crucial issues. They agree on the importance of generating precise models of complex phenomena that can then be matched to empirical data. They agree on the importance of areas such as phonology, morphology, and syntax for the construction of such models. Both groups realize that the problems of one approach are often the strengths of the other. Given this, it is surprising not to see researchers considering ways of integrating the classical and connectionist models. Presumably, the participants in this debate have decided that they could present their points more clearly by assuming a position of stark opposition. From the viewpoint of the history of science, this is useful. However, the consumer of both connectionist and classical views of language processing and acquisition should be warned that a reconciliation of connectionist and classical views may not be as impossible as many authors suggest.

This chapter will present a series of completed connectionist simulations of the acquisitions of morphology in German, English, and Hungarian and will show how these simulations successfully address a variety of problems unsolved in earlier work. Then we will examine connectionist accounts for the learning of word meanings and the processing of syntax. Before looking at the connectionist simulations, it is necessary to review earlier work in this area to understand its successes and its failures.

EARLIER MODELS OF MORPHOLOGICAL LEARNING

Modern investigations of the learning of morphology began with Berko's (1958) famous "wugs" experiment. Berko, Ervin-Tripp, Braine, Brown and others looked in detail at overregularizations such as "feets" or "bringed" as ways of understanding language learning more generally. This early work showed the extent to which language use is based on the productive application of patterns and not mere rote memorization. Although morphology is only a very small part of the general picture of language acquisition, it has some important properties that make it an ideal topic for detailed investigation. Above all, it is extremely easy to collect and quantify data on morphological productions, including both correct forms such as "jumped" and overregularizations such as "falled."

The first serious theoretical account of morphological learning across languages was provided by Slobin (1973). In a masterful overview of both experimental and diary data on the acquisition of dozens of languages, Slobin was able to propose a set of general operating principles that accounted for the most well-documented aspects of word formation by children. Some of the most important data in Slobin's account came from studies of plural and past tense formation in English and from nominal declension in Russian. Among the most crucial of Slobin's principles were those that led the child to:

1. pay attention to the ends of words,
2. realize that the phonological forms of words can be systematically modified,
3. pay attention to the order of words and morphemes,
4. avoid interruptions,
5. mark underlying semantic notions overtly and clearly,
6. avoid exceptions, and
7. try to make semantic sense out of grammatical markers.

From each of these general operating principles, Slobin derived a further set of universals that appeared to be true of the 40 languages for which data was then available. Slobin grounded these principles on fundamental psychological facts and an insightful view of language function.

Despite its widespread appeal, Slobin's synthesis failed to specify in more exact terms the ways in which the principles should interact. Without such specifications, it was difficult to make exact predictions regarding the course of morphological learning. Providing this type of specification was a top priority and the earliest account of this sort was the one worked out by MacWhinney (1978) on the basis of earlier proposals by Braine (1971). Because learning in this mode was based on a process of error correction much like the traditional Hegelian dialectic, the model was called the *dialectic model*. The six types of processing in the model were:

1. *Rote use.* Early production of forms such as "feet" and "fell" was considered to be by rote.
2. *Simple combination.* After analyzing out basic forms of affixes, the child could apply them to form patterns such as "foots" or "falled."
3. *General morphophonemic rules.* The control of vowel harmony patterns, voicing assimilations and other general alternations was based on the applications of fairly surface-oriented transformational rules.
4. *Morpheme-specific rules.* Minor rules were acquired by encoding archimorphemic alternations on both stems and suffixes. Such rules can be used to form irregulars such as "knives" and "sang."
5. *Paradigms.* When all else failed, the system began to hypothesize general word-formation paradigms.
6. *Analogy.* Paralleling the development of combination in levels 2–5, the child also was able to produce analogies such as "brang" as the past tense of "bring" or "rew" as the past tense of "row."

The dialectic model was successful in accounting for many detailed aspects of the acquisition of morphology in English, German, Hungarian, and Finnish. Indeed, it is still the most complete account available for the actual empirical findings in the learning of morphology. However, the account suffered from a fundamental inability to deal with analogic processing. We will discuss that issue in more detail shortly.

Several years later, Pinker (1984) constructed a revised account of morphological learning, which kept certain aspects of the dialectic model while rejecting others. Pinker's model is interesting for three reasons. First, by basing all learning on paradigm formation and analysis, it achieves a cleaner theoretical structure. Second, Pinker portrays the model as an elaboration of learnability theory—a framework that requires that all models of language learning be demonstrated to converge in finite time on target grammars. Third, Pinker and Prince (1988) refer to the model of Pinker (1984) as a prime example of a well-established account of language learning developed within the classical framework and one that is clearly superior to connectionist alternatives. Given these claims for the value of the model, it is important for us to consider exactly how much of an advance it represents over the dialectic model or over connectionist alternatives. Pinker's model can be summarized in terms of a series of paradigm building operations.

1. *Add columns.* Every time the child encounters a new form of a word with a new meaning, he can add a column to a word-specific paradigm.

		PERSON		
		1	2	3
TENSE	Present	go	go	goes

2. *Add rows.* When the child finds a new form of an old word that expresses a new dimension, he must add a new dimension to the paradigm. For example, a one-way paradigm can be made into a two-way paradigm by adding rows. This can also be done for dimensions such as phonological patterns. In general any relevant cue can be used as the basis for setting up new columns or rows.

		PERSON		
		1	2	3
TENSE	Present	go	go	goes
	Past	went	went	went

3. *Delete rows and columns.* If all of the cells in a given row or column have the same entries, eliminate the distinction.

4. *Find the stem.* The child is supposed to examine all the forms in the paradigm and extract the common phonetic material as the stem. This means that the stem will be the "least common denominator" rather than the "greatest common denominator." In this paradigm for the Latin noun *puella* "girl," the stem is *puell-* in the Pinker account.

	Singular	Plural
Nom	puella	puellāe
Acc	puellam	puellas
Gen	puellae	puellarum
Dat	puellae	puellīs
Abl	puellā	puellīs

5. *Create general paradigms from the affixes.* After extracting the stem from a word-specific paradigm, the remaining affixes constitute the general paradigm. For Latin first declension, the paradigm is

	Singular	Plural
Nom	-a	-ae
Acc	-am	-ās
Gen	-ae	-ārum
Dat	-ae	-īs
Abl	-a	-īs

For agglutinative forms such as Hungarian *ablak-od-nál* "window-yours-near," Pinker provides a recursive extraction procedure that would enter the suffix *-od* into the paradigm for the person suffixes and *-nál* into the paradigm for the case suffixes, while also constructing a word structure template of the form: *stem + person + case*.

6. *Use new forms to split old paradigms.* If there are any irregular forms or minor patterns in the language, repeated application of 4 and 5 can be used to split the general paradigm along "arbitrary" dimensions such as noun gender or verb conjugation in Indo-European. Alternatively, repeated application of 4 and 5 can be used to focus the child's attention on some otherwise ignored syntactic or discourse dimension not encoded in word-specific paradigms.

7. *Use the general paradigm to fill any remaining gaps in the word-specific paradigms.* If a particular word-specific paradigm is missing an entry, the child can use the general paradigm to fill that gap. For example, the child may not know the past tense of "fall." The general paradigm would tell him or her that it is "falled." Like MacWhinney, Pinker allows for a competition between the word-specific form and the general form.

Let us examine some of the technical problems that arise in Pinker's framework. Some of these problems also occur in MacWhinney's system, whereas others only arise in the Pinker account.

1. *New work or new cell?* When a child hears a new word, how does he or she decide whether it should be added to an existing paradigm or simply

entered as a new word into the lexicon? On the one hand, a child might decide not to related *went* to *go*, assuming they are too discrepant phonologically. On the other hand, the child might attempt to form a paradigm for words such as *thump, dump,* and *bump.* There are no sure principles in Pinker's system to guide the child through the Scylla and Charybdis of correct suppletion and erroneous paradigm formation. Since, in Pinker's system, word analysis cannot begin until general paradigms are formed, there is no way for the child to find stems in inflected words. Of course, a child could use meaning communalities to guide paradigm construction, but this is not a part of Pinker's proposal. The dialectic model has no problem with forms such as *go* and *went,* since it never puts them into paradigms in the first place. Later on, if it constructs unnecessary rules for alternations that do not really occur, those rules will simply be so weak that they will not survive.

2. *How does the child know which values belong to which dimensions?* In order to add a new value to a row or column, the child must know that the value belongs to a particular dimension. In order to add the value of dual to the dimension of number, the child has to understand that a given noun cannot be both plural and dual at the same time. In other words, the child must have already constructed the conceptual framework underlying the paradigm. Some contrasts, such as that between singular and plural, are obvious. Others, such as that between conditional and past or plural and dual are not so clearly nonoverlapping. Both the Pinker proposal and the MacWhinney proposal share the problem of basing paradigm construction on precisely the knowledge that is being constructed. However, the problem is worse for Pinker since his entire model relies on paradigm formation and MacWhinney only uses paradigm formation when all other forms of learning have failed.

3. *Should stems be reduced to the least common material?* As Braine (1987) has shown, Pinker's procedure runs into serious problems with strong morphophonological alternations. For example, for third declension nouns like *mīles* "soldier" the procedure would analyze out *mīl-* instead of the correct form *mīl(it)-*. In regard to the suffix, the procedure would yield a large array of inconsistent suffixes such as *-item, -inem,* and the like, all with stray pieces of the stem. In addition, there would be different ending forms for each of the different declensional types. In general, the Pinker solution adds a great deal of complexity and nonuniformity that is avoided in the proposals of MacWhinney (1978) and Braine (1987).

4. *How many words are needed to support a general paradigm?* Pinker tells us that new paradigms will not be set up when only a "small" number of forms are involved. Doing this leads to serious problems for irregular words in agglutinative languages. For example, Hungarian has several irregular noun groups with fewer than six members. According to the Pinker procedure, none of these groups could produce general paradigms. Within

the three large gender classes in German, there are about 20 further classes that show minor irregularities in the genitive, the dative plural, and elsewhere. What leads the child to treat these alternations as secondary and the major gender divisions as primary? Indeed, what evidence is there that minor rules and minor classes are treated in a fundamentally different way from major rules and major classes? Indeed, data from language history, language acquisition, and adult speech errors show that even the smallest paradigmatic groups have some productivity. Indeed, Malkiel (1968) showed that the single strong verb *dīcere* was able to play a major role in the shaping of the development of verbal conjugations in Romance.

5. *Should paradigms be used as the basis for extracting affixes?* The problem here is that Hungarian children pull out affixes from simple forms before they construct full paradigms. For example, they extract the first person singular definite *-om* from verbs such as *tudom* long before they construct the full six dimensional verb paradigm out of forms such as *tud-hat-gat-ná-tok* "know-potential frequentative-conditional-2PL". This is only a problem for Pinker's system, since the MacWhinney system orders analysis before paradigm formation.

6. *Learnability.* Despite his interest in learnability, Pinker provides neither learnability proofs for the model nor computational implementations to test the model's operation.

By attempting to provide a uniform treatment based on paradigms, Pinker has expanded on the most questionable part of the dialectic model and abandoned the part that was most fully motivated empirically.

Both MacWhinney and Pinker tried to emphasize the ways in which the child uses real semantic and phonological cues to predict morphological patterns. A rather different emphasis can be found in the work of Maratsos (1982). Maratsos analogized the learning of language to the learning of arbitrary patterns of etiquette. Why is the knife placed on the right of the plate and the fork on the left? According to Maratsos, there is no inherent reason. Why in German is *das Messer* "the knife" neuter, *die Gabel* "the fork" feminine, and *der Löffel* "the spoon" masculine? According to Maratsos, there is no good reason. Rather, language is arbitrary and language learning involves picking up arbitrary co-occurrence patterns between unmotivated form classes. The mechanism that Maratsos proposed to acquire these co-occurrences was one that would simply form classes out of things that go with other things. For example, in German, masculine nouns would be defined as ones which co-occur with *der*, *den*, and *dem*. Neuter nouns are defined as those that co-occur with *die* and *der*, and so on. Other categories are defined in similar ways. The nominative is the category of nouns occurring before verbs, with either *der*, *die*, or *das* and with no nominal endings and no preceding prepositions, and so on. Maratsos never stated exactly how these co-occurrences would be detected in a model.

These earlier models all had their strengths and their limitations. The Slobin account was empirically accurate, but inadequate mechanistically. The MacWhinney account was empirically accurate, but its mechanistic components were rather diverse. The Pinker account had greater symmetry, but paid a price in empirical adequacy. Maratsos makes many good points in emphasizing the arbitrariness of many aspects of language learning. However, his view fails to give enough attention to the other side of the coin—the predictable aspects of language patterns. Even for the seemingly clearcut example of German gender, it turns out that there is a great deal more predictability than Maratsos recognized (Köpcke & Zubin, 1983, 1984).

A CONNECTIONIST MODEL
OF MORPHOLOGICAL COMPETITION

All of the accounts examined here suffer from an inability to express both arbitrariness and predictability within a single comprehensive framework. The model examined next goes beyond these limitations. It is a connectionist network that is able to learn the basic properties of the German declensional paradigm. This model is a direct outgrowth of a variety of work within the competition model of MacWhinney and Bates (1989). Earlier reports on this line of research can be found in Taraban, McDonald, and MacWhinney (in press) and MacWhinney, Leinbach, Taraban, and McDonald (1989).

Before we look at the simulation itself, we need to review the way in which declensional facts are marked in German. The declensional paradigm is configured around the dimensions or number, case, and gender. Number is either singular or plural. Case is either nominative, accusative, genitive, or dative. Gender is either masculine, feminine, or neuter. The bulk of the work of marking gender, number, and case is done by the article or adjective that precedes the noun. A complete cross of the categories of gender, number, and case would yield 24 possible cells for the full declensional paradigm for the definite article. Fortunately for the German child, gender distinctions for the definite article disappear in the plural, reducing the paradigm to the 16 cells shown below.

	Singular			Plural
	M	F	N	
Nom.	der	die	das	die
Acc.	den	die	das	die
Gen.	des	der	des	der
Dat.	dem	der	dem	den

THE ACQUISITIONAL DATA

The two most comprehensive experimental studies of the learning of German declension are those done by MacWhinney (1978) and Mills (1986). The findings of these studies match well with nonexperimental observations from Park (1981) and the various other sources cited in MacWhinney (1978) and Mills (1986). Some of the most important findings of this literature are:

1. *Early acquisition of the nominative.* Children first achieve correct mastery of the use of the nominative case, often overgeneralizing it for the accusative (MacWhinney, 1978).
2. *Delayed acquisition of the genitive.* Of the four cases, it is the genitive that continues to cause problems for article marking. The dative plural is also a late difficult form, but this difficulty involves nominal marking rather than article selection.
3. *Children often omit the article.* Many of the cues to gender assignment are hard to detect and many are only imperfectly reliable. This forces the child to turn his or her attention to other ways of controlling gender categorization. One simple way of solving the problem is to omit the article. In fact, early on, omission of the article is very common and even later on, the article may be omitted when the child is in doubt about the correct gender assignment.
4. *Children often overgeneralize one gender.* Mills (1986) observed a tendency to overgeneralize the use of the feminine gender.
5. *Children make early use of the highly frequent -e cue.* Mills (1986) examined the role of some of the Köpcke-Zubin cues in the acquisition of Germany gender and found evidence for their use. MacWhinney (1978) conducted his work before the Köpcke-Zubin cues were available, but his experiment still included some of the cues. Both Mills (1986) and MacWhinney (1978) found early acquisition of the most highly available and reliable of the cues—the presence of final -*e* as a cue to feminine gender.
6. *Children make early use of highly reliable cues.* MacWhinney (1978) also found that children between the ages of 4 and 6 were able to make correct use of the morphological marking -*ei* as a cue to feminine gender and -*chen* as a cue to neuter gender. Schneuwly (1978) reports similar findings. These data indicate that children are indeed sensitive to the various phonological and morphological cues to gender and that the stronger these cues are, the earlier they are used consistently by children. Tucker, Lambert, and Rigault (1977) report on a set of careful and detailed studies of cue use in predicting French gender, which make it entirely clear that the higher the reliability of a cue, the stronger its use by adult subjects.

7. *Children can use paradigmatic marking cues to infer word classes.*
MacWhinney (1978) showed that 4-year-old children were able to
make reliable use of the pronoun as a cue to the gender of nonce
words. The experiment involved using the masculine form of the
accusative personal pronoun "him" *ihn* to refer to a nonce word
represented by a small toy. When the experimenter said, "I am
picking him *(ihn)* up in my hand," children were able to successfully
infer that the thing being picked up was masculine even though it was
an object they had never seen before with a name they had never
heard before.

THE SIMULATION

The behavior that the model is designed to simulate is the selection of one
of the six forms of the definite article given a noun and its case context. This
task is clearly a production task and not a comprehension task. We will
discuss comprehension-production relations later. The simulation relies
on the "back-propagation" architecture elaborated by Rumelhart, Hinton,
and Williams (1986). Like other connectionist models, the model consists
of a large number of densely interconnected "units" or "nodes" operating
in parallel. The model has three layers of units: input units, output units,
and intervening units, as can be seen in Figure 4-1. The network's "knowledge" is contained in the strength of the connections between the units in
the network. Nodes in the network can receive or send activation or both.
Activation is sent across connections. Receiving nodes update their activation as a function of the sum of their inputs. Each input is the product of the
activation of the sending node times the strength of the connection. The
input layer encodes the presence or absence of cues associated with a
particular noun and its sentential context. Each node on the input layer
represents a single cue feature. If the cue is present for a particular noun,
the input node is fully activated, and if it is not present the node remains
off. The words are represented as sets of cues. The activation of the input
layer produces activation on the internal layer(s), which in turn produces
activation on the output layer. Each of the six German definite articles is
represented by a unit on the output layer.

Input Units

The model uses a uniform coding of the phonological shape of input words.
As indicated in Figure 4-1 above, there are three types of input units: 143
phonological units, 5 semantic units, and 20 case context units. The 143
phonological units represent the full form of the noun in actual phonological features. These units are distributed over 13 slots with 11 features in
each slot. The 11 features are standard phonological distinctive features
such as [+labial], [+coronal], [+voice], [+high], etc. Diphthongs and affri-

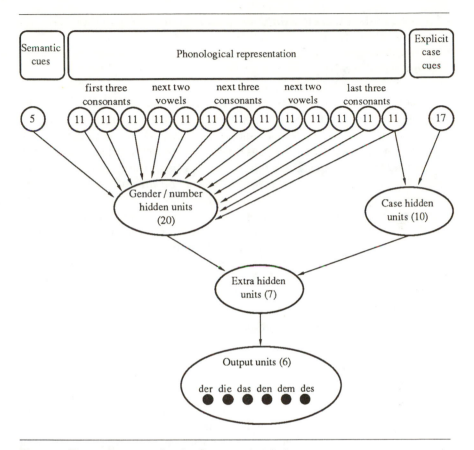

Fig. 4-1. The architecture for the German simulation.

cates are coded as pairs of phonemes. These features provide a unique 11-unit feature code for each German phoneme. The 13 slots are divided across various syllable positions. The 20 case context units code for seven prepositions, seven word order configurations (NNV, NVN, VNN, NN, first noun, second noun, third noun), and three verb types (verb of motion, copular verb, and plural verb). In addition, the hidden units that connect to the case context units also connect to the final phoneme of the word, allowing them to detect the presence of the case endings -s for masculine and neuter nouns in the genitive and -n for plural nouns in the dative.

The phonological and semantic units all project to a set of gender/number hidden units. The explicit case units and the phonological units for the final consonant of the stem all project to a set of case hidden units. The phonological information for the final consonant is used to code the presence of noun-final markers for the genitive and dative plural. Both sets of hidden units project to a third set of hidden units, which then activates the six output units.

Running the Model

Here is how the network was taught to perform the task. Initially, all the weights on the connections were assigned small random weights. A training set for the simulation was then presented to the network. The training set consisted of sets of cues for each word in the list and the correct article for that set of cues. During the training phase, the cues for each word were presented on the input layer and activated an output pattern. The activated output pattern was compared to the correct pattern and the difference between the two was used to compute an error measure. After a complete pass through all the words in the training set (an epoch), each weight in the network was individually strengthened or weakened so that during the next pass through the training set the activated patterns would be closer to the correct patterns (i.e., there would be less error). Each weight was changed according to the back propagation algorithm. The learning method was consistently applied to all the connections in the network, and there was no *ad hoc* intervention into the learning process.

The Training Set

The training set consisted of 102 different nouns selected from a frequency count of a spoken German corpus of over 80,000 words (Wängler, 1963). The higher frequency nouns were included several times for a total of 305 tokens in the training set. The network learned the training set completely by the end of 100 epochs of training.

GENERALIZATION ACROSS THE PARADIGM

Although the speed and accuracy of this learning is impressive, one could argue that the network simply developed a complicated rote-like representation of the data presented to it without really acquiring anything that corresponds to rule-like behavior. In order to see if the network had learned something beyond the specific associations between combinations of cues and definite articles present in the training set, two different tests of generalization were made. The first test checked how well the network was able to apply the declensional paradigm. The test set consisted of the same 102 nouns used in the training set, but each noun was paired with the subset of case contexts it had not been paired with in the training set. For example, a word that had occurred only in the dative singular in training was then tested in the nominative plural and the genitive singular.

This test was given to the network after it had achieved 100% performance on the training set. The results of this test were excellent. On the five generalization runs, the model had an average success rate of 94%. The chance level here would be 16%. This high level of performance provides strong evidence that the network was remarkably good at generalizing the overall paradigm to noun–case pairings that it was seeing for the first time. Many of the errors that the network made were caused by ambiguities in the paradigm. These are the kinds of errors children are expected to make. For example, if a noun occurred in the training set in the nominative *die*, the accusative *die*, and the genitive *der*, but did not occur in the dative, neither a child nor the network could know whether the noun stem was a feminine singular or a plural, since the plural takes the same articles as the feminine singular in these three cases. The ambiguity is even more confounded, since one of the most frequent cues to feminine, final *-e* on the noun, is also a plural marker. When a noun with final *-e* was presented in the dative case in the test, the network most often assigned it the article *der*—the marker of a feminine singular noun in the dative. Thus, plural nouns, which should take the article *den* in the dative, were sometimes assigned the incorrect article in the dative case in the generalization test. Another case of ambiguity in the training set occurred when a noun appeared in the dative case with *dem* and the genitive case with *des*, but did not occur in the nominative or accusative cases. In this situation it would be impossible to discriminate masculine singular from neuter singular nouns. Because of this overlap in the paradigm between masculine and neuter singular, the network often confused or conflated the two.

PREDICTION OF THE GENDER OF NEW NOUNS

In order to test the ability of the network to predict the gender of new nouns, the next simulation used a much larger input set. This set included all the 2095 high frequency German nouns in the Wängler corpus. From these, 199 nouns were picked at random and reserved for generalization testing. The remaining 1896 nouns constituted the training set. For this test the architecture of the system was simplified in various ways. The five semantic cues were eliminated, as well as the dimensions of case and number from the simulation, using only the articles *der, die,* and *das* of the nominative. This simplified architecture allowed the ability of the network to acquire cues for predicting gender to be seen more clearly. The results were exactly as expected. The simulation was able to predict the gender of new nouns with over 70% accuracy. Since there are only three articles used in this simulation, chance is 33%. The nouns for which the simulation chose the wrong gender were generally ones that resembled patterns of another gender. The model was not expected to achieve perfect or even near perfect performance in this task, since even native German speakers cannot achieve perfect accuracy in predicting the gender of new words. However, the strong performance of the model on this very large data set in this simplified architecture indicates that there are indeed many powerful cues to the prediction of German gender and that a connectionist network is a good tool for picking up these cues.

COMPARISON TO THE DEVELOPMENTAL LITERATURE

Finally, the model's errors at various points were examined during its learning of the training set. The results from these further analyses uniformly matched the first six major phenomena noted in the developmental literature. Early acquisition of the nominative, delayed acquisition of the genitive, omissions of the article, overgeneralizations of the feminine gender, early use of the strong *-e* cue, early use of the reliable *-chen* cues and others like it were found. The earlier simulation had already shown the model's ability to use the "paradigm" to infer word classes. This last finding is perhaps the most remarkable, given the fact that there was no direct representation of a paradigm anywhere in the model. Although the model used no formal inferential logic, it was able to behave as if it were making this inference.

The model provides an interesting alternative to the information-processing account of morphological learning presented first in MacWhinney (1978) and later in Pinker (1984). Within a single network, the processes of rote, combination, analogy, and paradigm application are all expresssed in terms of patterns of associations between cues. The ad hoc nature of the processes proposed in the earlier accounts is entirely eliminated. Whereas earlier research on morphological systems such as that of Tucker, Lambert, and Rigault (1977) or MacWhinney (1978) was forced to think of generalization in terms of rule use, generalization can now be thought about in terms of cue acquisition. The model also allows merging of the insights of the co-occurrence model of Maratsos and Chalkley (1980) with the cue-based learning emphasized in the competition model (MacWhinney, 1987). Within a single network can be found prediction of form class on the basis of both co-occurrences and cues. The network was able to deal successfully with both arbitrary relations and cue-based predictable relations.

Finally—and this is no small matter—this is the first real operational simulation of morphological learning that has ever been fully completed.

GENERALIZING THE MODEL

The architecture used in the simulation discussed so far was designed to model a very specific aspect of German language production. Given a noun and its case context, the simulation could activate the correct form of the definite article. Using a slightly different type of architecture, it is possible to simulate the processes of production and comprehension within a single network. To explore this possibility, the next study focused on the learning of nominal case marking in Hungarian. A set of 92 Hungarian nouns, each having ten different declined forms, was chosen. These ten different cases are what Hungarian grammarians call *ragok*. They include the accusative, the plural, the inessive, the dative, the benfactive, various possessive forms, and so on. Each inflected form is produced by combining a nominal stem with an affix. During the process of suffixation, both stem and suffix can undergo a variety of transformations that are described in detail in MacWhinney (1978, 1985). For example, when the stem *bokor* ("bush") combines with the suffix *-ok*, the resultant form is *bokrok*. The actual shape of the suffix varies depending on the phonological shape of the stem. For example, the various possible forms of the plural suffix include *-k, -ok, -ak, -ek* and *-ök*. Here is a very small piece of the Hungarian nominal paradigm.

Nom-Sg	Nom-Pl	1PSposs-Acc	Acc	Allative	Super
ló	lovak	lovamat	lovat	lóhoz	lóvon
ablak	ablakok	ablakomat	ablakot	ablakhoz	ablakon
madár	madarak	madaramat	madarat	madárhoz	madáron
epér	eprek	epremet	epret	epérhez	epéren
ötös	ötösök	ötösömet	ötöst	ötöshöz	ötösön

The complete paradigm has about 30 rows and at least 96 columns. Our current simulation sampled only 10 of the columns and 8 of the rows.

The goals of the simulation were (1) to model production by producing the phonetics of a declined form, given the semantics of the noun and the semantics of the desired declination, (2) to model comprehension by generating the semantics of a noun and the semantics of its declination type, given the phonetics of its declined form, and (3) to be able to improve performance on both of these tasks through training on the *other*. All of these goals were achieved with surprising success.

The structure of this network, as with the German simulation, was quite simple. Three layers of units were used—an input layer, an intermediate "processing" layer, and an output layer. Training was again carried out using the back propagation algorithm described above. In this simulation, however, both the input and output layers were used to represent the same thing—a semantics/phonetics pair that fully described the declined form of a noun, as indicated in Figure 4-2. The semantics of a declined form were represented by a random unique pattern specific to the noun, followed by a pattern across a set of 14 meaningful units which together expressed the meaning of a declination type. The phonetics of a declined form were simply represented as a string of the phonemes of that form, each phoneme

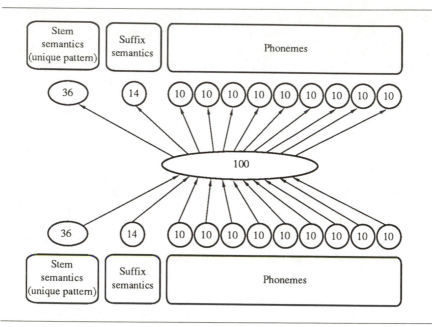

Fig. 4-2. An architecture that relates comprehension and production.

being represented by a pattern across 10 feature units that together specified the desired phoneme.

Training was conducted in two modes. During comprehension training, the network was taught to generate a complete semantic and phonological description, given just the phonological form. The idea here is that children can often infer the meanings of words from context. They hear the word and can then check to see if what they thought the word might mean actually corresponds to what the context indicates. During production training, the network was taught to generate a complete semantic and phonological description of a declined form, given just the semantics of that form. One third of the nouns were randomly selected to have one of their declined forms (randomly chosen) excluded from training (both comprehension and production). The ability to produce and comprehend these unseen forms was then tested, once the network had learned correctly to produce and comprehend all of the forms it was trained with. The purpose of this test was to ensure that the network was actually using appropriate rules of comprehension and production, and not simply memorizing which output patterns went with each input patterns. The results indicated that the network had in fact learned some excellent rules for these tasks. When asked to comprehend the untaught forms, the resulting semantic descriptions of the forms were better than 99% correct in terms of the stem semantics and 100% correct in terms of the declination-type semantics. When asked to produce the unseen forms, the resulting phoneme strings were 98.3% correct.

The network also demonstrated an interesting interplay between comprehension and production. The observation that the language learner is better prepared to produce a word if he or she has already learned to comprehend it was also captured by this network, as hoped. This was made possible by the "full-description" word representations that were used as output targets. These representations forced the network to learn not only how to produce semantics from phonology and phonology from semantics, but also to reproduce semantics from semantics and phonology from phonology. In doing so, each task generated middle-level representations that were useful to the other task. The comprehension task generated middle-level representations that were useful for producing phonological output (generally useful for performing production), and the production task generated middle-level representations useful for producing semantic output (generally useful for performing comprehension). This meant that, if the network had already learned one of these tasks, when attempting to learn the other, it could exploit this previously learned ability. This is apparently what the network did. Figure 4-3 shows the network's ability to

Fig. 4-3. Savings from prior comprehension training.

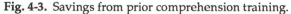

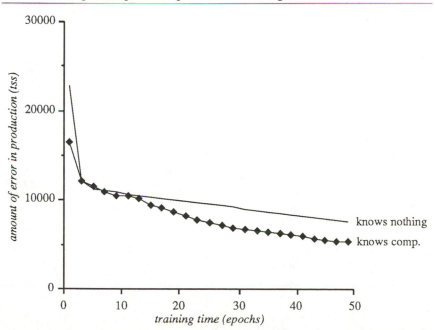

remove error from its production performance over time, in each of two conditions. Clearly it is much more adept at learning the production task if it has already learned to comprehend the words it is trying to produce.

This architecture could also be applied to the German declination system, providing a much more robust consideration of the many processes involved there. Such a project and a project involving the declination of English verbs into various tenses are currently underway. These projects will all use a uniform phonological architecture, a uniform network topology, and a uniform learning rule to model morphological learning in these very different languages.

MODELS IN OTHER DOMAINS

The next three sections examine ways of constructing connectionist models for phonological, lexical, and syntactic competition. These proposals are still largely speculative, although some simple simulations in these areas have already been constructed. The reader needs to remember that models of morphological processing are inherently easier to develop than models of semantic processing. Morphology is a small, tightly defined domain for which empirical data are relatively easy to obtain. The development and processing of word meaning, on the other hand, is a much larger area without the same sharp data and tight definitions. Despite these practical differences, there are reasons to believe that the same connectionist concepts developed for the study of morphological development will also be useful in studying learning in these other domains.

MODELING PHONOLOGICAL COMPETITION

McClelland and Elman (1986) have constructed a connectionist account of phonological processing called the trace model. However, that model did not have a learning component and is not well adapted to use in language acquisition studies. However, the architecture being used in our current simulations for morphology can also be adopted to the study of phonological development, if certain modifications are made. The first modification is the replacement of semantic features in the network with phonological features. Thus, instead of trying to go from phonological features to semantic features, the network will try to go from phonetic features to words as characterized by phonological features and then back to phonetic features. In this way, the network produces a unique phonological code that could be used for further connectionist processing without having to compute at the same time the largely arbitrary mapping from sound to meaning. Figure 4-4 indicates the possible shape of such a model.

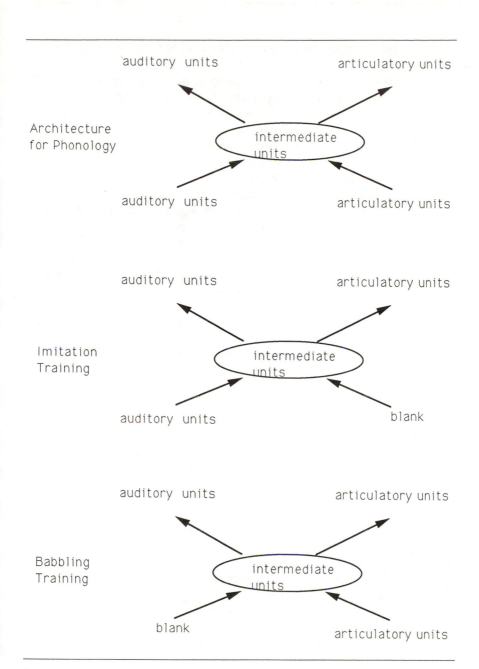

Fig. 4-4. A model for phonological learning.

MODELING LEXICAL COMPETITION

The most basic type of semantic competition is lexical competition. This type of competition arises during production when one is trying to decide what word to use to refer to a particular object or activity. Consider a set of competing words like "cup," "mug," and "demitasse." In the competition model account, these three forms are seen as occupying neighboring parts of a multidimensional semantic topography. For simplicity, imagine that the crucial attributes distinguishing these three forms are size, thickness, and cylindricality. Figure 4-5 illustrates the core semantic territory for each of the three words on these three dimensions. For the adult, objects that fall within the core territories are clear cases of cups, mugs, and demitasses. Objects that fall outside the core will be attracted to one of the three neighboring semantic clusters depending on a feature-weighting algorithm. The closer they are to strong cues of a particular neighbor, the more likely they are to be pulled into the semantic influence of that neighbor. Thus the cue of cylindricality can be in competition with the cue of size for a smallish cylindrical object. Although most demitasses are not cylindrical and most mugs are, the size cue would probably win over the shape cue for most adults. As a result, a very small cup would be called a demitasse, even if it is cylindrical.

Fig. 4-5. Semantic space for "cup," "mug," and "demitasse."

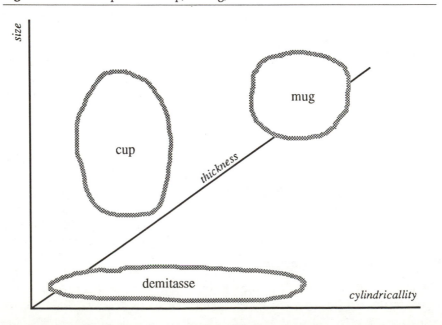

Cues are sometimes not available when we need them to make distinctions between competing forms. For example, the attribute of heat-resistance might often be used to distinguish mugs from cups. However, it may not be possible to judge whether a given drinking utensil is capable of holding hot liquids until it is actually used. Even if this cue is available, it still may not be entirely reliable, since many porcelain cups are as capable of holding hot liquids as are mugs.

The three-level connectionist networks used for work with morphology can also be used to study interactive effects in lexical competition. Figure 4-6 shows a network of this type for the domain of eating utensils. The input to the network would include perceptual and functional properties of the type discussed above—properties such as cylindricality, size, thickness, heat-resistance, and so on. The category inputs would be words like "cup" or "mug." The intervening or hidden units would detect nonlinear interactions between the properties or categories. The network could be used to predict categories from properties, as in production, or to predict properties from categories, as in comprehension. This type of network is easy to build. However, detailed coding of the features themselves is a laborious process and can only be handled reasonably for small domains. Lexical fields where connectionist simulations could make interesting contacts with current semantic theory include locative prepositions, transfer verbs, verbs of covering, reversible actions, and quantifiers.

POLYSEMIC COMPETITION

The previous section discussed the competition that occurs during production when we attempt to choose among totally different words. However, there is a level of semantic competition that occurs below the level of the word. This is the competition that occurs during comprehension when we have to select among alternative meanings or polysemes. When we hear a word such as "palm," we must decide whether to think of it as a tree or as a part of a hand. This competition between alternative meanings of the same word is an extremely pervasive aspect of human language. When a lexical item is detected, it automatically activates each of its polysemes (Swinney, 1979). These polysemes are then placed into competition (Small, Cottrell, & Tanenhaus, 1988). The polyseme supported by the strongest cues wins. Like the competition between words, the competition between polysemes is determined by a process of cue strength summation. The notion of a multidimensional semantic topography is a useful way of understanding the way in which alternative meanings compete. This topography makes distinctions not just between words, but also within words.

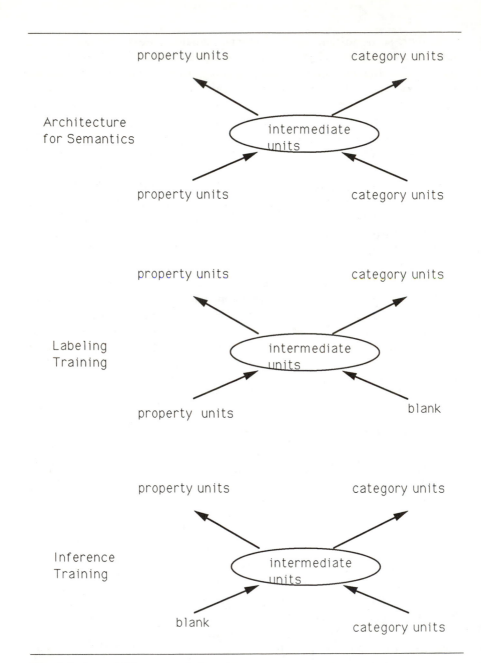

Fig. 4-6. A model for semantic learning.

Consider a word like "ball." Webster's Third contains three major entries for "ball." The first major entry is for a noun that describes round physical objects; the second is for a verb that involves forming things into balls; the third is for a noun describing a formal gathering for social dancing. Within each of the major entries is a series of minor readings or polysemes. For example, the third entry for "ball" has one polyseme for "a formal gathering" and a second for "a good time." Or the first entry has polysemes for things like "odd ball," "a ball game," "a fast ball," "testes," or "keep the ball rolling," along with the basic meaning of "a round object."

Within a given minor polyseme, further polysemy can be found. For example, within the basic polyseme for the first entry of "ball," there are 15 minor polysemes. Various types of round objects called "balls" include the ball of the foot, a baseball, the ball of the earth, an eyeball, a fall of fudge, and so on. Even within the minor polyseme for objects that bounce or roll, there is a long list of types, including baseballs, footballs, golf balls, and so on. Nor does polysemy really end at this level. Within the interpretation of "ball" as "football," specific objects such as "nerf football," "mini football," and "regulation football" can be further distinguished.

The word "ball" may refer to any one of these many different polysemes at the various levels. It is the listener's job to try to decide which of the many competing options is the one which is currently intended. If the listener wants to understand the message at all, it is almost always important to pick out the correct major polyseme. If the listener heard that Cinderella "went to the ball," he would have a very strange idea of what happened if he thought of her as approaching a round object. If he had heard "the baby threw the ball," he would need to avoid thinking of a baby throwing a wad or hot candy or the bone in someone's foot. He would certainly want to focus in on the reading of "round object for throwing or bouncing." However, within this general minor polyseme, it might not yet be possible to distinguish between a beach ball, a volley ball, or a nerf ball. There may be no further information in the discourse or in the discourse context that could tell him which of these particular objects is being thrown by the baby. If there is further disambiguating information, he will attempt to use it. A series of studies by Anderson and Ortony (1975), Anderson et al. (1976), and Anderson, Reynolds, Schallert, and Goetz (1977) demonstrated the degree to which discourse context influences the final interpretation of lexical items. For example, in a sentence such as "The Coca-Cola poured all over the table, and then the container was empty," subjects tend to interpret "container" as a "bottle." However, in a sentence such as "The apples rolled all over the table, and then the container was empty," subjects tend to interpret "container" as "basket." There are three major types of cues for resolving the competition between polysemes.

Connectionist networks can be applied to the problem of processing polysemy. The simplest type of network would have all of the possible polysemes of a single word as output and all of the cues that are likely to be important in the polysemic processing as possible inputs. For example one could build a network for the processing of the polysemes of the word "ball." In order to activate the reading of "ball" as a dance, the input could includes features such as "music" or "costumes." These features would be turned only if there are words containing these features in the actual input. The inputs could activate intervening units that might be generally useful for collecting evidence regarding the concept "dance." Other intervening units would be more activated by meanings of "ball" that have to do with candymaking, and so on. There are four major problems with networks of this type.

1. Word-specific nets of this type would fail to capture the interrelatedness of the lexicon. Given the word "ball," the easiest way to activate the "golf ball" interpretation over the "basketball" interpretation and other competitors, is to activate the "golf" concept. However, if our networks only resolve competitions for single words, this interrelatedness is missed.
2. Isolated single-word networks also fail to capture general polysemic competitions such as metonymies, personifications, and the like. The same extensional logic that allows us to talk about "having a ball" can be used to talk about "having a spin." If the polysemes of "ball" and "spin" are processed in total separation, these effects cannot be captured.
3. Isolated single-word networks cannot, by themselves, resolve lexical competition of the type discussed earlier for "cup," "mug," and "demitasse."
4. In reality, some words are more important than others in determining the polysemic competition. In particular, as seen below, words tend to exert the greatest pressure on other words with which they have syntactic relations.

One straightforward way of dealing with these limitations is to build bigger nets. Nets can be constructed that model both the major lexical competitions for a given semantic domain and all of the polysemic competitions within that domain. Such nets could relate comprehension and production in the way outlined for the simulations of Hungarian morphology above. These richer nets would need to have more input features. For example, in the domain of "cup" and "mug," one would want to add to the cues of shape and function various cues to distinguish between "mug" as a drinking vessel and "mug" as a derogatory term for a person's visage. Of course, the cues for the latter polyseme of "mug" are really ones that are more relevant to the competition between "face," "mug," "visage," and "puss." Each of the first three problems mentioned above points out the need for constructing really large nets to capture any of the interesting aspects of lexical processing. The fourth problem noted above points in yet another direction to be explored in the next section.

MODELING SYNTACTIC PROCESSING

Languages differ markedly in the way they use grammatical cues to govern attachment competitions. As Bates and MacWhinney (in press) have shown, the cue of preverbal positioning is the strongest cue in English to identification of the subject role. Given a sentence like "The eraser are chasing the boys," English-speaking subjects show a strong tendency to choose "the eraser" as the subject and, hence, the actor. This occurs despite the fact that the noun "boys" has the cues of verb agreement, animacy, and humanness all on its side. These three weak cues are just not enough to counterbalance the strength of the preverbal position cue in English. In Italian, however, the corresponding sentence is *la gomma cacciano i ragazzi* in which *la gomma* "the eraser" has support from the cue of preverbal positioning and *i ragazzi* "the boys" has support from the cues of agreement, animacy, and humanness. As Bates et al. (1984) have shown, agreement is a much stronger cue in Italian than it is in English. In Italian, the strongest cue is verb agreement and the second strongest cue is preverbal positioning. Thus Italians interpret this sentence as meaning "The boys are chasing the eraser."

How can a connectionist model account for this type of competition for syntactic attachment? It would be easy enough to construct a net for a particular sentence. The inputs to the net would be cues such as preverbal positioning, verb agreement, case marking, animacy, and so on. The output units would be the competing nouns. There must also be a way of identifying or keeping track of each competing noun. For example, in the sentence "the dogs are chasing the cat" the first noun phrase would be "the dogs" and the second would be "the cat." The net would be designed specifically to resolve the competition between the *first noun* and the *second noun* for the role of subject of the verb. The cues that would be used include noun animacy, agreement, stress, and certain semantic features of the verb. Having set up the network in this way, it provides a faithful connectionist rendition of the basic syntactic claims of the competition model in regard to the competition between nouns for grammatical roles.

In a sense, the main function of the syntactic net is not to determine syntactic relations, but to resolve ambiguity in the meanings of the words being related. Consider the word "run." The phrase "another run," as in "let's take another run," forces the verb "run" to behave like a noun. If one talks about wanting "a deeper blue," the adjective "blue" is forced to behave like a noun. This use of syntactic combinations to push words into other part-of-speech categories can be called *pushy polysemy*. What is interesting about pushy polysemy is that it only works between words that are syntactically related through the type of valence relation discussed earlier. In this example, it is the word "another" that is forcing the word "run" to behave like a noun.

Pushy polysemy is strong enough to overcome most of the standard categorizations of words into parts of speech and subclasses of the parts of speech. It can easily force a mass noun to assume a reading as a common noun. For example often it is said that "sugar" is a mass noun and that phrases such as "another sugar" are ungrammatical (Gordon, 1985). From this, it follows that the sentence "I'd like another sugar, please" is also ungrammatical. However, if someone is asking for a small packet of sugar and using the contents of the packet to refer to the whole (metonynmy), the extension is quite reasonable and even conventional. Or it could be that someone is working in a chemistry lab analyzing the reactions of various sugars such as fructose, sucrose, and glucose. In this case, "another sugar" refers to another type of sugar. This extensional pathway uses a word to refer to a member of a taxonomic class. One can say that only words like "sugar" can do this because of the special circumstances mentioned. However, even so unlikely a sentence as "I'd like another sand, please" can be interpreted in similar ways. Much like the interpretation of "another sugar" as referring to a packet of sugar, "another sand" might be referring to a bag of sand used either for construction or for sand-bagging a swollen river. Just as one could imagine a chemist working with various sugars, one could imagine a situation where geologists are describing the sand content of a new formation. They have used sieves to sort out the various types of sand in the formation and then placed these sands into jars. One of them asks the other for "another sand" for testing, meaning either another bottle of sand or another type of sand.

Proper nouns can also be converted into common nouns. Usually, we are told that a determiner such as "a" cannot precede a proper noun such as "Reagan." However, there is nothing wrong with a sentence, such as "A wiser Reagan returned from Rejkjavik," if "Reagan" is being though of not just as a single man, but also as a man who can assume various states or values. Virtually any proper noun can be extended in this way. Another extensional path allows conversion of adjectives into nouns, as in the sentence "the green is nicer than the red." This type of conversion works best if new deadjectival nouns can be conceived as members of a collection or ensemble.

Pushy polysemy is also at the heart of co-occurrence learning. It is polysemic processing that allows the "abduction" of semantic facts on the basis of formal regularities. For example, given a sentence such as "the man niffed the plate at the fence," the child can abduce some of the semantics of "niff" on the basis of co-occurrence pattern. The child does this by attending to the underlying system of connections between semantics and verb frames. This system tells us that "niff" takes a subject and an object and that the action of the subject on the object is like that in "hit" and "slam." The importance of a mechanism of this type has been stressed by MacWhinney (1987), Maratsos and Chalkley (1980), Bowerman (1982), and Schlesinger (1977). There is evidence that even very young children are able to infer the class of a word from co-occurrence data. For example, Katz, Baker, and Macnamara (1974) found that, beginning around 17 months, girls who were given a proper name for a doll learned this name better than girls who were given a common noun. In the proper noun frame, girls were told that the doll was called "Zav"; in the common noun frame they were told that the doll as "a zav." Thus, even at this early age, children seem to realize that names with articles are common nouns and names without articles are proper nouns. This ability to infer the semantics of words on the basis of co-occurrence continues to develop. Werner and Kaplan (1950) were able to show in their classic "corplum" experiment that by age 8, children could acquire many aspects of the semantics of abstract nouns from highly abstract sentence contexts.

The connectionist model of McClelland and Kawamoto (1986) does a good job of simulating this abductive learning. Words that behave formally like other words begin to be treated like those words. For example, in a sentence such as "the doll hit the ball" the simulation has a tendency to begin to attribute animacy to "the doll" on the basis of its status as the subject of "hit." In fact, this learning is not unproductive, because in both fantasy and fiction dolls are often treated as animate.

The eventual goal of this type of a connectionist analysis of verbs and case roles is to go from a set of semantic features to a set of valence descriptions. Such a system will allow for the emergence of generalities on the basis of semantic features, while still tolerating exceptions for high frequency items (Stemberger & MacWhinney, 1986). Within an inheritance network that processes valence and polysemy, more detailed features of the predicate may activate more detailed features of the valence description. For example, if the predicate is "big," the feature [+measurable] is activated for the argument. Of course, virtually any object can be treated as measurable, but the point is that the presence of the word "big" would force focus on the size properties of its argument.

Making valence descriptions subject to semantic features of the predicate and its argument has some further interesting consequences for extensional uses of verbs. For example, the first argument of the verb "polish" is usually an animate actor and the second argument is usually an inanimate object. However, when an inanimate occurs as the first argument in pre-predicate position, as in "this table polishes easily," its presence forces the verb to take on the features [+potential] and [+state] and to drop the feature [+activity]. This general change can apply to any action verb, such as "this phone dials easily" or "this micro programs easily." Such forms can be produced and comprehended without any prior experience with them, indicating that the valence descriptions involved cannot be frozen forms, but must arise from some general process. In fact, this general process is exactly what is captured by the valence description network.

Nouns have valence descriptions that simply require them to be the argument of other predicates. Thus, all nouns expect to be either the argument of some verb or preposition. However, common nouns have an additional expectation of being the first argument of a modifier with the feature [+delimiting], such as "another," "one," "a," or the plural suffix. Thus, one cannot say "I like dog" without treating "dog" as a mass noun. To treat it as a mass noun, it would have to be thought of in terms of, say, "dog meat."

CLUSTERING

The view of language processing sketched out so far is well within the scope of the types of issues that can be dealt with by current connectionist models. Although many of these phenomena will require very large and complex models, there is little in what we have said so far that lies beyond the scope of connectionist processing. However, there is a fundamental issue that has been carefully concealed under the rug up to this point—the problem of the relation between polysemic processing and the formation of larger structural units. When the predicate "another" combines with the argument "beer," it forms a new structural unit that can then be further combined with additional predicates or can be referred to anaphorically. Here it will be referred to as a *cluster*. Clustering is the fundamental nonconnectionistic process that lies at the heart of the competition model approach to syntactic processing, as sketched out in MacWhinney (1987, 1989). Clustering takes an argument and a predicate, merges their semantic features, and outputs a new syntactic and semantic unit. Consider how clustering works to process a simple sentence, such as "the cat is on the mat." First, "cat" links with "the" to form a new cluster. Then "the cat" links with "is" to form a partially saturated verb. Then "on" links with "the mat" to form an adverbial phrase which then attaches to "is" and the processing is complete. The final clustered structure is:

$$((the \rightarrow cat) \leftarrow sat \rightarrow (on \rightarrow (the \rightarrow mat))).$$

This account of the processing of "the cat is on the mat" ignores any possible competitions for attachments and assumes that each lexical item assumes its default polysemic value. At various points in the left-to-right processing, there are often words not yet attached. The processor must be able to store these words temporarily. It must also be able to take the output of the polysemic processors and pass them on to new competitions. All that is really required here is the ability to keep track of lexical items and new clusters.

CONCLUSIONS

This chapter has presented detailed findings from connectionist models of morphological processing along with more speculative claims about the design of a general connectionist system. Although connectionist accounts of language processing are very new, they offer a variety of advantages over earlier noninteractionist accounts. One major strength of connectionist approaches is the ability of networks to learn in a general way. The same basic mechanism of learning on error can be used to model the acquisition of declension in German or Hungarian, the development of lexical fields, and the learning of case role frames in English verbs of transfer. The other important property of connectionist networks is their ability to enforce mutual constraint satisfaction. In the area of sentence processing, one can see how pushy polysemy interacts with attachment competition. Although current connectionist models require an external process to keep track of the identity of the competing lexical forms, it may be that future models will be able to express even control processes within a uniform connectionist architecture.

REFERENCES

Anderson, R., & Ortony, A. (1975). On putting apples into bottles—a problem of polysemy. *Cognitive Psychology, 7,* 167–180.

Anderson, R., Pichert, J., Goetz, E., Schallert, D., Stevens, K., & Trollip, S. (1976). Instantiation of general terms. *Journal of Verbal Learning and Verbal Behavior, 15,* 667–679.

Anderson, R., Reynolds, R., Schallert, D., & Goetz, E. (1977). Frameworks for comprehending discourse. *American Educational Research Journal, 14,* 367–382.

Bates, E., & MacWhinney, B. (In press). Functionalism and the competition model. In B. MacWhinney & E. Bates (Eds.), *The crosslinguistic study of language processing.* New York: Cambridge University Press.

Bates, E., MacWhinney, B., Caselli, C., Devescovi, C., Natale, F., & Venza, V. (1984). A cross-linguistic study of the development of sentence interpretation strategies. *Child development, 55,* 341–354.

Berko, J. (1958). The child's learning of English morphology. *Word, 14,* 150–177.

Bowerman, M. (1982). Reorganizational processes in lexical and syntactic development. In E. Wanner & L. Gleitman (Eds.), *Language acquisition: the state of the art.* New York: Cambridge University Press.

Braine, M. D. S. (1971). The acquisition of language in infant and child. In C. Reed (Ed.), *The learning of language.* New York: Appleton-Century-Crofts.

Braine, M. D. S. (1987). What is learned in acquiring word classes—a step toward an acquisition theory. In B. MacWhinney (Ed.), *Mechanisms of language acquisition*. Hillsdale, NJ: Erlbaum.

Gordon, P. (1985). Evaluating the semantic categories hypothesis: The case of the count/mass distinction. *Cognition, 20,* 209–242.

Katz, N., Baker, E., & Macnamara, J. (1974). What's in a name? A study of how children learn common and proper nouns. *Child Development, 45,* 469–473.

Köpcke, K., & Zubin, D. (1983). Die kognitive Organisation der Genuszuweisung zu den einsilbigen Nomen der deutschen Gegenwartssprache. *Zeitschrift für germanistische Linguistik, 11,* 166–182.

Köpcke, K., & Zubin, D. (1984). Secks Prinzipien für die Genuszuweisung im Deutschen: Ein Beitrag zur natürlichen Klassifikation. *Linguistische Berichte, 93,* 26–50.

MacWhinney, B. (1978). The acquisition of morphophonology. *Monographs of the Society for Research in Child Development, 42,* 1–122.

MacWhinney, B. (1985). Hungarian language acquisition as an exemplification of a general model of grammatical development. In D. I. Slobin (Ed.), *The crosslinguistic study of language acquisition: Vol. 2, Theoretical issues*. Hillsdale, NJ: Erlbaum.

MacWhinney, B. (1987). The Competition Model. In B. MacWhinney (Ed.), *Mechanisms of language acquisition*. Hillsdale, NJ: Erlbaum.

MacWhinney, B. (1989). Competition and teachability. In M. Rice and R. Schiefelbusch, (Eds.), *The teachability of language*. Baltimore: Brooks-Cole.

MacWhinney, B. (In press). Competition and connectionism. In B. MacWhinney and E. Bates (Eds.), *The crosslinguistic study of sentence processing*. New York: Cambridge University Press.

MacWhinney, B., & Bates, E. (In press). *The crosslinguistic study of sentence processing*. New York: Cambridge University Press.

MacWhinney, B., Leinbach, J., Taraban, R., & McDonald, J. (1989). Language learning: Cues or rules? *Journal of Memory and Language, 28,* 255–277.

Malkiel, Y. (1968). The inflectional paradigm as an occasional determinant of sound change. In W. Lehmann & Y. Malkiel (Eds.), *Directions for historical linguistics*. Austin: University of Texas Press.

Maratsos, M. (1982). The child's construction of grammatical categories. In E. Wanner & L. Gleitman (Eds.), *Language acquisition: The state of the art*. New York: Cambridge University Press.

Maratsos, M., & Chalkley, M. (1980). The internal language of children's syntax: The ontogenesis and representation of syntactic categories. In K. Nelson (Ed.), *Children's language: Vol. 2*. New York: Gardner.

McClelland, J., & Elman, J. Interactive processes in speech perception: The TRACE model. In J. McClelland & D. Rumelhart (Eds.), *Parallel distributed processing: Vol. 2. Psychological and biological models*. Cambridge: MIT Press.

McClelland, J. & Kawamoto, A. (1986). Mechanisms of sentence processing: Assigning roles to constituents. In D. Rumelhart & J. McClelland (Eds.), *Parallel distributed processing*. Cambridge: MIT Press.

Mills, A. (1986). *The acquisition of gender: A study of English and German*. Berlin: Springer.

Park, T.-Z. (1981). *The development of syntax in the child with special reference to German*. Innsbruck: Amoe.

Pinker, S. (1984). *Language learnability and language development*. Cambridge: MIT Press.

Pinker, S. & Prince, A. (1988). On language and connectionism: Analysis of a parallel distributed processing model of language acquisition. *Cognition, 28,* 73–193.

Rumelhart, D., Hinton, G., & Williams, E. (1986). Learning internal representations by error propagation. In D. Rumelhart & J. McClelland (Eds.), *Parallel distributed processing: Explorations in the microstructure of cognition: Vol. 1, Foundations.* Cambridge: MIT Press.

Rumelhart, D., & McClelland, J. (1986). On learning the past tenses of English verbs. In J. McClelland & D. Rumelhart (Eds.), *Parallel distributed processing: Explorations in the microstructure of cognition: Vol. 2, Psychological and biological models.* Cambridge: MIT Press.

Rumelhart, D., & McClelland, J. (1987). Learning the past tenses of English verbs: Implicit rules or parallel distributed processing? In B. MacWhinney (Ed.), *Mechanisms of language acquisition.* Hillsdale, NJ: Erlbaum.

Schlesinger, I. M. (1977). *Production and comprehension of utterances.* Hillsdale, NJ: Erlbaum.

Schneuwly, B. (1978). *Zum Erwerb des Genus in Deutschen: eine mögliche Strategie.* Manuscript, Max-Planck Institut, Nijmegen.

Slobin, D. I. (1973). Cognitive prerequisites for the development of grammar. In C. A. Ferguson and D. I. Slobin (Eds.), *Studies of child language development.* New York: Holt, Rinehart, & Winston.

Small, S., Cottrell, G., & Tanenhaus, M. (Eds.). (1988). *Lexical ambiguity resolution.* San Mateo, CA: Morgan Kaufmann.

Swinney, D. (1979). Lexical access during sentence comprehension: (Re)consideration of context effects. *Journal of Verbal Learning and Verbal Behavior, 18,* 645–660.

Taraban, R., McDonald, J., & MacWhinney, B. (In press). Category learning in a connectionist model: Learning to decline the German definite article. In R. Corrigan (Ed.), *Linguistic categorization.* Amsterdam: Benjamins.

Tucker, R., Lambert, W., & Rigault, (1977). *The French speaker's skill with grammatical gender: An example of rule-governed behavior.* The Hague: Mouton.

Wängler, (1963). *Rangwörterbuch hochdeutscher Umgangssprache.* Marburg: Elwert.

Werner, H., & Kaplan, (1950). The development of word meaning through verbal context: An experimental study. *Journal of Psychology, 29,* 251–257.

CHAPTER 5

Diverse Conversational Contexts for the Acquisition of Various Language Skills

CATHERINE E. SNOW

Researchers in language development have over the last 25 years developed certain fairly standard ways of assessing children's language development (e.g., mean length of utterance [MLU] and provision of morphological markers during spontaneous speech), as well as performance on certain tests of language comprehension and vocabulary. These measures, like any assessment instrument, reflect a theory of what constitutes language proficiency, in this case, a generally unexpressed and therefore unexamined theory. This chapter will argue that the notion of language proficiency widely relied upon within the field of developmental psycholinguistics requires modification. Furthermore, work with language handicapped and with multilingual populations is a particularly powerful source of ideas that should enrich and modulate the traditional notion of language proficiency derived from work on the early language development of nonhandicapped monolingual children.

The author would like to acknowledge the Spencer Foundation, the Office for Educational Research and Improvement through the Center for Language Education and Research, and the Ford Foundation for support of research discussed in this chapter, and the NICHHD which supported preparation through HD 23388.

SOURCES OF AN ALTERNATIVE
MODEL OF LANGUAGE PROFICIENCY

The default model of what language is and how it develops that has gone largely unquestioned by mainstream language development researchers views language as essentially a single system, one in which the interesting behaviors all derive from a single underlying competence that can be adequately reflected with one or only a few developmental indices. Any impact of contextual factors is seen as related to performance only, and thus as of relatively little interest. Assessment simply requires finding a context for observing spontaneous speech in which the child's performance is optimal, and thus presumably reflects as closely as possible the underlying competence.

The alternative model of language proficiency to be presented here rejects these claims, making the counterclaims that language proficiency consists of a complex of somewhat separate components. This componential view implies that more than one developmental index is needed in describing language, and that researchers need to go beyond a single (whether or not optimal) context for collecting speech samples to an analysis of the effect of context and task itself upon performance. The alternative model, then, is firmly based on interest in and attention to performance. Furthermore, it is based on the notion that linguistic performance is not the product of *linguistic* competence alone, but also of cognitive, affective, and social competencies; thus, the study of language development has to be re-embedded in an understanding of development in these other areas. Finally, the alternative model sees language proficiency as including the full range of language competencies required to perform the wide array of real-world language tasks—telling stories, giving explanations, telling and getting jokes, understanding the special conventions of classroom discourse, reading, writing, learning to speak, read, write, and comprehend second languages, and so on.

DOMAIN MODELS OF LANGUAGE

One part of this alternative model, the claim that language proficiency consists of analyzable, separable components, is not entirely novel, nor is it completely divorced from mainstream views within developmental psycholinguistics. There is a familiar componential view of language reflected in Figure 5-1 that might be called the domain model of language proficiency. It holds that knowing a language consists of knowing the rules of phonology, morphology, syntax, speech act expression, conversation, and discourse, and certainly admits the possibility (though often not explicitly) that development in these different domains may be somewhat

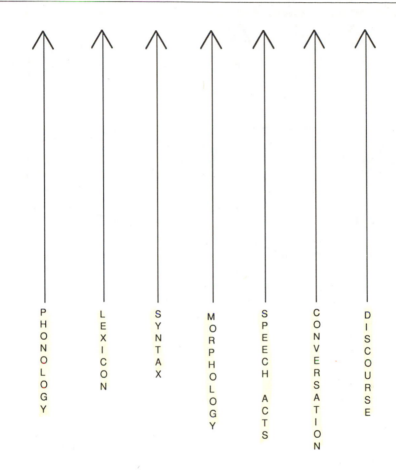

Fig. 5-1. A model of separable paths of development for components of language skill.

independent (e.g., Miller, 1981). In fact, it has been suggested that (a) various populations of language-handicapped children show their own peculiar developmental profiles of strengths and weaknesses across these various domains (Tager-Flusberg, 1987), whereas (b) children from "normal populations" typically show a fairly high level of cross-domain predictability, but (c) that in a few cases essentially normally developing children with relatively retarded development in one domain can generate a picture of language deviance because of the resulting cross-domain asynchronies.

Figure 5-2 presents possible profiles of two normally developing chil-

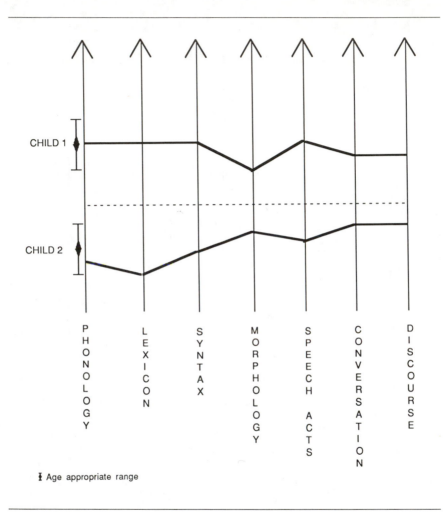

Fig. 5-2. Language development profiles for two normally developing children with different patterns of strengths and weaknesses.

dren. As presented here, child 1 shows a pattern of relative strength in phonology, lexicon, and syntax, but relative weakness in morphology, conversation, and discourse, whereas child 2 shows the opposite pattern. While these profiles are merely exemplary, the possibilities of such divergent patterns are clearly real. Preliminary use of a new method for assessing morphological sophistication with 20-month-olds has revealed a generally high and significant positive correlation with MLU; however, there are also a few outlier children who show relatively long utterances but very little morphological marking, and others who are providing a high proportion of morphological markings already in one-word utterances (Pan & Elkins, 1989). It has been suggested that "noun-loving" or referential children will show relatively large vocabularies and "clean" phonology but no particular strengths in the acquisition of conversational skill, whereas expressive children may show more control over the conversational system, and may display more morphological marking as well, relative to their vocabulary development. While all these results are quite tentative, they suggest that one should not expect an absolutely flat profile across domains for any child. However, for normally developing children one might expect the profile to fall within a certain window, ensuring a certain degree of predictability from the developmental level in any one domain to the developmental level in any other.

Figure 5-3 presents conceptual profiles based on descriptive data collected by researchers sympathetic to the domain model of language proficiency. Child 3 is like the one described by Ingram (see Chapter 3 in this volume), some aspects of whose phonological development were sufficiently slowed down that a deviant order of development occurred, particularly since lexical and grammatical development were proceeding relatively normally. Child 4 might be one of the Down Syndrome children described by Miller (1987, see also Chapter 10, this volume) or Hopmann (1986), whose vocabulary size and conversational skills are quite advanced compared to their capacities in the domains of phonology, syntax, or morphology. Finally, Figure 5-4 suggests a possible profile for an autistic child (child 5) and a specifically language-impaired child (child 6), based on extrapolation from linguistic descriptions and reported clinical impressions (e.g., Loveland, Landry, Hughes, Hall, & McEvoy, 1988; Tager-Flusberg, 1981; Wetherby & Prutting, 1984).

The ultimate value of a domain model of language proficiency will not be testable until there exists some basis for assessing developmental level in each of the relevant domains, and for comparing relatively large groups of children matched on any one domain for their level of performance in the other domains. Clearly researchers are a long way from being able to do this—the largest group of children of a particular age for whom there are even a few of the relevant domain-specific measures is very small, and for some of the domains specified there are not even any measures! Nonetheless, the potential of this sort of model seems clear, and the centrality of data on language-handicapped populations to its development and to the task of testing it further is undeniable. One goal of this chapter is ultimately to integrate the domain model with a more recently developed model that gives a different componential view of language proficiency and language development.

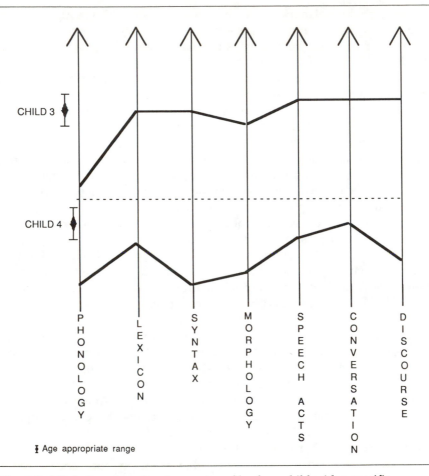

Fig. 5-3. Likely language development profiles for a child with a specific phonological disorder (child 3) and a Down syndrome child (child 4).

THE TASK MODEL

Although the domain model of language proficiency has clear interest and considerable initial credibility, it is not the componential model to which this author's research has been directed over the last several years. The model being tested shares with the domain model the presumption that the various components of language are theoretically separable for all children and empirically separable for some, and that developmental progression through the various components might occur at very different rates for a single child. However, it defines the components not in terms of the linguistic rule systems which they reflect, but in terms of the tasks being performed and the particular demand characteristics of those tasks.

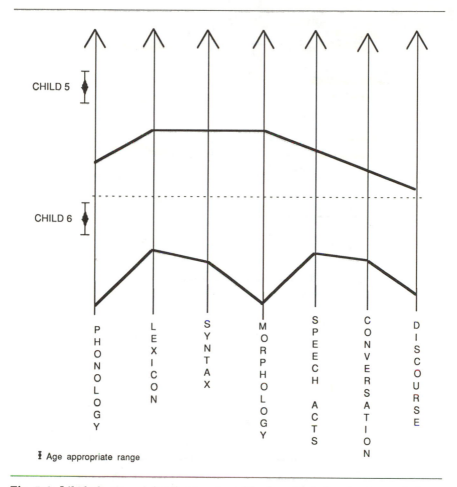

Fig. 5-4. Likely language development profiles for a high-functioning autistic child (child 5) and a specifically language-impaired child (child 6).

The three dimensions initially proposed as relevant to defining the demands of language production tasks (Snow, 1987, in press, b) were degree of audience participation, presumption of shared background knowledge, and message complexity (Figure 5-5). Whereas message complexity clearly relates to task complexity, the first two dimensions were conceived of as being relevant not to the difficulty of the task, but to the type of task demand being made. Thus, for example, having a highly participatory audience requires that speakers monitor the audience, use conversational devices to maintain their own turns and to solicit interlocutor turns, acknowledge and respond to the content of interlocutor turns, and so on. Speaking to a distant or nonparticipatory audience makes a different, not

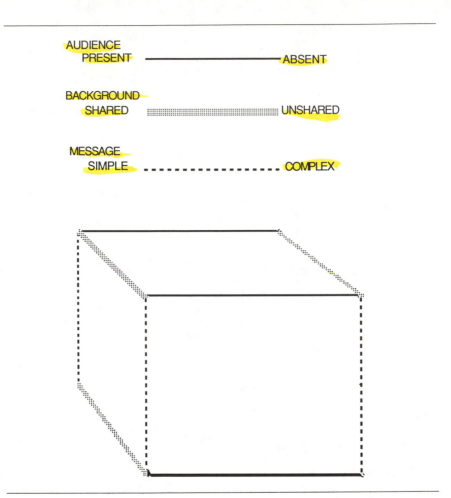

Fig. 5-5. A model of three-dimensional space in which language tasks can be placed as a function of the demands they make upon the speaker.

necessarily more serious, set of demands—that the speaker self-monitor for comprehensibility rather than relying on audience responses, that the information be presented in a sufficiently explicit and preplanned way, that information not available to the audience not be presumed, and so on. Similarly, both sharing a great deal of background information with the audience and sharing very little make particular demands on the speaker, and it is not clear that either situation is automatically easier. (Admittedly, the second is the one that very young children typically encounter, and might thus be assumed to be easier; however, parents are usually sufficiently entranced by what their children say that they don't mind when children ignore the task demands of shared background knowledge and repeat things already known. Nonparental interlocutors are often less forgiving.)

For the last five years research with my collaborators David Dickinson, Herlinda Cancino, Mary Dolbear, Matthijs Koopmans, Sara Schley, Patricia Velasco, and others has involved a series of research projects designed to assess the correctness of the task model of language proficiency. In particular, studies were designed to assess the correctness of the following claims of that model:

1. That children's abilities to perform certain language tasks would be well predicted only by their performance on other language tasks that shared many of the same task demands, not by language tasks that were very distant in the language space defined in Figure 5-5.
2. That very different language tasks could be conceived of as having independent developmental pathways (i.e., both different levels of achievement and different sets of social or linguistic facilitators).

The research has been carried out with children who could be tested for their language performance in more than one language, both because bilingual children who had learned their languages in different settings could provide a better test of the effect of various social/linguistic facilitators, but also because the pattern of transfer across languages of the specific language skills identified was of interest.

THE RESEARCH UNDERTAKING

RESEARCH STRATEGY

The research has been undertaken with three populations of bilingual children and two groups of monolingual, English-speaking children:

1. A small sample of middle-class and of working-class English-speaking kindergartners all attending the same schools.
2. A small middle-class sample of native speakers of French or English attending a private elementary French-English bilingual school called the Ecole Bilingue.
3. A much larger sample of mostly middle-class children attending second through fifth grades at the United Nations International School (UNIS), an English-curriculum school with a strong multicultural focus and an extensive French foreign language program. About 45% of this sample consists of native speakers of English, all of whom were taking French as a foreign language. A small group in the sample were children who spoke French at home as well as studying

it at school. The other children were native speakers of some language(s) other than French or English. Some of these had received intensive ESL instruction at UNIS or at schools previously attended. About half were participating fully in the English curriculum and were also taking French as a foreign language.

4. A large sample of working-class Puerto Rican children in grades 2 to 8. The children came from families with generally low educational attainment and low incomes, and attended transitional Spanish-English bilingual classrooms in New Haven, Connecticut.

These groups of children were tested on a variety of language tasks designed to sample the "task-space" defined in Figure 5-5 as widely as possible, in at least two languages in every case. The results expected, if the model being tested was correct, were (a) low correlations across tasks within language, (b) high correlations within task across languages that had been learned in similar settings, (c) but low within-task cross-language correlations for languages that had been learned and used in very different social contexts, and (d) differential predictions from the various tasks to reading or other measures of academic achievement.

THE TASKS

Most of the data analyzed so far comes from three tasks. The first, picture description, was designed to manipulate explicitly the variable of shared background knowledge. In one instructional setting, children were asked to describe a picture to the adult, who was seated next to the child and could also see the picture. This situation, called "contextualized," was contrasted to the "decontextualized" instruction, in which the child was asked to describe a picture "so that another child, listening to your tape, could draw a picture that looks just like this one, just from hearing what you say about it." Adapted instructions were also used for some of the children in a written version of the task. Descriptions of pictures that were glued to the paper on which the description was written were compared to descriptions given in response to "write a description so that another child could draw a picture just like this one, just from reading what you write."

The second task, giving definitions, was designed to allow the child the option of interpreting the task as one involving a distant audience and little shared background knowledge, or as an interactive task in which audience participation could be relied upon and shared background knowledge could be presumed. Children were asked to define simple, well-known nouns. The task was not designed as a vocabulary measure, so difficult words were not used and cases where the child did not know the meaning of a word were deleted from the analysis. The form in which the child responded to the question "What does xxx mean?" was analyzed to determine the extent to which it conformed to the structure of a formal definition, which presumes a minimum of shared knowledge between speaker and listener. Furthermore, the child's use of conversational features (appeals to the interlocutor, gestures, questions, turn-taking markers, etc.) was assessed during the task.

Finally, a task was used to assess the child's conversational skills. Language in the context of conversation is often considered to be the best reflection of the child's language ability because the adult conversational partner provides maximal support to the child's display. A more challenging conversational task, one in which the child had to do more of the work to keep the conversation going, was used in this study. The four-minute talk show, first used by Bryan, Donahue, Pearl, and Sturm (1981), served our purposes perfectly. The child is reminded of television interview shows, and then told that s/he will be the host of his/her very own show. The adult offers to play the role of guest—a celebrity guest if the child desires. The child is told that s/he must keep the conversation going for four minutes, "until the first commercial," and is reminded that topics like work, books, movies, and trips might be good things to talk about. This task proved quite challenging for some children, even in their native languages, and generated an enormous range of individual differences in terms of degree of success in filling up the four minutes without more than minimal polite responses from the adult.

Each of these tasks generated a number of different measures. Details of coding and scoring each task can be found in Davidson, Kline, and Snow (1986), Dickinson and Snow (1987), Koopmans (1988), Ricard and Snow (in press), Snow (in press, a) and Snow and Dolbear (1989). For the reader's ease an overview of tasks and scores is given in Table 5-1.

SOME RESULTS

CROSS-TASK CORRELATIONS

The first prediction was that relatively low correlations would be obtained within languages across tasks that differed considerably in their task demands. Table 5-2 shows correlations across measures from the definitions and the picture description task for the 33 kindergartners (from Dickinson & Snow, 1987), and Table 5-3 shows similar data for the UNIS sample tested in English (from Schley, Snow, & Dolbear, 1989). In general, while the scores on formal definitional quality (FDQ) correlate negatively with those on informal definitional quality (IDQ), there are only low correlations from definitions even to measures of explicitness in the picture description task (from Ricard & Snow, in press). The kindergartners' PPVT scores also showed no significant correlations to definitions, though story comprehension scores were correlated with FDQ at r = .46.

Table 5-1. Overview of tasks and measures

DEFINITIONS OF FAMILIAR NOUNS

FDQ   (Formal Definitional Quality): A summary score based on both the syntactic and the semantic characteristics of the definitions given.

FDS   (Formal Definitional Supplement): A summary score indicating additional information provided in a formal definition.

IDQ   (Informal Definitional Quality): A summary score of the amount of information provided in definitions with no formal definitional syntax.

CF   (Conversational Features): Frequency of use of conversational features like gestures, questions to examiner, etc., during the definitions task.

CA   (Communicative Adequacy): A rating on a four-point scale of the adequacy of a definition.

%FD   (Percent Formal Definitions): Of the noun definitions given, the percent that contained formal definitional syntax and/or a superordinate.

PICTURE DESCRIPTIONS (CONTEXTUALIZED OR DECONTEXTUALIZED)

Length and Complexity Measures: Number of words, number of utterances, mean length of utterance, number of verbs per utterance.

Explicitness measures: Lexical NPs/total NPs, adjectives/words, specific locatives/utterances, clarificatory markers/utterances.

Content measures: Identification of main event, number of characters mentioned, number of details mentioned, number of different colors mentioned.

Narrativity measures: Presence of narrative opening or closing, naming of characters, reference to characters' internal states, focus on events, identification of cause or motives.

FOUR-MINUTE TALK SHOW

Sophistication of conversation strategies: Percent of child utterances that were topic-starters, percent open-ended or wh-question topic-starters, ratio of child to adult topic starting.

Responsiveness: Percent of adult utterances to which child gave a response, percent of child turns that included both a response and a topic-starter, percent responses that were on the topic of the adult's preceding turn, frequency of child back-channels.

Dysfluency: Frequency of hesitations, of filled and unfilled pauses, of false starts, and of self-corrections on word choice or grammar.

Monotony: Frequency of child self-repetitions, of incoherent utterances, and of interruptions by the child of the adult.

The pattern of interpretable relations among scores on the definitions task and the picture description task contrast sharply with comparisons of the other tasks to scores on the talk show. The only significant correlations found for the UNIS children tested in English were between frequency of self-corrections in the picture description and the talk show tasks, and between use of conversational features in the definitions task and sophis-

Table 5-2. Correlations across definitions and picture description scores for 33 kindergartners

Picture Description	Narrativity	FDQ	IDQ	CF	CA	PPVT
Explicitness	.14	.11	−.16	.24	−.01	.01
Narrativity		−.14	.02	.04	.01	.18
FDQ			.79**	.66**	.21	.20
IDQ				−.56*	−.05	.15
CF					.30	.02
CA						.18

**p < .01
* p < .05
Source: Dickinson & Snow, 1987.

Table 5-3. Correlations across definitions and picture descriptions scores for UNIS sample

Picture Description	Clarificatory Markers	FDQ	IDQ	CF	CA
Locatives	.35*	.26*			.29*
Clarificatory markers		.22*			.26*
FDQ			−.04	−.10	.56**
IDQ				.14*	.06
CF					−.03

**p < .01
* p < .05
Source: Ricard & Snow, in press.

tication of topic-starting in the talk show. These correlations should be interpreted somewhat cautiously since they emerge from very large correlation matrices and might well constitute chance effects. However, they do seem both interpretable and reasonable. Interestingly, the highly correlated measures in both cases reflect better performance on one task (self-corrections on picture description and sophistication of topic-starting in the talk show) but worse performance on the other (self-corrections in the talk show and conversational features in the definitions).

DEVELOPMENTAL PATTERNS

Another way to detect a lack of relationship across different language measures is to see different developmental patterns. The case can be made very strongly for the various definitions scores, for example, that though derived from exactly the same task they show different patterns of growth and thus must be developing somewhat independently. Table 5-4 shows scores on the English definitions task for the UNIS sample (these data come from Snow [in press, a] and from Snow, Cancino, De Temple, & Schley [in press]). Both %FD and FDQ, as well as CA, show growth between grades 2 and 4, with some leveling off between grades 4 and 5. However, IDQ, a measure of the amount of information given in nonformal definitions, shows no grade effect at all, indicating that it has already reached its ceiling by grade 2.

The talk show measures look much more like IDQ than like FDQ or %FD; they show large individual differences that are almost entirely unrelated to age (Table 5-5). This result is quite surprising when one considers how difficult a task it is to keep an interlocutor talking for four minutes. Nonetheless, it seems not to be a task which most children get better at during the early and middle elementary years.

Table 5-4. Scores on English definitions for 2nd through 5th graders at UNIS

Grade	2	3	4	5	Grade Effect
%FD	49%	66%	79%	79%	.001
FDQ	6.6	7.3	8.2	8.4	.001
IDQ	2.2	2.5	2.2	2.1	n.s.
CF	.06	.05	.03	.08	n.s.
CA	.99	1.33	1.58	1.64	.001

Source: Snow, Cancino, De Temple, & Schley, in press.

Table 5-5. Scores on conversational composite variables in English (E) and French (F)

Grade		2	3	4	5
Sophistication	E	1.42	1.31	1.15	1.38
	F	5.96	3.76	4.03	3.25
Responsiveness	E	.13	.09	.20	.18
	F	1.56	2.17	2.35	2.15
Dysfluency	E	.20	.22	.22	.25
	F	1.08	.57	1.29	1.22
Monotony	E	1.77	1.72	2.03	2.10
	F	7.49	3.43	3.11	11.09

CROSS-LANGUAGE CORRELATIONS

A second prediction of the task model of language proficiency is that identical tasks would correlated highly across languages. The first test of this hypothesis, with the Ecole Bilingue sample, was very encouraging; FDQ in English and French correlated .76 (Davidson, Kline & Snow, 1986). We were somewhat discouraged, then, to find rather lower correlations from English to French for the UNIS children (see Table 5-6 taken from Snow, Cancino, De Temple & Schley, in press). However, further analysis of the cross-language correlations from the UNIS sample suggested that correlations as low as these are to be expected from children still mostly at relatively early stages of acquiring French. Furthermore, definitions are a language form that is encountered most frequently in content lessons in most classrooms. The Ecole Bilingue children were having content lessons in both English and French, and thus might be expected to show similar skills at definitions in their two languages, since the context of acquisition was similar. The UNIS children learned and/or used English in content instruction, but most learned and only used French in the foreign language classroom. Thus, it is perhaps not so surprising that they show much lower cross-language correlations. These results do suggest, however, that transfer across languages of the ability to perform specialized language tasks is not automatic, but requires both some minimum level of proficiency in the second language and some opportunity to learn how to perform the language task in question in the second language.

Given these considerations, the cross-language correlations for the New Haven children were predicted to be higher than those for the UNIS children, since in New Haven students were receiving instruction in both Spanish and English, but lower than for the Ecole Bilingue sample, since the level of proficiency in L2 was not as high for the New Haven sample. Indeed, FDQ from English to Spanish correlates .46, and IDQ .21, just as predicted.

Furthermore, cross-language correlations on measures indicating de-contextualization in the picture description task were quite high for the New Haven sample (Velasco & Snow, in prep.; Table 5-7), again indicating

Table 5-6. Cross-language correlations on definitions scores for UNIS children

	%FD	FDQ	FDS	IDQ
r	.27	−.03	.20	−.27
p	<.05	n.s.	<.05	<.05

Source; Snow, Cancino, De Temple, & Schley, in press.

Table 5-7. Cross-language correlations on picture description scores for New Haven children

Variable	r	p
Adjectives	.71	.0001
Clarificatory markers	.25	.03
Revisions	.47	.0001
Communicative revisions	.51	.0001
% lexical NPs	.57	.0001
Number of NPs	.55	.0001
Specific locatives	.53	.0001
Number of verbs	.61	.0001
Nonpresent verbs	.73	.0001

Source: Velasco & Snow, in preparation.

that if children are attending school in both their languages, their patterns of strengths and weaknesses in language use will tend to be quite similar across the two languages. Furthermore, children with very strong academic language skills in Spanish may look relatively stronger in academic tasks in English compared to oral, conversational tasks in English (Lanauze & Snow, in press).

DIFFERENT RELATIONSHIPS TO READING?

Another prediction of the model presented above is that some language tasks predict reading and other literacy skills as well, whereas others show little or no relation to reading in the same or the other language. This prediction has been confirmed for both the UNIS and the New Haven population. At UNIS, the measures of reading that were available were the children's scores on the California Achievement Test (CAT). The %FD, the FDQ, and the CA scores showed generally significant and positive correlations to the reading subtests of the CAT, whereas the IDQ scores showed no relation and the CF scores showed negative correlations (Snow, Cancino, Gonzalez & Shriberg, 1989). In the New Haven population, 3rd and 5th graders selected as poor readers based on the Spanish California Test of Basic Skills showed a much lower percentage of formal definitions in both Spanish and English than age-matched good readers (Velasco, 1987), and a composite score reflecting listener orientation in the picture description task explained more than 40% of the variation on reading comprehension in a regression analysis (Velasco, 1989). These results contrast sharply to the findings from the talk-show procedure, which showed no significant correlations to CAT scores for the UNIS population.

DIFFERENT SOURCES OF FACILITATION?

A major question that analyses carried out so far have only begun to address is whether the various language skills hypothesized by the task model, which the correlational analyses reported above help to distinguish, can be shown to have different sources of facilitation. Some results already available suggest strongly that the answer is yes.

First of all, significant and rather large differences were found on both the definitions task and the picture description task as a function of social class among monolingual kindergartners (see Dickinson & Snow, 1987). These differences suggest that factors that differentiate middle-class from working-class homes have an impact on the development of the skills specific to doing well on these decontextualized tasks.

Results from the older children attending UNIS, however, suggest that school exposure to the language of testing influences ability at decontextualized tasks much more strongly than home exposure. Regression analyses were used to test the impact of home versus school exposure to English on English definitions scores, and of home exposure to French on French definitions scores (Snow, in press, a). It was found that school exposure to English explained a much larger proportion of the variance on FDQ and %FD scores than home exposure to English, suggesting that the skills necessary to do well on these measures were largely acquired in school. Home exposure to French explained a significant amount of the variance only on IDQ scores in French. In French, as in English, for children in this older age range home exposure enabled the children to talk more, but did not help them develop the specific skills of analysis and planning that enabled them to succeed at giving formal definitions.

An even more strikingly specific effect of language acquisition context on task performance comes from a comparison of French and English performance on the talk-show task for the UNIS children. Using principal components analysis, the many variables that reflected the children's performance in the talk-show task were reduced to four composites: sophistication, responsiveness, dysfluency, and monotony, with the first two positive and the second two negative indicators of conversational skill. Table 5-6 shows the scores for UNIS children in grades 2 through 5 who could be tested in both English and French on each of these four composites. It can be seen that the children score significantly higher in French on all four composites—those that indicate skill as well as those that indicate failure at the task. It is not surprising that these children should be more dysfluent and more boring in French—after all, they are for the most part relative beginners at the language. What is surprising is that they score higher on measures of responsiveness to the interlocutor and on the sophistication of their means for initiating topics in French than in English.

Why should they do better at these things in their poorer language? The answer must be sought, I think, in an analysis of the specific skills the children were learning in their foreign language classroom. The foreign language curriculum at UNIS, as at most elementary schools, is based heavily on the learning of dialogues. Children in the talk-show task are asked to take on the relatively novel role of interviewer, with responsibility for maintaining the conversation. Clearly, well-practiced dialogues can be a resource to be relied upon in such a task, and specific conversational devices learned and practiced in those dialogues (e.g., language specific ways of marking conversational responsiveness, such as *alors* and *eh bien*) are available for use during the task. What is odd is that children who use their dialogue skills in French do not automatically transfer this strategy for solving the task into their stronger language, English, which would enable them to score at least as well in English as in French.

A NEW AND BETTER MODEL OF LANGUAGE PROFICIENCY

The results reviewed here and others collected over the last five years have confirmed the value of the task-analysis approach to thinking about language proficiency. This approach has important implications for educational practice and for assessment and remediation with language-impaired children of school age. However, it is also clear that the domain model discussed in the first part of this chapter has considerable heuristic and theoretical value. Clearly, these two models should be integrated in a fuller conception of language proficiency. Perhaps one example will give a hint of how that integration might proceed.

Conversation constitutes one of the language domains that could be argued to show a separate developmental path. Conversation is included as a domain (despite its obviously somewhat less mainstream status than, for example, phonology or syntax) because it clearly is rule-governed, and there is ample evidence that the rules for conversational turn-taking, for establishing conversational relevance, for applying the various Gricean maxims, and for assigning responsibility to speaker versus listener for successful communication are language-specific. Thus, one can assume that the child acquires these rules in the process of learning a native language. In addition to knowing (something about) the rules for conversation, a typical child will be faced with a variety of conversational tasks in the course of growing up—engaging in dinner-table conversation with parents, chatting on the phone to relatives, amusing oneself and one's siblings during long car rides, perhaps even being asked to entertain parental dinner guests while cocktails are being prepared. Performing effectively in these various tasks requires considerably more than knowing the language-specific rules for conversation. It requires integrating that rule-knowledge with the systems for syntax, morphology, lexical retrieval, and so forth. It requires analyzing the social and cognitive demands of the specific situation. It may depend very heavily on having practiced components of the skills required to perform the task, so that the processing load is reduced. Results summarized above suggest, furthermore, that it benefits from having practiced those skills in the language in which they are to be displayed—that knowledge of how to perform a conversation task skillfully is not abstracted from the language system but is embedded in the language in which it has been acquired and practiced, at least at first.

These results also suggest that children who develop exceptionally good control over certain linguistic domains might restructure tasks so as to utilize their own strengths. Thus, for example, children from UNIS, who had received excellent and extensive instruction in story-writing, often interpreted the picture description task as one requiring a narrative. Children who were particularly effective in the talk-show task often interpreted the definitions task as a conversation, and effectively recruited the experimenter to collaborate in generating better definitions.

REFERENCES

Bryan, T., Donahue, M., Pearl, R., & Sturm, C. (1981). Learning disabled children's conversational skills: The 'TV Talk Show.' *Learning Disability Quarterly, 4,* 250–259.

Davidson, R., Kline, S., & Snow, C. E. (1986). Definitions and definite noun phrases: Indicators of children's decontextualized language skills. *Journal of Research in Childhood Education, 1,* 37–48.

Dickinson, D. K., & Snow, C. E. (1987). Interrelationships among prereading and oral language skills in kindergartners from two social classes. *Research on Childhood Education Quarterly, 2,* 1–25.

Hopmann, M. (1986). An ethological approach to language development: Conversations between adults and children with Down Syndrome. Paper presented at Symposium on Research in Child Language Disorders, Madison, Wisconsin, June.

Koopmans, M. (1988). Reasoning in two languages: An assessment of the effects of language proficiency on the syllogistic performance of Puerto Rican bilinguals. Doctoral dissertation, Graduate School of Education, Harvard University, Cambridge.

Lanauze, M., & Snow, C. E. (In press). The relation between first- and second-language writing skills: Evidence from Puerto Rican elementary school children on the Mainland. *Linguistics and Education.*

Loveland, K., Landry, S., Hughes, S., Hall, S., & McEvoy, R. (1988). Speech acts and the pragmatic deficits of autism. *Journal of Speech and Hearing Research, 31,* 593–604.

Miller, J. F. (1981). *Assessing language production in children.* Baltimore: University Park Press.

Miller, J. F. (1987). Language and communication characteristics of children with

Down Syndrome. In A. Crocker, S. Pueschel, J. Rynders, & C. Tinghey (Eds.), *Down syndrome: State of the art*. Baltimore: Brooks Publishing.

Pan, B. A., & Elkins, K. (1989). A new method for assessing morphological development. Paper presented to the New England Child Language Association, Northeastern University, May.

Ricard, R. J., & Snow, C. E. (In press). Language skills in and out of context: Evidence from children's picture descriptions. *Journal of Applied Developmental Psychology*,

Schley, S., Snow, C. E., & Dolbear, M. (1989). Components of conversation skill. Manuscript, Harvard University.

Snow, C. E. (1987). Beyond conversation: Second language learners' acquisition of description and explanation. In J. Lantolf & A. Labarca (Eds.), *Research in second language learning: Focus on the classroom*. Norwood, NJ: Ablex.

Snow, C. E. (In press, a). The development of definitional skill. *Journal of Child Language*.

Snow, C. E. (In press, b). Towards a definition of language proficiency. In H. Dechert & G. Appel (Eds.), *Contemporary Psycholinguistics*. Amsterdam: Benjamins.

Snow, C., Cancino, H., Gonzalez, P., & Shriberg, E. (1989). Giving formal definitions: An oral language correlate of school literacy. In D. Bloome (Ed.), *Classrooms and literacy*. Norwood, NJ: Ablex.

Snow, C. E., Cancino, H., De Temple, J., & Schley, S. (In press). Giving formal definitions: A linguistic or metalinguistic skill? In E. Bialystok (Ed.), *Language processing and language awareness by bilingual children*. New York: Cambridge University Press.

Snow, C. E., & Dolbear, M. (1989). The relation of conversational skill to language proficiency in second language learners. Manuscript, Harvard University.

Tager-Flusberg, H. (1981). On the nature of linguistic functioning in early infantile autism. *Journal of Autism and Developmental Disorders, 11*, 45–56.

Tager-Flusberg, H. (1987). On the nature of a language acquisition disorder: The example of autism. In F. Kessel (Ed.), *The development of language and of language researchers: Essays in honor of Roger Brown*. Hillsdale, NJ: Erlbaum.

Velasco, P. (1987). Oral decontextualized language skills and reading comprehension in bilingual children. Paper presented to Boston University Child Language Conference, October.

Velasco, P. (1989). The relationship of oral decontextualized language and reading comprehension in bilingual children. Doctoral Dissertation, Harvard Graduate School of Education.

Velasco, P., & Snow, C. E. (In preparation). Decontextualized language skills of Spanish-English bilingual good and poor readers. Manuscript, Harvard University.

Wetherby, A. M., & Prutting, C. (1984). Profiles of communicative and cognitive-social abilities in autistic children. *Journal of Speech and Hearing Research, 27*, 364–377.

CHAPTER 6

Event Knowledge and the Development of Language Functions

KATHERINE NELSON

This chapter presents a functional perspective on problems of language development, based on broad considerations of language functions from an evolutionary perspective, both phylogenetic and ontogenetic, as well as more fine-grained views of the functions of particular language genres and utterances in terms of an event knowledge system, and then considers the evolution of language functions in child-language systems. In the end I will suggest how this perspective may relate to problems of language delays and disorders.

OBJECT KNOWLEDGE AND EVENT KNOWLEDGE

In the functional perspective taken here it is assumed that the basic structure of the child's knowledge—and language that is used in expressing that knowledge—is organized around events. This contrasts with the usual departure point of considering the child's knowledge of objects and object categories as basic. Clearly, object categories are important to both language and cognition, but I believe we can best understand how children begin to make sense of language if we consider that their underlying conceptual organization is derived from their experientially based knowledge of events. (See Nelson, 1985, 1986 for extensive argumentation of this point of view.)

In contrast to this point of view, it is frequently claimed that objects are the very foundation stones of language, for the child as for the species. Indeed, it seems that humans, at least Western humans, are obsessed with objects. Western philosophies, as well as psychologies, are organized around objects. Gentner (1982), for example, has made a case that objects and object names are universal primes in the child's language system; and both Terrace (1985) and Seidenberg and Pettito (1987) have claimed that the reason that chimpanzees cannot learn human language is because they do not pay enough attention to objects and thus do not learn names for things as children do. The only objects chimps seem to be interested in are foods; thus they view objects instrumentally and not as things that are of interest in their own right as, it is claimed, human children do.

In response to these claims, I take a perspective that emphasizes evolutionary continuity between primate species, which will shed light on ontogenetic development as well. This perspective leads to the question, What is the nature of the primate knowledge base?

Anthropologists in general agree that the most reasonable evolutionary account is that language emerged as a communicative system (Givon, 1989; Margolis, 1987; Wilson, 1980). Its relation to human cognition is then a byproduct of its communicative function. If language emerged for communication, its foundation must rest in the function of expressing the needs, problems, and plans of our primitive ancestors, reflecting their organization of knowledge about the world in relation to these practical ends. Their knowledge organization was probably not different in kind from the organization that other primates, (such as our close relatives the chimpanzees) employed. It is a reasonable assumption that the important organizing conceptions for primate groups are those that involve conspecifics and relations among them, modes of food-gathering and -sharing, modes of ensuring safety from predators, modes of protecting and nurturing the young, and so on. In other words, their cognitive representations would be organized around goals and in terms of general event types. Objects as such are important in such knowledge schemes only as they enter into important event types, for example, as foods or as tools. Before long (in the evolutionary time scale) objects seem to have become valued in their own right as having decorative or symbolic significance. Continuity, then, is apparent in these respects from very primitive human groups to our own society.

Language in these early human groups no doubt was functionally oriented around using words to communicate messages about the organization of social activities. Language forms could then enter into individual consciousness to organize and reify (that is, to stabilize) thoughts about these topics. Thus languages developed to the point of being used to analyze reality, construct tales, solve problems, and constitute cultural realities; toward these mature cultural ends, object names might take on particular significance.

What this account amounts to is the claim that the referential function of language, its utility in terms of pointing to and organizing things in the world, emerged from its instrumental and expressive functions. The point of this speculative excursion into the dark ages of human history is to shore up the notion that both phylogenetically and ontogenetically experientially derived knowledge may be organized in ways that seem primitive to linguistically tuned minds. Not only chimpanzees, but little children really are different from adult humans: that is, they don't have as much language as adults do, and to understand how language develops, it is necessary to understand what cognition without language is like. The evolutionary perspective on language is consistent with the proposal that in ontogenetic development representation of knowledge of the world is in the first instance primarily *in terms of important events,* and that more static and abstract knowledge is derived from this initial dynamic and interactive event knowledge base.

What kind of knowledge is event knowledge? When one begins to think in terms of events, rather than only in terms of objects, it becomes necessary to frame the discussion in terms of events situated in a *social context,* as well as within a temporally and spatially *particular* situation. Events are always *socially and culturally meaningful.* This is especially the case for very young children whose world is arranged by adults, and for whom important events are framed and carried through to a large extent by adults. Children are *first of all participants* in other people's activities and *secondarily actors* on their own. They must therefore learn the parts played by others and how those parts relate to their own role in the activity. (This is not to deny the active role that children play in organizing their own knowledge, as Piaget emphasized. But the child's activity is framed within larger activities—or events—that are organized by adults.) At the outset event knowledge *is* social knowledge and social knowledge *is* event knowledge.

In addition to its social component, to have knowledge of an event is to have some reasonably abstract organized knowledge of a *sequence* of actions, that is to represent the *temporal order* in which the components of the event takes place, and the *causal relations* among actions within an event. These have been shown in previous research (e.g., Nelson, 1986) to be important aspects of the representations of even very young children, and recent research by Bauer and Mandler (1989) indicates that such knowledge is available to children as young as 15 months and probably even earlier.

The basic assumption here then is that the infant-becoming-child mentally represents experiences of events which may be episodic and specific, but which may also be quite general and abstract. Very young children appear to have quite well-structured general ideas about how events of the day should go—what follows what, how mealtimes, bedtimes, simple games, and so on are sequenced. And it makes sense that children *should* remember how events in their world go so that they can participate smoothly in those events.

The question is, what kind of a support for language does such event knowledge afford? What evidence is there that children come to understand and use language within their organized event knowledge system? What bearing might that have on children who have trouble with language? Halliday's (1973; 1975) taxonomy of the functions of early language will help address these questions, but it is necessary to go beyond it to show how language itself enables the child to advance to new functions. The underlying model here is a dialectical one in which language and cognition play alternating roles, each influencing the other as the systems develop.

FUNCTIONS OF LANGUAGE

Thus far I have argued that language evolved in the first place as a communicative system, and that additional functions that serve both individual and social cognitive and aesthetic needs emerged as linguistic systems became elaborated. A number of different descriptions of language functions have been put forth. The scheme that Halliday (1973; 1975) worked out for the analysis of his son Nigel's developing language emphasizes the child's underlying goal in using language, and is easily related to individual cognitive functions.

Halliday divided the child's functions during the early phases of development (roughly 10 to 24 months) into two broad classes, Mathetic and Pragmatic. These were both defined in terms of their communicative intent. However, Mathetic functions may be useful beyond the primitive communicative needs of the child and enter into more independent cognitive functions, reflecting an implicit developmental hierarchy of language functions, which Halliday himself suggested. I will first lay out and illustrate from my own data the communicative functions that Halliday described and will subsequently indicate more advanced functions that language may come to serve for the child.

The data relied on for the examples here come from transcripts of parent-child talk at bedtime, followed by child monologues in the crib after the parents left the room. The child in question, Emily, was tape-recorded at bedtime periodically between the ages of 21 and 36 months and the transcripts were subsequently analyzed from several different perspectives (Nelson, 1989).

The pre-sleep situation presents a specific context for talk that has many peculiarities (just as any given conversational context presents its own peculiarities). In the bedtime situation it becomes clear very quickly that parents and child have competing goals. The parents wish to provide a pleasant occasion of settling the child down to sleep and departing relatively quickly without fuss. The child's goal is to keep the parents in the room as long as possible and to delay their leave-taking. The parents therefore express love and good wishes for a pleasant sleep and also provide pleasant accounts of what the child can look forward to after nap or the next day. The child, however, rarely picks up on these pleasant themes. Rather, she engages in various stratagems for delaying their departure, including requesting drinks, toys to take to bed, extensions of goodnight routines such as lying down and having a blanket put over her, demanding that the shades be lowered, announcing her own defiant actions (e.g., "I standing up"), and when all else fails, breaking into tears.

It is clear from Emily's contributions to the bedtime routine that they reflect her well-organized knowledge of how this event type is structured, which in turn enables her to manipulate that structure through language. Within this general goal orientation the specific functions described by Halliday that are served by each of her utterances can further be identified. These may be thought of as examples of specific tactics within her overall strategy. Although the general strategy determines what functions are most frequently expressed in the dialogues, examples can be found there of each of Halliday's types over the early months of these recordings toward the end of her second year and the beginning of her third.

COMMUNICATIVE FUNCTIONS

Pragmatic

There are three early developing pragmatic functions in Halliday's scheme: Instrumental, Regulatory, and Interactional. In addition, there is an early developing Personal function, which expresses comments on the child's own activities and thus seems to fall more logically into the Mathetic category. However, its early use seems to be primarily for practical ends, drawing attention to the self.

Instrumental. With the instrumental function the child uses words to gain ends. Prior to language the child might have used nonverbal and verbal gestures for the same purposes. An example from Emily at 22 months: "I need more juice." Here she expresses a desire for a particular commodity. In this situation the statement is addressed to the parents who have it in their power to provide the juice or not. However, she does not directly invoke their help in obtaining it, which distinguishes the instrumental use from the regulatory.

Regulatory. This function employs language to regulate the actions of others, going beyond the instrumental by specifically involving another person, often to accomplish an end that the child cannot accomplish by herself. An example from Emily at 23 months: "put blanket on!" directing her father to carry out his part of their bedtime routine.

Interactional. This function is used to establish or maintain the bond between the child and others. As already noted, in the pre-bed dialogues with her parents Emily rarely uses language for this purpose, although her parents initiate many expressions of love and hopes for a good sleep and so on. Emily's contributions, however, tend to the instrumental, regulatory, and personal. Occasionally she makes satisfied noises ("hm, hm," etc.) presumably indicating interpersonal warmth. Although she rarely responds in kind to her parents' expressions of love and good will, on a few occasions at 21 months she echoes her father's "good night, Em" with "bye, Daddy," or "night-night." The dearth of expressions of the interactional function in these transcripts may be an individual idiosyncracy tied to Emily's attempt to keep her parents in the room through regulatory and instrumental demands, but it might more generally reflect the possibility of expressing interactional functions through nonverbal means (cries, verbal gestures, hugs, and so on), thus obviating the need to express this function in language. Its expression in conventional language terms may be a late-developing function.

Personal. With this function the child comments on her own states and actions, without the expressed intention to achieve any other end. An example from Emily at 21 months: "I standing up!" announced at the point in the bedtime routine when she should be lying down. This statement may be interpreted as a challenge, which Emily expects to be met by a counter from her father (Gerhardt, 1989), but its specific overt function is simply to announce and thereby to draw attention to her behavior.

Mathetic

Halliday (1973) identified two functions in the early phases as Mathetic. By *mathetic* is meant broadly using language in the service of knowing and learning. This label suggests the potential for complex cognitive uses, but its beginnings are quite limited, as Halliday's discussion indicated.

Heuristic. Halliday viewed the emergence of the mathetic function in general and the heuristic function in particular as an important impetus toward the acquisition of vocabulary. This function uses language as a means of learning about the environment, of making and recalling observations. The new words in the expanding vocabulary function "mainly as a means of categorizing observed phenomena.... The child is constructing a heuristic hypothesis about the environment, in the form of an experiential semantic system." (Halliday, 1975, p. 251). By the time of these recordings Emily had already acquired a large vocabulary and was no longer in the phase of simply categorizing through naming. Rather her heuristic functions can be identified as those statements that describe or place items in context. For example, one of the pre-bed verbal routines at 22 months was to name the people who were napping or "going night-night," thus impressing on Emily the fact that everyone was going to sleep, not just Emily. On one occasion she states, in response to her mother's "Now you have a really good nap and we'll see you later": "that Carl napping, that Carl napping." Her parents pick up the refrain, listing other friends and relatives who are going to nap and ending "and Mommy too." Emily responds with "Mommy tired" then "Mommy go nap." This exchange illustrates the way in which information about people's routines, states, and actions gets entered into the child's repertoire in what Halliday would categorize as heuristic.

Imaginative. The imaginative function is invoked when the child leaves the here-and-now and enters into a pretend mode. It is illustrated in Emily's conversation with her parents about playing ring-around-the-rosie. There is a picture over her crib of children playing and she often refers to it, saying, for example, at 21 months "Carl playing ring-a-rosie."

Both the heuristic and the imaginative are more evident in Emily's monologues than in her dialogic speech, as will be illustrated later, whereas the pragmatic functions dominate the dialogic discourse.

Informative

The informative function uses speech to impart information to others. This is the function that appears to most adult users (and adult analyzers) to be the pre-eminent function of language, as Halliday noted. For Halliday, mastery of this function was seen as an important milestone toward mature language use. The child could not master the informative function, he argued, until he grasped the "fundamental nature of the communicative process" which entails grasping the principle of dialogue. The dialogic principle is critical in Halliday's view as the foundation for the establishment of the adult functional system. Within the adult functional system, each utterance encodes ideational, interpersonal, and textual functions together. It is clear from these transcripts that by 21 months Emily had entered into the dialogic mode with her parents, and thus examples of the informative function in the dialogues may be expected.

Although far outnumbered by her strategic use of the pragmatic functions, there are some clearly informative uses in the dialogues. For example, at 22 months Emily declared that she wanted her stuffed toy mouse in the crib, but her parents, not being able to find it, tried to distract her with other toys. She insisted on the mouse, and her mother, realizing that it would be better to provide it than to provoke the child further, set out to look for it. Emily called out, "In Daddy's room." Mother: "Is it in Daddy's room? Okay, I'll check there." And, indeed, that is where she found it. Here Emily seems to have recalled the location of the mouse and imparted the information to her mother who did not know of it otherwise. This is a not very advanced form of the informative function, but it indicates that Emily has grasped the important fact that language can be used to impart information as well as to regulate others and to clarify one's understanding of apparent objects and relations in the world.

These examples (summarized in Table 6-1) Halliday's scheme has been followed to describe the use of language in communicative situations involving Emily's pre-bed dialogues with her parents. Her uses there are embedded in the bedtime routine, an event that is well structured and well understood by Emily. Therefore her uses of language in that context are somewhat limited, routinized and predictable from one occasion to another. Of greater interest is how she adapts these functions to other cognitive uses as displayed in her crib monologues. The crib monologues contained a variety of different types of talk, or genres (Nelson, 1989), including some play with dolls, some stories, some calling out requests for attention. For the most part, however, pragmatic functions were not prevalent, nor would the talk be classified as informative, there being no interlocutor present to receive information. The focus here then is on the development of the mathetic functions—the heuristic and imaginative—as they are displayed in the monologues over the 15 months of this study.

The general claim here is that the functions that are first used in communicative contexts are recruited for the child's purposes in organizing cognitive representations of reality. That is, what was at first primarily communicative takes on primarily cognitive utility. However, Emily's monologues reflect far more complex cognitive functions than have been illustrated thus far based on Halliday's account of the early stages of Nigel's speech.

COGNITIVE FUNCTIONS

The mathetic function is elaborated beyond its simple heuristic component (i.e., categorizing by naming) by the time the child has reached the level of linguistic sophistication that Emily had attained by 2 years. Crib monologues provide a unique context for examining these functions because they lack any explicit interactive context. The child is alone, cast onto her

Table 6-1. Communicative Functions

Functions	*Examples* *(Emily 21–24 Mo.)*
PRAGMATIC	
Instrumental	I need more juice
Regulatory	Put blanket on!
Interactional	Night-night!
Personal	I standing up!
MATHETIC	
Heuristic	Mommy tired, mommy go nap
Imaginative	Carl playing ring-a-rosie
INFORMATIVE	[Mouse is] in Daddy's room

Source: Adapted from, Halliday 1975.

own resources for organizing her talk. What is remarkable about that talk is that it exhibits both more formal and more functional sophistication than was apparent in her dialogic speech (Nelson, 1989). In the monologues the following types of advanced mathetic uses are evident: narrating, generating generalities, generating possibilities, generating necessities, generating categories, inferencing, and acquiring information. Each of these will be illustrated in turn.

Narrating

Narrative accounts of her specific life experiences constitute a large portion of Emily's crib monologues. Two examples will provide a flavor of these. The first is a portion of an account at 23 months of being wakened at her babysitter's:

1. When my slep and, and, Mormor came. Then Mommy coming then get up, time to go ho-o-ome. Time to go home. Drink P-water [Perrier]. Yesterday did that. Now Emmy sleeping in regular bed.

Next is a narrative at 32 months about buying a doll:

2. We *bought* a baby, cause, the well because, when she, well, we *thought* it was for Christmas, but *when* we went to the s-s-store we didn't have our jacket on, but I saw some dolly, and I *yelled* at my mother and said I want one of those dolly. So after we were finished with the store, we went over to the dolly and she *bought* me one. So I have one.

In both of these cases the narrative is produced spontaneously, that is, it was not talked about in the pre-bed dialogues, and according to the mother's notes, it had not been the focus of parent-child conversation in other contexts. There is a notable progression over the months of the study in Emily's ability to organize a coherent and cohesive story and to use appropriate linguistic devices for doing so, for example, through the use of anaphoric pronouns (Bruner & Lucariello, 1989; Levy, 1989).

In the beginning, her narratives are loosely organized, repetitive tales in which it is difficult to understand the intended relation between the events recounted. By 23 months the narratives are more tightly organized and various narrative devices are employed toward that end. Note especially in (1) the beginning contrast of verb tenses, even though the verb system is still in the process of being acquired, and the finale: "Yesterday did *that*; now Emmy sleeping in regular bed." Here Emily manipulates the temporal contrast not only through the verb forms (irregular past versus progressive) but by the use of temporal adverbs and the anaphoric "that" used to refer to the entire event recounted. By 32 months she tells a brief, well-organized tale of persuading her mother to buy her a doll. This account is a model of conciseness. Eavesdroppers can understand it perfectly although it was not produced for a listener. Rather, these productions (and many others like them) were apparently told for her own purposes. Those purposes I have argued involve comprehension through active organization of the memory of an experience, in order to get the account straight (Nelson, 1989). The progression in form can be seen as serving the cognitive organizing function. For example, in (1) at 23 months the account is repeated five times with variations, each apparently an attempt to put things in order. It is not clear whether she felt in the end that she had achieved a "correct" order, but presumably she was satisfied with the final version. By 32 months one brief account of the episode was enough; there was still a sense of savoring this tale, but it was apparently sufficiently well understood so that it did not need to be repeated.

Generating Generalities

A different kind of account is one that generalizes from experience. Such accounts have been studied extensively in pre-school children (Nelson, 1986), and a number are found in Emily's monologues. An early generalization (24 months) is as follows:

3. I can't go down the basement with jamas on. I sleep with jamas. Okay sleep with jamas. In the night time my only put big girl pants on. But in the morning we put jamas on. But, and the morning gets up . . . of the room. But, afternoon my wake up and play. Play with Mommy, Daddy.

By 2¹/₂ Emily produced several accounts of how her day goes, beginning with "Tomorrow morning when I wake up we go down and have breakfast, like we usually do ... " Time and space constraints prohibit reprinting these long accounts here, but it must be emphasized that formulating general event narratives was as central to her crib talk as were the specific episodic narratives.

Generating Possibilities

One of the most fascinating types of Emily's monologic productions involved her mulling over of possibilities within future expected events. These began to appear when she was just 2. An example from that period:

> 4. I don't, I don't know what boy bring book tomorrow. Maybe Lance. I don't know which boy bring book today. Maybe Danny or maybe Carl, maybe my, maybe Lance, maybe (too-wee). How about Lance bring book.

In this monologue Emily bases her speculations on general knowledge about the event in question. She apparently has a well-organized script of the day-care routine, and understands that each day someone brings a book to be read to the children. The question to be pondered is, Who will bring the book tomorrow and what will the book be? There seem to be as many possibilities as there are children.

Generating Necessities

In Emily's emerging model of the world some things are variable and therefore produce possibilities. Other things are predictable and therefore are apparently viewed as necessary, as seen in the following at 28 months:

> 5. If ever we go to the airport we have to get some luggage. If have to go to the airport, hafta take something for the airport, to the airport or you can't go.

This "rule" was derived on the basis of her two airplane trips to visit relatives over the summer. From the adult's point of view it is logically in error, confusing existential with deontic modality. It can be assumed therefore that it is a genuine original creation by Emily.

Generating Categories

An early example of Emily's formation of the food category is the following from 22 months:

6. Emmy like cornbread and toast. I don't like [?] apples and [?] I like toast and muffins. Food I like and [muffins] too. I don't like anything . . . cept for that, that bread daddy has . . .

These kinds of lists are not frequent in the monologues. However, a number of categories are constructed in the dialogues with her parents, including especially foods to be eaten at breakfast, and colors of her blankets. It appears that Emily is not particularly concerned with forming general superordinate categories for her own cognitive purposes, although she seems to enjoy and enter into the game happily with parents. (Of course, she generates basic level categories referenced by object names.) It may be speculated that superordinate category construction is an activity fostered by adults, one that children come to participate in as they use the language with adults on a higher more abstract cognitive level. Emily participated in such abstract uses with her parents at the age of 2 (probably earlier than most children) but they were not a prevalent theme in her monologues for herself.

Making Inferences

In contrast to category formation, making inferences, filling in gaps in information was often apparent in Emily's monologues. The examples of generating possibilities and necessities illustrate this activity. Other examples include the following, based on her parents' promise of an expedition to the beach on the following day:

7. We'll have to go in the green car, cause that's where the car seats are. Um, I can be in the red car, but, see, I be in the green car. But you know who's going to be in the green car . . . both children . . . I'm going to be in the green car in my car seat.

Her parents had projected a fairly detailed account of the beach episode but had said nothing about which car to take. The conjecture was Emily's, based on the fact that the car seats had been moved that day to the green car. The conjecture was wrong, although the inference was logical.

Another example a month later illustrates the complexity of her thought processes by 2 ½. Here she has set up a fantasy of pretending that she is Carl, her best friend, whose mother's real name is Chris:

8. No I'm Carl, it's Emily that sleeps. I'm no, there are two Chrises, I'm Emily, no, um I'm Carl . . . and Chris is my mother here and there's another Chris at Carl's house, there's one Chris for me . . . [???] and there's one Chris for the other Carl, the regular Carl.

Emily's logic here is straightforward: if she is Carl her own mother's name must be Chris, and there must be two Chrises, one at her house and one at (the regular) Carl's.

Learning through Language

From the beginning, Emily's parents in their pre-bed talk tell her about what will happen the next day or after nap, and talk to her about other things as well. At first, she attempts to repeat these accounts to herself, but manages only fragmentary and inaccurate renditions. Gradually, she begins to hold on to longer portions, and to fill in the accounts, as in the car seat example (7). Initially these depend on her own prior event knowledge about how things are and what should happen. An example that involves not her own activity, for which she has a direct experiential base, but someone else's activity (namely her father's) is the following from 32 months:

9. Today Daddy went, trying to get into the race but the people said no so he, he has to watch it on television. I don't know why that is, maybe cause there's too many people. I think that's why, why he couldn't go in it . . . So he has to watch it on television.

This account is a pretty good rendition of what her father had told her about his attempt to run in the New York City marathon. It is not based on any experience that Emily herself has had.

Up to this point all of the functions described are based on her own pre-existing event knowledge, knowledge built up on direct experience of individual events, or generalized knowledge of repeated events. Here is a new level, where the child can construct a representation of a possible event on the basis of what someone else has told her about an event with which she has no prior experience. Acquiring information through the linguistic medium is the other side of imparting information to others, which was achieved by Emily by 2 years as illustrated earlier. But learning from others through language is cognitively much more complex.

In some ways this process is equivalent to hearing and remembering a story, which even very young children seem to be quite good at. Emily repeated story fragments from the time she was 2 years old. But stories for young children are accompanied by pictures which provide a context for organizing and remembering the material. In addition, the narrative format matches the temporal-causal scheme of the child's own event knowledge system. In contrast, the account of her father's race (and others like it) rests solely on information conveyed through the linguistic medium (there are no pictures to evoke context), and there is very little narrative structure to it; thus it seems to require a higher level of abstract representational capacity.

Emily's ability to take in this information and to speculate with it in the same way that she does with accounts that involve her own activity more directly indicates that she has achieved an important new functional level of mathetic language. This level involves taking in information conveyed by another through the communicative function and using it oneself in cognitive operations. This level of mathetic function is a fundamental but revolutionary achievement of human language, one that has made culture and the advancement of knowledge possible. This level is not achieved simply with initial mastery of the language system, but only as a leap forward after the integration of language and experientially based representations has been established. After this point, new mental representations can be set up simply on the basis of what someone else describes.

LANGUAGE IN EVENTS AND EVENTS IN LANGUAGE

I will now draw together the strands of my story to delineate the relation between event representations and language functions in development. The functions considered to this point are outlined in Table 6-2 in terms of a developmental progression.

Halliday's functional description of Nigel's language begins even before conventional linguistic forms are acquired. The pragmatic functions emerge with pre-lexical forms. This level, as noted earlier, is but a small advance over nonverbal communication. In Halliday's view the achievement of the mathetic functions (chiefly categorizing) is an advance over the purely pragmatic, but these functions as well can be realized in single-word speech, as when the child points to things and names them. For Halliday the major achievement comes toward the end of the second year when three developments are (almost) simultaneously observed: the explosion of vocabulary, the onset of grammatical speech, and the establishment of dialogue.

In my view these developments at the end of the second year reflect a new understanding on the part of the child that language can be used to reference one's own conceptual representations and to share those concepts and experiences with others who speak the language (Nelson, 1985). Language becomes more than a communicative tool; it becomes a medium of expression and exchange of thoughts. This development leads inexorably onto the next. Engaging in dialogue that reveals common understandings about the world may lead the child to the attempt to organize and comprehend on a new level her own experiences whether or not they are specifically discussed with others. Certainly this is what we seemed to

Table 6-2. Development of Language Functions

Level	Usual Age of Achievement	Functions of Language
I	10–20 months	Simple pragmatic: instrumental, regulatory
II	15–24 months	Simple mathetic: Heuristic (projecting basic categorical knowledge); Imaginative (transforming basic knowledge structures)
		Interactional
III	20 mo.–3 years	Dialogue (sharing knowledge with others)
		Informative (imparting knowledge to others)
IV	2–5 years	Narrative construction of experienced events
		Generalizing event knowledge
		Projecting possibilities
		Forming higher-level categories
		Forming rules
		Making inferences
		Understanding stories
V	3 years–adult	Learning from language

observe in Emily's monologues. Thus language moves from a tool for referencing concepts embedded in representations of events, to a mode of talking with others about those representations, to a medium for the organization, comprehension, and re-presentation of experience. Already it is obvious that the relation of communication and cognition through language is not one-way: it moves first from a mapping of cognition onto language, then to communication of cognition through language, and from there to reflective use of language in cognition.*

The more advanced level proposed here represents the integration of communication and cognition through language. At this level, dialogue with others effectively establishes new representations, new (learned) knowledge, new possibilities within the child's own mental representational system, which initially was constrained to the representation of direct experience. Although the beginnings of this level in Emily's monologues appeared before she was yet 3, it seems probable that this level is not reached in general or well established for most children until late in the preschool years.

---

*I do not intend to neglect in this brief account the important fact that language does not simply map neatly onto prelinguistic cognition. Cognition is altered by language at the same time that language is used to exchange knowledge and beliefs between individuals. But that is a separate story too complex to relay here.

IMPLICATIONS FOR LANGUAGE DELAY AND LANGUAGE DISORDERS

Emily is a precocious child, quite the opposite of children who have difficulty with language. However, I believe that an account based on evidence from her language use can be helpful to understanding children less capable than she. Emily's rapid progress provides a way of seeing the many uses to which language may be put from the very simple to the very complex.

If the preceding analysis is correct, it has important implications for how professionals view and ultimately treat children whose entry into language is difficult or severely delayed. Most intervention programs are focused on Levels 1 and 2 of the scheme shown in Table 6-2. But at these levels the child is still at the point of either using the language to reference her own primitive event representations, expressing desires and needs, or using language to categorize according to categories imposed by adults. Given the present analysis it seems to be important in intervention efforts to establish conditions under which it becomes possible for the child to *share* knowledge of events with others, thus opening up the path toward spontaneous organization of event knowledge to accord with the common views of the language community. These steps are essential before the child can conceive of using language to establish new knowledge, which must be the ultimate goal of any language program, as it is the essential function of all schooling.

REFERENCES

Bauer, P. J., & Mandler, J. M. (1989). One thing follows another: Effects of temporal structure on 1- to 2-year-olds' recall of events. *Developmental Psychology, 25,* 197–206.

Bruner, J. S., & Lucariello, J. (1989). Monologue as narrative recreation of the world. In K. Nelson (Ed.), *Narratives from the crib.* Cambridge: Harvard University Press.

Gentner, D. (1982). Why nouns are learned before verbs: Linguistic relativity versus natural partitioning. In S. A. Kuczaj II (Ed.), *Language development: vol. 2, Language, thought, and culture.* Hillsdale, NJ: Erlbaum.

Gerhardt, J. (1989). Monologue as speech genre. In K. Nelson (Ed.), *Narratives from the crib.* Cambridge: Harvard University Press.

Givon, T. (1989). *Mind, code and context: Essays in pragmatics.* Hillsdale, NJ: Erlbaum.

Halliday, M. A. K. (1973). *Explorations in the functions of language.* London: Edwin Arnold.

Halliday, M. A. K. (1975). *Learning how to mean.* London: Edwin Arnold.

Levy, E. (1989). Monologue as development of the text-forming function of language. In K. Nelson (Ed.), *Narratives from the crib.* Cambridge: Harvard University Press.

Margolis, H. (1987). *Patterns, thinking, and cognition.* Chicago: University of Chicago Press.

Nelson, K. (1985). *Making sense: The acquisition of shared meaning.* New York: Academic.

Nelson, K. (1986). *Event knowledge: Structure and function in development.* Hillsdale, NJ: Erlbaum.

Nelson, K. (1989). *Narratives from the crib.* Cambridge: Harvard University Press.

Seidenberg, M. S., & Pettito, L. A. (1987). Communication, symbolic communication, and language: Comment on Savage-Rumbaugh, McDonald, Sevcik and Rupert (1986). *Journal of Experimental Psychology: General, 116,* 280–287.

Terrace, H. (1985). In the beginning was the "name." *American Psychologist, 49,* 1011–1028.

Wilson, P. J. (1980). *Man the promising primate.* New Haven: Yale University Press.

SECTION III

Language Disorders

CHAPTER 7

Associations and Dissociations in Language Development

ELIZABETH BATES AND DONNA THAL

For more than 100 years, aphasiologists have tried to determine how language is put together by examining all the different ways that it comes apart under conditions of focal brain damage. This includes a search for *dissociations* (which aspects of language can be selectively impaired?) and *associations* (which aspects of language are invariably spared or impaired together, as though they were separate manifestations of the same underlying skill?). The *sine qua non* of research within this tradition is the *double dissociation*. It is not enough simply to demonstrate that *A* can be damaged while *B* is spared, because *A* might turn out to be nothing more than a rather difficult version of the same mental skill that is responsible for the spared function *B*. A patient weakened by illness may have trouble lifting a 40-pound weight, despite the fact that s/he can still lift any weight under 5 pounds. This fact tells us little about the natural boundaries of motor processing. Similarly, if a patient retains the ability to add and subtract but loses the ability to carry out differential equations, it would be most unwise to conclude that arithmetic and higher algebra are handled by separate brain centers. Suppose, however, that another patient is found who can still handle differential equations despite a marked deficit in basic arithmetic. This is a most unlikely scenario, but if it did occur then we might be on safer ground in ascribing arithmetic and algebra to partially dissociable components of the mind/brain. Using the same logic, aphasiologists have explored the architecture of language and the brain by seeking double dissociations between language and cognition, together with more subtle double dissociations within the language processor itself.

The successes and failures of this long-standing endeavor can provide useful insights to those who are engaged in studying language development under normal and abnormal conditions. Conversely, the study of associations and dissociations in language development can also shed light on some controversial issues in neurolinguistic research, providing information that cannot be obtained by studying brain-damaged adults. We will try to defend and illustrate these complementary claims, in this chapter, organized as follows:

1. A brief review of three phases in the history of research on adult aphasia, emphasizing the different ways that investigators have tried to characterize the components of language that come apart under focal brain damage.
2. A discussion of how research on normal and abnormal language development can help us to overcome fundamental limitations in research on adult aphasia.
3. An overview of associations and dissociations in language development, in three different groups of children: (a) children in the normal range; (b) children who are acquiring language at an abnormal rate, despite the apparent absence of any medical or neurological abnormalities (i.e., "early talkers" and "late talkers"); (c) infants with focal brain lesions, acquiring language for the first time despite forms of brain damage that are associated with fluent or nonfluent aphasia in adults.

THREE PHASES IN THE STUDY OF ADULT APHASIA

PHASE 1: SENSORIMOTOR DISSOCIATIONS

Paul Broca and Carl Wernicke, the founders of modern aphasiology, tried to characterize the selective impairments they uncovered in brain-damaged adults by mapping dissociable components of language directly onto the known sensorimotor areas of the brain (Broca, 1861; Eggert, 1977; Head, 1926). Damage to anterior regions of the left hemisphere (i.e., frontal and temporal cortex, in particular a region called Broca's area) seemed to result in a nonfluent aphasia, with marked impairment in language production despite relative sparing of language comprehension. This profile makes excellent neuroanatomical sense, insofar as the regions implicated in this so-called motor aphasia lie close to primary motor cortex. Conversely, damage to posterior regions of the left hemisphere (i.e., particularly parietal cortex, including a region called Wernicke's area) seemed to result in a form of aphasia characterized by moderate to severe deficits in language comprehension; although patients with this syndrome do display serious problems in finding particular words, their speech is still surprisingly fluent and well-formed. This so-called sensory aphasia also fits well with known facts about the sensorimotor organization of the brain, because the areas that appear to be implicated in fluent syndromes lie in or near sensory cortex and/or sensorimotor association areas (in particular, auditory cortex).

As described by Henry Head (1926) in his critical history of this phase in aphasia research, the "diagram makers" were so confident of their input-output analyses that they went on to postulate the existence of fibers connecting sensory and motor language areas, fibers that could be selectively disconnected to produce *conduction aphasia*, a syndrome in which repetition is selectively impaired despite sparing of spontaneous comprehension and/or production (a syndrome that would be difficult to detect in normal circumstances, unless the clinician were expressly looking for it to test a theory of this kind). The picture was neatly rounded out with the postulation of *transcortical sensory aphasia* (sensory aphasia in patients with spared repetition skills) and *transcortical motor aphasia* (impairments in spontaneous output despite a sparing of repetition skills). Patients were found who seemed to fit each of these postulated disconnection syndromes, and new syndromes displaying the same logic were soon reported for reading and for writing (doubly dissociated, with or without disturbances in acoustic-articulatory language skills).

The diagram makers had an ample number of contemporary critics, well before Head's influential critique. These include Pierre Marie (1906), who pointed some serious flaws in Broca's original case studies, and Sigmund Freud (1891), a man who was never easy on his opponents. These scholars, like Goldstein (1948), Hughlings Jackson (1931) and Luria (1966) several decades later, pointed out that the components of language must operate together in real time; one cannot snip out one component without seriously compromising the activities carried out throughout the system as a whole. This approach has sometimes been caricatured as a *holistic* view, implying a certain homogeneity in brain tissue and brain function. However, if one actually returns to read the original works, one finds that the so-called holists actually espoused a complex theory of the brain as a highly differentiated dynamical system, in which thoughts are transformed into the spoken word (and vice-versa) in a cascade of intricate interactions across the whole brain (see also Brown, 1977). Alas, these subtle theories had little in the way of empirical evidence to sustain them, requiring the analysis of real-time brain physiology at a time when it was difficult to study anything other than brain anatomy in patients who arrive at autopsy.

It is perhaps not surprising that these alternatives to diagram-making did not survive. The view of aphasia that is expressed in most twentieth-century medical textbooks still reflects the sensorimotor disconnections first proposed by Broca and Wernicke (i.e., disconnections involving comprehension, production and repetition).

PHASE 2: LINGUISTIC DISSOCIATIONS

Disconnection syndromes were given a new intellectual life in the 1960s, when Norman Geschwind and his colleagues attempted a persuasive reinterpretation of Wernicke's diagrams in modern linguistic and psycholinguistic terms (Geschwind, 1965). While roundly criticizing the holists for their (supposed) oversimplification of brain architecture, Geschwind also criticized the original diagram makers for ignoring some fundamental differences between Broca's and Wernicke's aphasics that are hard to explain in sensorimotor terms. For example, he underscored the fact that fluent aphasics do indeed suffer from serious limitations in language production; these include word-finding problems that can in their most serious form result in substitutions, neologisms, empty and disrupted speech that is in many respects far more difficult to understand than the limited output of a so-called motor aphasic. In the same vein, Geschwind's colleagues at the Boston Veterans Administration Hospital went on to provide evidence against a motor-output characterization of Broca's aphasia. For example, Zurif and Caramazza (1976) demonstrated that Broca's aphasics suffer from specific comprehension deficits revolving around the interpretation of inflections and function words—precisely the same elements that are missing or impaired in their spontaneous speech (see also Caramazza & Berndt, 1978; Heilman & Scholes, 1976; Von Stockert & Bader, 1976).

A new view of language breakdown in aphasia began to emerge in the 1970s, in which the double dissociations represented by fluent and nonfluent aphasia were reinterpreted in linguistic rather than sensorimotor terms. Broca's aphasia was now viewed as a kind of *agrammatism* (i.e., a selective disruption in grammatical knowledge and/or grammatical processing that should in principle be manifest in all performance domains, including both comprehension and production) (Berndt & Caramazza, 1980). Conversely, the two symptoms that characterize Wernicke's aphasia (i.e., word-finding problems and comprehension deficits) could be explained parsimoniously by a single impairment in lexical semantics. In principle, this central semantic deficit should extend to all those performance domains that call upon the putative lexical-semantic processor. But what about the so-called repetition syndromes? Selective impairment and/or sparing of repetition could also be characterized in linguistic terms, if it is assumed that the language faculty contains a partially dissociable phonological component that is responsible for turning the combined outputs of the respective grammatical and semantic components into a string of sounds.

This view of the language faculty fits very well with Chomsky's proposal that language is a "mental organ" (Chomsky, 1965, 1980), composed of several distinct and autonomous components or "modules" (see also Fodor, 1985). And it is of course no accident that the new approach to aphasia emerged in the Boston community, the cradle of MIT-style generative grammar. Indeed, the linguistic study of aphasia appeared to hold such great promise during the 1970s and early 1980s that several linguists trained within the MIT generative grammar tradition turned their full-time efforts to a characterization of aphasic speech (Caplan and Hildebrandt, 1988; Grodzinski, 1986a, 1986b; Kean, 1979).

It was never entirely obvious how or why the brain ought to be organized in just this way (e.g., why Broca's area, the supposed seat of grammar, ought to be located near the motor strip), but the lack of a compelling link between neurology and neurolinguistics was more than compensated for by the apparent isomorphism between aphasic syndromes and the components predicted by current linguistic theory. Several recent textbooks on neuropsychology and/or neurology reflect this view, offering a characterization of language breakdown in aphasia in terms of linguistic modules corresponding roughly to grammar, semantics, and phonology.

PHASE 3: LEVELS OF PROCESSING

As a colleague of the authors once stated ruefully, "Never test a good theory." Despite its intellectual appeal, the linguistic approach to language breakdown in aphasia has recently fallen on hard times. A great deal of evidence has accumulated to suggest that there is no such thing as central agrammatism. And if the doctrine of central agrammatism falls, then the grammar/semantics/phonology division described above becomes very difficult to maintain, because we no longer have the requisite double dissociations in place.

Briefly summarized, four classes of evidence have arisen across the 1980s to place the existence of central agrammatism in doubt. First, a number of case studies have been published demonstrating expressive agrammatism in patients who appear to have perfectly normal control over grammar in tests of comprehension (Caramazza & Berndt, 1978; Von Stockert & Bader, 1976). Second, an even larger body of evidence has emerged to show that receptive agrammatism can occur in patients who show no signs of grammatical breakdown in their expressive speech (Bates, Friederici & Wulfeck, 1987; Bates & Wulfeck, 1989, in press; Smith & Bates, 1987; Talay & Slobin, 1988). Third, cross-linguistic studies have demonstrated large and reliable differences in comprehension and production among agrammatic aphasics, differences that can only be explained if it is assumed that these patients retain knowledge of their premorbid language (Bates & Wulfeck, 1989, in press; Goodglass & Menn, 1985; Menn & Obler, in press). Fourth and finally, several studies have now shown that many so-called agrammatic Broca's aphasics can make remarkably subtle judgments of grammatical well-formedness—even in sentences that they themselves cannot understand (Linebarger, Schwartz & Saffran, 1983; Shankweiler, Craine, Gorrell, & Tuller, 1989; Wulfeck, 1988). This last finding is perhaps the cruelest blow to neurolinguists working within the generative grammar tradition, because the ability to make grammaticality judgments is the hallmark of competence in one's native language.

Evidence of this kind has left the neurolinguistic community in considerable disarray, and it is difficult to discern a new consensus to replace the modular view of language breakdown in aphasia. Some original proponents of central agrammatism have responded to these events by arguing that all clinical syndromes be abandoned in favor of an approach in which individual cases (without labels) are studied in isolation to test theories derived from the normal literature (Badecker & Caramazza, 1985; Caramazza, 1986; Caramazza & Berndt, 1978; Caramazza & Zurif, 1976). The bitterness inherent in this view is well illustrated by the following quote from Miceli, Silveri, Romani and Caramazza (1989), who describe the heterogeneity that is evident in a large sample of agrammatic patients and then go on to conclude that:

The observed heterogeneity in the production of grammatical morphemes among putatively agrammatic patients renders the clinical category of agrammatism, and by extension all other clinical categories from the classical classification scheme (e.g., Broca's aphasia, Wernicke's aphasia, and so forth) to more recent classificatory attempts (e.g., surface dyslexia, deep dysgraphia, and so forth), *theoretically useless* [p. 447].... These empirical facts can no longer be ignored just for the *obstinate protection of a fictional category of dubious theoretical value* [p. 475, italics ours].

Other aphasiologists maintain that a coherent linguistic characterization of agrammatism is still possible, but they insist that such a characterization will turn on very subtle details of current grammatical theory (Caplan & Hildebrandt, 1988; Grodzinski, 1986a, 1986b, in press; Lapointe, 1985; Rizzi, 1985). Unfortunately, these details tend to change so rapidly that it is hard for neurolinguistic researchers to keep up. Perhaps more important, it is difficult to see how such subtle linguistic accounts of grammatical breakdown could be reconciled with the heterogeneous symptoms that lead Miceli and colleagues to the despairing conclusion cited above.

A unifying account of the heterogeneous linguistic symptoms observed in aphasia may still be possible, if it can be shown that the contrasts among aphasic syndromes reflect horizontal modules (processors that cut across content domains) instead of vertical modules (processors that deal exclusively with one kind of information—see Fodor, 1983, & Bates, Bretherton & Snyder, 1988, for extended discussions). Because such horizontal modules bear only an indirect relationship to language proper, they may be associated with considerable individual variability in the linguistic content of aphasic symptoms. But what kind of processing account might this be? There can be no return to the comprehension-production-repetition approach espoused by the original diagram makers, because it is now quite clear that there is no such thing as a "pure" comprehension deficit or a "pure" impairment in expressive language (other than, perhaps, a very peripheral deficit in oral-motor activity). What other possibilities are there?

An alternative processing account has begun to emerge in the current neurolinguistic literature, based on results obtained with so-called on-line methods for investigating real-time language use. A number of investigators (including some who were once active proponents of the Geschwind view) now invoke terms such as *automatic* versus *controlled*, and *global* versus *local* to describe the contrasting profiles displayed by fluent and nonfluent aphasics in such on-line experiments (Baum, 1989; Swinney, Zurif & Nicol, in press; Tyler, 1985; Zurif, Gardner, & Brownell, in press; Zurif & Grodzinsky, 1983). For example, Broca's aphasics seem to demonstrate little evidence for the kind of linguistic facilitation or "priming" that occurs so rapidly in normal language processing; this limitation has now been demonstrated in several different linguistic domains (i.e., semantics, phonology, grammar), and it shows up in patients who nevertheless demonstrate good "off-line" metalinguistic skills. By contrast, Wernicke's aphasics display normal or even hyper-normal profiles in priming experiments, suggesting that the more "automatic" excitatory/facilitatory aspects of language processing are still intact; the same patients perform very poorly when the same aspects of language must be processed "off-line" (e.g., in metalinguistic judgment tasks).

This new double dissociation is difficult to interpret, but it seems to bear a nontrivial resemblance to the contrast between automatic and controlled processing proposed by Shiffrin and Schneider (1977), Posner and Snyder (1975), and/or Norman and Shallice (1980) to account for qualitative differences in modes or levels of processing in normal human attention and performance. The neural basis for such a dissociation is still quite obscure, and may ultimately turn on facts of brain physiology that are only indirectly related to specific neuroanatomical regions (i.e., variations in excitation, inhibition, and rates of processing). Indeed, this may be the right time to revive the dynamical systems approach to brain and language first proposed by Goldstein, Jackson, Luria, and other theorists in the much-maligned (and misnamed) Holistic School, making use of new techniques for studying brains in action (e.g., event-related brain potentials; positron emission tomography) that were not available when these theories first appeared.

For present purposes, the point here is that aphasiology has reached an historical crisis. Researchers have been forced to discard a number of convenient characterizations of language breakdown in aphasia. The original sensorimotor approach of Broca and Wernicke (i.e., a division into comprehension, production, and repetition) made good neuroanatomical sense, but apparently cannot account for the full range of adult data. The more recent division of the language processor into linguistic modules (e.g., grammar, semantics, and phonology) maps beautifully onto linguistic theory, but unfortunately it does not fit nearly so well with the realities of linguistic performance in aphasia. The proposed new division into levels or modes of processing (e.g., automatic versus controlled) may ultimately provide a better account of real-time processing in brain-damaged adults, but this approach is currently lacking in *both* neurological and linguistic appeal. Surely relief from any quarter would be welcome in the current crisis; some advantages of developmental psycholinguistic research as a source of information about associations and dissociations among the processors responsible for language will be considered below.

SOME ADVANTAGES OF THE DEVELOPMENTAL APPROACH TO THE STUDY OF DISSOCIATIONS

The study of language development forces one to factor the complex issue of change over time into an already complex series of questions about brain and language. This may be one reason why so many neurolinguistic researchers have traditionally preferred to concentrate on language break-down in adulthood, when correlations between brain and behavior have presumably reached some kind of "steady state." However, there are a number of serious limitations on the interpretation of dissociations in adult aphasia, limitations not encountered (or encountered to a lesser degree) when associations and dissociations in language development are studied.

1. *Lesions do not respect organic boundaries.* The associations and dissociations seen in adult aphasics are usually the result of insults to brain tissue (i.e., stroke, closed head trauma, tumor, projectile wounds) that cut across the "natural" organic boundaries of the mind/brain. Even if there is a lawful topographic relationship between linguistic functions and specific brain regions (a conclusion that is by no means certain), the code connecting the two is likely to remain elusive as long as the search is restricted to such gerrymandered preparations.

From this point of view, normally developing children provide important complementary information. If it is found that two aspects of language can develop out of synchrony, across different environmental conditions, then it may be inferred with some confidence that this asynchrony reflects a natural boundary. Specifically, the authors suggest that such individual differences reflect variation in rate of development among two or more of the mental/neural mechanisms responsible for language acquisition and language use (Bates et al., 1988).

2. Adults are capable of sophisticated adaptations that obscure brain/language relationships. The research reviewed earlier shows that most aphasic patients retain considerable knowledge of their native language; studies of grammaticality judgments show that they are also capable of reflecting on that knowledge. In addition, many of these patients (especially Broca's aphasics) are painfully aware of their condition; they have to fill many hours of fear, frustration, and/or boredom trying to deal with serious limitations on the language capacity that they took for granted for so many years, and they are perfectly capable of developing a self-fulfilling theory of those aspects of language that are "easy" or "hard" for them. Under these circumstances, one must be prepared for the possibility that the symptom patterns displayed by an adult aphasic reflect sophisticated and often idiosyncratic adaptations (Kolk & Heeschen, 1985). Hence the cause-and-effect relationship between brain and behavior in a stable aphasic patient may be very indirect.

The situation is quite different in a young child acquiring language for the first time. Small children are indeed capable of a certain amount of metalinguistic reflection (Gleitman, Gleitman & Shipley, 1972; Crain & Fodor, 1987; Shankweiler, et al., 1989), and they also have some awareness of their own limitations (Clark & Clark, 1977). But they lack the sophistication required to build complex adaptations to their current condition; and, in any case, the "current" linguistic condition of a very small child changes so rapidly that adaptations of this sort would rapidly become moot. For this reason, the authors suggest that the dissociations observed in the early stages of language acquisition provide a more direct view of the relationship between mental/neural mechanisms and linguistic performance, compared with the dissociations observed in an adult who is (or was) a mature native speaker.

3. *Automaticity is a product of experience.* In an adult speaker with many years of experience, some aspects of language (especially grammar and phonology) may become relatively automatic, requiring little investment of attention and/or other cognitive resources. When cognitive resources are diminished through focal or diffuse brain damage, those aspects of language that have attained this automatic status may be "protected," resulting in patterns of selective sparing and impairment that bear only an indirect relationship to the localization of language functions in the brain (Kempler, 1984).

In small children acquiring their language for the first time, it can be assumed with some confidence that this kind of "modularity through automaticity" has not yet occurred. Hence the patterns of selective sparing and impairment seen in children with focal brain lesions may provide a more direct view of the degree to which brain regions are specialized for particular language functions.

Evidence for associations and dissociations in early language development will be reviewed below and comparisons made with the patterns of language breakdown in aphasia just described (i.e., sensorimotor dissociations, linguistic dissociations, and dissociations based on levels or modes of processing). These developmental patterns force reconsideration of a sensorimotor characterization of mental/neural architecture, while providing little comfort for those who seek an architecture based on language modules. Comparing these results with the new levels-of-processing approach to language breakdown in adults, one can see the outlines of a truly developmental view in which the relationship between brain and language changes with experience and expertise.

DEVELOPMENTAL DISSOCIATIONS

Evidence from the Normal Range

This section will focus on those components of language that can "pull ahead" or "lag behind" in normally developing children. With relatively large samples, associations and dissociations of this kind are usually assessed through correlational analysis: high positive correlations reflect developments that "hang together" over time, while low correlations mean that the measures in question are developing on separate schedules. Of course this research strategy has some well-known pitfalls, and high or low correlations can be obtained for uninteresting reasons (see Bates et al., 1988, chapter 3 for a detailed discussion). For example, low correlations (and apparent dissociations) can be obtained by using an unreliable measure (e.g., a measure that correlates poorly with itself). To avoid spurious results, researchers look for patterns that are consistent across many different measures of the same function (e.g., parental report, free speech, structured observations); if the same associations and dissociations replicate across multiple fallible measures, then it is justifiable to draw inferences about the mental/neural systems that underlie this pattern.

Within this methodological framework, there is now a sizeable literature exploring the componential structure of language and cognition during the early stages of language development, in normal and atypical children (see Bates et al., 1988; Thal & Bates, in press, for reviews). At every age level, and in every content domain (i.e., lexical, grammatical, phonological, pragmatic), two distinct clusters or "strands" have been documented. Because there are some striking similarities across studies in the nature of these two extremes, it is tempting to conclude that the same mechanisms are responsible in every case.

Table 7-1 summarizes some dimensions of variation in rate and style of language development that have been described in this literature to date. The table is organized into two columns, reflecting the two stylistic extremes that are described in virtually all these studies. Strand 1 reflects an approach to language learning that was originally called referential style; strand 2 reflects a complementary approach that was originally called *expressive style* (Nelson, 1973). Children in Strand 1 share an analytic approach to breaking the language code which they apply at all levels of language learning, focusing on the extraction and consistent production of small units (Peters, 1983). For example, at the extreme end of this style, prespeech sounds and early words are restricted to a small but consistent repertoire of consonant-vowel segments (Dore, 1974; Ferguson, 1984; Vihman, 1981; Vihman & Carpenter, 1984). In the early one-word stage (from 1–50 words), vocabularies are composed primarily of names for common objects (Nelson, 1973). Early word combinations tend to be telegraphic utterances with few inflections or function words, for example, "Daddy car" or "Adam cookie" (Bloom, Lightbown & Hood, 1975). Chidren at the extreme end of Strand 2, on the other hand, produce long strings of prespeech babble that sound very much like the intonation contours of adult sentences. However, there is considerable heterogeneity and inconsistency in the way individual phonetic segments within these utterances are pronounced (Dore, 1974; Ferguson, 1984; Vihman, 1981; Vihman & Carpenter, 1984). The early vocabularies of children at this extreme also tend to be heterogeneous, including some multiword formulae or routines such as "Dat mine" or "Wan dat" (Nelson, 1973; Peters, 1983). These children tend not to produce telegraphic utterances, but to include pronouns and other function words in their first word combinations (Bloom et al., 1975). However, there is reason to believe that this "precocious" use of inflections and function words reflects rote production, with little analysis of the grammatical forms and/or functions that these morphemes convey in adult speech. Indeed, there appears to be a negative correlation between the use of function words at 20 months and productive control over the same terms 8 months later (Bates et al., 1988). Findings like these have led some investigators to conclude that these two strands reflect a partial dissociation between two learning mechanisms: an analytic/segmenting mechanism (dominant in referential-style children) and a rote/holistic mechanism (dominant in expressive-style children). Both mechanisms are necessary for the complete acquisition of a natural language, but children may rely on one or the other to a different degree.

Bates et al. (1988) set out to test the two-strand model, in a longitudinal study of 27 middle class infants observed at 10, 13, 20, and 28 months of age (i.e., the period from first words to grammar). Within each age level, they

Table 7-1. Individual differences in early language development: summary of claims in the literature

Referential/Nominal	Expressive/Pronominal
SEMANTICS	
High proportion of nouns in first 50 words	Low proportion of nouns in first 50 words
Single words in early speech	Formulae in early speech
Imitates object names	Unselective imitation
Greater variety within lexical categories	Less variety within lexical categories
Meaningful elements only	Use of "dummy" words
High adjective use	Low adjective use
Context-flexible use of names	Context-bound use of names
Rapid vocabulary growth	Slower vocabulary growth
GRAMMAR	
Telegraphic in Stage I	Inflections and function words in Stage I
Refers to self and others by name in Stage I	Refers to self and others by pronoun in Stage I
Noun-phrase expansion	Verb-phrase expansion
Morphological overgeneralization	Morphological undergeneralization
Consistent application of rules	Inconsistent application of rules
Novel combinations	Frozen forms
Imitation is behind spontaneous speech	Imitation is ahead of spontaneous speech
Fast learner	Slow learner
PHONOLOGY	
Word-oriented	Intonation-oriented
High intelligibility	Low intelligibility
Segmental emphasis	Suprasegmental emphasis
Consistent pronunciation acros word tokens	Variable pronunciation across word tokens
PRAGMATICS	
Object-oriented	Person-oriented
Declarative	Imperative
Low variety in speech acts	High variety in speech acts

Source: Adapted from Bates, Bretherton & Snyder (1988), p. 54.

applied principle component analysis to a representative set of language measures. If the two-factor model is correct, then two factors (roughly equivalent to those implied by Table 7-1) should be necessary and sufficient to account for individual differences at that age level. Then, to determine whether or not the "same" factors carry over from stage to stage, correlational analyses of these factor scores were carried out between each time point. Their results suggest that the two-factor model is not sufficient to explain language development between 10 and 28 months. At least three partially dissociable mechanisms may be necessary to account for patterns of variation in the transition from first words to grammar. Furthermore, these patterns bear some resemblance to sensorimotor components proposed by the classical aphasiologists: a division into comprehension, production, and repetition.

At the 10–13 month level, the Bates et al. factor analysis yielded two orthogonal components. These two components were defined primarily by a split between comprehension and production. However, like the comprehension/production dissociations displayed by adult aphasics, these dissociations defy a straightforward sensorimotor explanation. In particular, referential/analytic aspects of production loaded highly on the comprehension factor; the independent production factor was defined primarily by rote and/or imitative speech.

This implicit three-way split reached significance at 20 months, when three components fell out of the analysis: a comprehension factor, and two production factors reflecting the contrast between analyzed and rote/imitative speech. This is the point at which the strongest parallels with the classic aphasia literature are found: three dissociable mechanisms that are roughly equivalent to comprehension, production and repetition.

Another comprehension/production dissociation emerged in the principle component analysis at 28 months of age. Interestingly, this dissociation cut across lexical and grammatical measures (e.g., children who are high comprehenders and low producers in the lexical domain display the same profile in measures of grammatical development). However, the rote factor that emerged so clearly at 13 and 20 months seems to have disappeared by 28 months. Because this is the age level at which all normal children must carry out the analyses required for productive control over grammatical morphology, it may be that rote processes play a minimal role in this phase of language acquisition. However, it is entirely possible that the rote "strand" will reappear later on, in line with observations by Horgan (1981), Peters (1977), and Fillmore (1979), among others.

To what extent can it be concluded that a continuous set of processes are operating from one age level to another? Cross-age correlations in the Bates et al., study suggest that there are intimate interactions among these three putative mechanisms: dissociations come and go, and today's independent variance may be woven back into the shared fabric of linguistic knowledge at a later point. Figure 7-1 depicts the cross-age relationships that were observed in this study. One major continuous pathway runs from comprehension and analyzed production at 13 months, through isolated analyzed production at 20 months, to both general comprehension and general production at 28 months. However, there are also two smaller

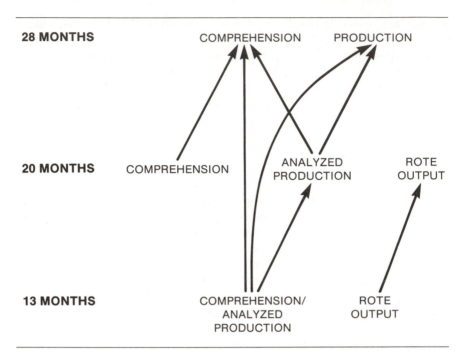

Fig. 7-1. Cross-age relationships among comprehension, analyzed production, and rote production in 27 middle-class infants between 13 and 28 months of age. Adapted from Bates et al., 1988. p. 227.

routes taking the child from first words to grammar as well. One of them is the rote production factor which is connected between 13 and 20 months (from first words to first word combinations), and the other is a pure comprehension factor which is linked between 20 and 28 months (operating across lexical and grammatical measures).

Nowhere in this developmental picture is there any sign of a dissociation between linguistic components (e.g., grammar versus lexical semantics). Indeed, lexical and grammatical development are strongly correlated in rate and style (e.g., a correlation of +.83 between vocabulary at 20 months and mean length of utterance (MLU) 8 months later). Putting these patterns of association and dissociation together, there is some support for a mind/brain architecture that is organized along sensorimotor lines (comprehension, production, repetition) and little support for an architecture organized into linguistic modules (grammar, semantics, phonology). Hence, returning to the divisions that have been proposed in the literature on adult aphasia, the developmental evidence appears to favor some version of the classical input-output view.

However, the reasons why modern aphasiologists have abandoned the classical view must also be remembered: so-called motor aphasics do demonstrate subtle receptive language problems, and so-called sensory aphasics display severe word-findings problems and other expressive language symptoms. By the same token the cross-age patterns uncovered in the Bates et al. (1988) study point out that there are dynamic interactions among the partially dissociable mechanisms that underlie individual differences in language development. Today's comprehension feeds into tomorrow's production (and, perhaps, vice-versa). The apparent advantage gained by children who rely heavily on rote production (sounding very precocious at 20 months) may turn into a disadvantage when internal segmentation of morphemes is required for further progress. And so forth, *mutatis mutandem*.

To fill out this picture (and, perhaps, arrive at a rapprochement with today's aphasia literature), the chapter will now turn to the dissociations observed in two unusual populations: neurologically intact children who are acquiring language earlier or later than usual, and children who must acquire language with focal brain lesions that prevent normal language functioning when they occur in adults.

EVIDENCE FROM ATYPICAL POPULATIONS

LATE AND EARLY TALKERS

The comprehension/production disparities described above have also been demonstrated in studies of late and early talkers (Thal & Bates, 1988a, 1988b). Late talkers are defined as children between 18 and 28 months of age who are in the bottom tenth percentile for expressive vocabulary development as indicated by a series of parental report instruments developed and validated in our laboratories (Bates, Snyder, Bretherton & Volterra, 1979; Dale, Bates, Reznick & Morisset, 1989; Reznick & Goldsmith, 1989). Early talkers are defined as children between 11 and 22 months who are in the top tenth percentile on the same measures. In each group, there are children who are equally late (or equally precocious) in both comprehension and production. However, there are also a number of children who demonstrate a dissociation between comprehension and production. Those children are indistinguishable from age-matched controls on measures of receptive vocabulary (including parental report and structured testing in the laboratory) despite their delay or precocity in expressive vocabulary. This finding led to the exploration of the relationship between language and cognition in a slightly different way, by asking how the nonverbal correlates of language (summarized in Table 7-1) align with comprehension and production in these two atypical groups.

To date, the data suggest that most nonverbal measures correlate with the child's current level of comprehension. It looks as though language and cognition are most closely related at the level of language understanding;

that is, what the child *knows* rather than what he or she *does*. However, for children with expressive vocabularies under 50 words (before the vocabulary burst), specific measures of symbolic gesture do align quite closely with the child's current level of language production. In particular, recognitory gestures (i.e., gestures that are associated with common objects and their functions, such as drinking, combing, and telephoning) elicited one at a time out of context, with little or no support from the object itself (e.g., drinking from a wooden block, combing with a toy spoon) are reliably correlated with language production in both groups of children. This general deficit may be viewed as a kind of anomia (see also Kempler, 1988) because of the resemblance to relationships reported between anomia (difficulty with object naming) and ideomotor apraxia (difficulty with gestural pantomime) often reported in the literature on brain-damaged adults (Duffy, Duffy, & Pearson, 1975; Gainotti & Lemmo, 1976; Goodglass & Kaplan, 1963).

The analytic-holistic distinction is also seen in the exceptional groups. The best example can be seen in a case study of two children who are extraordinarily precocious in expressive language (Thal & Bates, 1988b). M was a 21-month-old with an expressive vocabulary of 627 words; S was a 17-month-old with an expressive vocabulary of 596 words. Both children were also quite advanced in comprehension, although less so than their expressive precocity would lead one to expect. Both produced a wide array of verbs and adjectives as well as nouns, a development that typically signals the onset of grammar. They had also begun to master English grammatical morphology, producing contrasting endings on at least a few nouns and verbs (e.g., "walk" versus "walking"). The one clear difference between these two exceptional children revolves around sentence length: S had a mean length of utterance (MLU) in morphemes of 2.39, equivalent to a 30-month-old child; M had just begun to combine words, with an MLU of 1.19, exactly what would be expected for a child of her age. Because these two children are not measurably different in their mastery of noun and verb endings, one would not want to conclude that they demonstrate a dissociation between vocabulary and grammar. Nor would one want to conclude that S is advanced in syntax, since her long sentences contain very little evidence for transformation, extraction, inversion, or any of the operations that define and characterize the syntactic components of grammar. We have suggested instead that M and S vary markedly in the size of the unit that they are able to store and produce at any given time. This interpretation is supported by the fact that S had a repertoire of idioms like "No way, José!" and "You little monkey!" Her ability to manipulate and even blend these units is illustrated by the expression "No way you monkey!" which she produced for the first time in our lab. In short, it is possible that M and S represent an analytic-holistic dissociation with levels of comprehension and expressive vocabulary held constant.

To summarize the work to date on early and late talkers, two kinds of dissociations have emerged: a sharp dissociation between comprehension and production, and a further split within comprehension between lexical development and word combinations. The latter dissociation may reflect a particularly interesting variant of the analytic/rote distinction described earlier. If this analysis is correct, then the dissociations displayed by children at the extremes of normal development confirm the patterns that have emerged in work on individual differences across the normal range.

INFANTS WITH FOCAL BRAIN INJURY

It has been known for some time that children can recover to a remarkable degree from unilateral brain injuries that have devastating and irreversible effects when they occur in adulthood (Hecaen, 1976, 1983; Lenneberg, 1967; Woods & Teuber, 1978). Subtle deficits can be detected in the victims of early injury (Aram, 1988; Dennis and Whitaker, 1976; Vargha-Khadem, O'Gorman & Watters, 1985), but the degree of recovery and/or reorganization that does occur in young brain-injured children provides a strong challenge to any theory of cortical specialization for language in the human species. Furthermore, there are also interesting qualitative differences between children and adults in the patterns of dissociation that are observed immediately after focal brain injury. For example, young children rarely display the fluent aphasias that are associated with posterior brain damage in adults; instead, nonfluent patterns typically result (with or without comprehension deficits) if there are substantial lesions anywhere in anterior or posterior cortex (Hecaen, 1983). There is also some reason to believe that unilateral right hemisphere damage results in short-term language deficits that are not observed in right-hemisphere damaged adults (Aram, Ekelman, Rose, & Whitaker, 1985; Aram, Ekelman, & Whitaker, 1986, 1987; Riva & Cazzaniga, 1986; Riva, Cazzaniga, Pantaleoni, Milani, & Frederizzi, 1986). These facts pose an important developmental question: what is the process by which specific regions of cerebral cortex take on the specialized functions that are responsible for the patterns of language breakdown observed in adult aphasia?

A team of researchers at UCSD has taken a *prospective* approach to this problem, examining the first stages of language development in infants with focal brain injury, concentrating on a group of infants with well-defined focal brain injury acquired prenatally or within the first 6 months of life. To date, there is a combination of cross-sectional and longitudinal data for 15 infants, ranging across the developmental transition from prespeech to the onset of early grammatical skills. So far, the dissociations observed are not qualitatively different from the patterns that emerge in research across the normal range. However, at least a few hints about the developing (and changing) neural basis for these patterns have been found (Marchman, Miller and Bates, 1989; Thal et al., 1989).

First of all, dissociations between comprehension and production have been observed in some of the children between 12 and 16 months of age; in the few children for whom longitudinal information exists, these patterns seem to persist through the 16–24 month age range. In the research to date, this disparity between near-normal word comprehension and markedly delayed expressive vocabulary is restricted entirely to children with some form of left hemisphere damage; by contrast, right hemisphere lesions are associated with deficits in comprehension that are greater than or equal to delays in production. Although the results for infants with right hemisphere damage are based on very small numbers, the production-ahead-of-comprehension pattern is so rare and so surprising that it warrants further investigation. (Remember that these patterns are based on *percentile* scores; they do not mean that children with right hemisphere lesions have a larger absolute *number* of words in their expressive vocabulary.)

These brain-injured children also display atypical patterns of vocabulary composition, extreme versions of the patterns that are usually associated with analytic versus holistic style in normal children. For example, two out of 6 children examined between 27 and 35 months of age used an extremely high percentage of nouns to the exclusion of other word classes; thus, they demonstrated an exaggerated nominal/analytic pattern. Three others (of the same 6) used abnormally high proportions of closed-class words; this pattern looks like an extreme version of expressive/holistic style.

Correlations between behavior and lesion site in a sample of only six children must be taken with more than one grain of salt. However, there are some tantalizing and surprising trends in these data, trends that stand in direct contrast to the brain-behavior correlations observed in adult aphasics. Adults with left posterior lesions tend to display fluent but empty speech (i.e., Wernicke's aphasia); adults with left anterior lesions tend to produce nonfluent, telegraphic speech (i.e., Broca's aphasia). The developmental data directly reverse this trend: the two children who displayed a particularly marked telegraphic style have lesions in left posterior cortex; the extremes of expressive/pronominal style occur both in one child with left anterior damage and two children with lesions restricted to the right hemisphere.

Putting these results together with the comprehension/production patterns described above results in the suggestion that there may indeed be a certain amount of regional specialization for particular language functions during the early stages of language development. For example, the right hemisphere may play a particularly important role in the early stages of word comprehension, and the left posterior cortex may be integrally involved in every aspect of early language production (lexical and grammatical). However, these patterns of specialization change with maturation and/or with linguistic experience. Lexical comprehension may become so "automatic" that right hemisphere contributions are no longer necessary. And certain aspects of language production (e.g., phonology and grammar) may come under the control of anterior brain regions after they reach a certain level of proficiency. One can speculate about the reasons for this progressive "anteriorization"; for example, after a lifetime of experience with a limited set of lexical and grammatical frames, those frames may be produced as prepackaged motor schemes. Like other well-practiced skills (e.g., driving, typing), these motor schemes can be adjusted quickly and unconsciously to new local demands; in other words, they are productive. But they no longer require the kind of effort that was necessary in the early stages of lexical and grammatical development. Hence they have been "handed forward," from sensorimotor association areas to primary motor cortex. In very young children, this kind of "automatic" status can be seen in a few relatively unanalyzed and nonproductive sentence formula, but rote production may play an increasingly important role in the later stages of language use.

CONCLUSION

Evidence has been presented here for patterns of association and dissociation in early language development in three different groups: children who are developing at a normal rate, very early or very late talkers, and children with focal brain lesions. The same basic patterns emerged in every group: dissociations between comprehension and production, and dissociations between productive/creative speech and rote/repetitive speech. By contrast, there is little evidence in the early stages for dissociations defined in linguistic terms: phonology, lexical semantics, and early grammatical development are correlated in both rate and style across the transition from first words to grammar.

Furthermore, the data for infants with focal brain lesions suggest that the areas governing these aspects of language are quite different at the early stages of development, compared with the literature on language breakdown in adults. Comprehension/production disparities may reflect a left/right distribution rather than the anterior/posterior distribution associated with similar comprehension/production dissociations in adult aphasics. Furthermore, it appears that early lesions to left posterior cortex are associated with telegraphic speech; by contrast, specific deficits in the production of function words are more common among adults with lesions to left anterior cortex. In short, there appear to be developmental changes in the neural structures that support language.

There is not yet enough evidence from any quarter to permit strong conclusions about the developing relationship between brain and language. However, one can discern the beginnings of a rapprochement between adult aphasia and the study of normal and abnormal language development. The sensorimotor characterization of aphasia offered by Broca and Wernicke is undoubtedly much too simple to account for the subtle and complex deficits displayed by an adult aphasic. But perhaps some version of the sensorimotor classification scheme can explain the early stages of development. The human brain may start out with a rough sketch: a set of input-output biases and potential dissociations that follow a basic sensorimotor blueprint that the human species shares with many others. The "special" organization for language found in an adult brain (e.g., the now-popular dissociation between automatic and controlled processing) may come into existence only after many years of experience with this "special" cognitive skill. In other words, brain development may involve a transition from sensorimotor organization, to an organization that more closely reflects the processing dimensions that are needed for adult language use.

Speculations of this magnitude must be subjected to a much more rigorous empirical test, but the possibilities are tantalizing. This chapter began by arguing that the study of associations and dissociations in language acquisition can inform understanding of the mental/neural architecture that is responsible for language in the mature adult. But the relationship between these two domains of inquiry may be even stronger. For too long, researchers have assumed (implicitly or explicitly) a unidirectional link between brain maturation and behavioral change (i.e., that the basic milestones of language development are *caused* by changes in the brain). Instead, the authors suggest that language acquisition and brain organization are tied together by an epigenetic process with bidirectional causal links. To some extent, linguistic experience may help to *create* the correlations between brain and behavior that are revealed by the study of language breakdown in adult aphasia.

REFERENCES

Aram, D. (1988). Language sequelae of unilateral brain lesions in children. In F. Plum (Ed.), *Language, communication, and the brain.* New York: Raven.

Aram, D., Ekelman, B., Rose, D., & Whitaker, H. (1985). Verbal and cognitive sequelae following unilateral lesions acquired in early childhood. *Journal of Clinical and Experimental Neuropsychology, 7,* 55–78.

Aram, D., Ekelman, B., & Whitaker, H. (1986). Spoken syntax in children with acquired unilateral hemisphere lesions. *Brain and Language, 27,* 75–100.

Aram, D., Ekelman, B., & Whitaker, H. (1987). Lexical retrieval in left and right brain-lesioned children. *Brain and Language, 28,* 61–87.

Badecker, W., & Caramazza, A. (1985). On considerations of method and theory governing the use of clinical categories in neurolinguistics and cognitive neuropsychology: The case against agrammatism. *Cognition, 24,* 277–282.

Bates, E., Bretherton, I., & Snyder, L. (1988). *From first words to grammar: Individual differences and dissociable mechanisms.* New York: Cambridge University Press.

Bates, E., Friederici, A., & Wulfeck, B. (1987). Comprehension in aphasia: A crosslinguistic study. *Brain and Language, 32,* 19–67.

Bates, E., Snyder, L., Bretherton, I., & Volterra, V. (1979). The emergence of symbols in language and action: Similarities and differences. *Papers and Reports on Child Language Development, 17,* 106–118.

Bates, E., & Wulfeck, B. (1989). Comparative aphasiology: A crosslinguistic approach to language breakdown. *Aphasiology, 3,* 111–142.

Bates, E., & Wulfeck, B. (1990). Crosslinguistic studies of aphasia. In B. MacWhinney and E. Bates (Eds.), *The crosslinguistic study of sentence processing.* New York: Cambridge University Press.

Baum, S. (1989). On-line sensitivity to local and long-distance syntactic dependencies in Broca's aphasia. *Brain and Language, 37,* 327–338.

Berndt, R. S., & Caramazza, A. (1980). A redefinition of the syndrome of Broca's aphasia: Implications for a neuropsychological model of language. *Applied Linguistics, 1,* 225–278.

Bloom, L., Lightbown, L. & Hood, L. (1975). Structure and variation in child language. *Monographs for The Society for Research in Child Development, 40* (Serial No. 160).

Broca, P. (1861). Remarques sur le siege de la faculte du langage articule, suivies d'une observation d'aphemie. *Bulletin et Memoires de la Société anatomique de Paris, 2,* 330–357.

Brown, J. W. (1977). *Mind, brain and consciousness.* New York: Academic.

Caplan, D., & Hildebrandt, N. (1988). *Disorders of syntactic comprehension.* Cambridge: MIT Press.

Caramazza, A. (1986). On drawing inferences about the structure of normal cognitive systems from the analysis of patterns of impaired performance: The case for single-patient studies. *Brain and Cognition, 5,* 41–66.

Caramazza, A., & Berndt, R. (1978). Semantic and syntactic processes in aphasia: A review of the literature. *Psychological Bulletin, 85,* 898–918.

Caramazza, A., & Zurif, E. (1976). Dissociation of algorithmic and heuristic processes in language comprehension: Evidence from aphasia. *Brain and Language, 3,* 572–582.

Chomsky, N. (1965). *Aspects of the theory of syntax.* Cambridge: MIT Press.

Chomsky, N. (1980). *Rules and representations.* New York: Columbia University Press.

Clark, H., & Clark, E. (1977). *Psychology and language: An introduction to psycholinguistics.* New York: Harcourt Brace Jovanovich.

Crain, S., & Fodor, J. (1987). Simplicity and generality of rules in language acquisition. In B. MacWhinney (Ed.), *Mechanisms of language acquisition* (35–62). Hillsdale, NJ: Erlbaum.

Dale, P., Bates, E., Reznick, S., & Morisset, C. (1989). The validity of a parent report instrument of child language at 20 months. *Journal of Child Language, 16,* 239–250.

Dennis, M., & Whitaker, H. (1976). Language acquisition following hemidecortication: Linguistic superiority of the left over the right hemisphere. *Brain and Language, 3,* 404–433.

Dore, J. (1974). A pragmatic description of early language development. *Journal of Psycholinguistic Research, 4,* 423–430.

Duffy, R., Duffy, J. & Pearson, K. (1975). Pantomime recognition in aphasics. *Journal of Speech and Hearing Research, 18,* 115–132.

Eggert, G. H. (Ed.) (1977). *Wernicke's works on aphasia: A sourcebook and review.* Paris: Mouton.

Ferguson, C. (1984). From babbling to speech. Invited address to the International Conference on Infant Studies, New York, April.

Fillmore, L. (1979). Individual differences in second language acquisition. In C. Fillmore, D. Kempler, and W. Wang (Eds.), *Individual differences in language ability and language behavior.* New York: Academic.

Fodor, J. A. (1983). *The modularity of mind.* Cambridge: MIT Press.

Fodor, J. A. (1985). Multiple book review of *The modularity of mind. Behavioral and Brain Sciences, 8,* 1–42.

Freud, S. (1891). *Zur auffassung der aphasie.* Wien: Deuticke.

Gainotti, G., & Lemmo, M. (1976). Comprehension of symbolic gestures in aphasia. *Brain and Language, 3,* 451–460.

Geschwind, N. (1965). Disconnection syndromes in animals and man. *Brain, 88,* 237–294.

Gleitman, L., Gleitman, H., & Shipley, E. (1972). The emergence of the child as grammarian. *Cognition, 1,* 137–164.

Goldstein, K. (1948). *Language and language disturbances: Aphasic symptom complexes and their significance for medicine and theory of language.* New York: Grune & Stratton.

Goodglass, H., & Kaplan, E. (1963). Disturbance of gesture and pantomime in aphasia. *Brain, 86,* 703–720.

Goodglass, H., & Menn, L. (1985). Is agrammatism a unitary phenomenon? In M. L. Kean (Ed.), *Agrammatism.* New York: Academic.

Grodzinsky, Y. (1986a). Language deficits and the theory of syntax. *Brain and Language, 27,* 135–159.

Grodzinsky, Y. (1986b). Cognitive deficits, their proper description, and its theoretical relevance. *Brain and Language, 27,* 178–191.

Grodzinsky, Y. (in press). Aphasic syndromes and theories of syntactic representation and processing. In H. Whitaker and A. Caramazza (Eds.), *Studies in neuropsychology.* Hillsdale, NJ: Erlbaum.

Head, H. (1926). *Aphasia and kindred disorders of speech.* Cambridge: Cambridge University Press.

Hecaen, H. (1976). Acquired aphasia in children and the ontogenesis of hemispheric functional specialization. *Brain and Language, 3,* 114–134.

Hecaen, H. (1983). Acquired aphasia in children: Revisited. *Neuropsychologia, 21,* 581–587.

Heilman, K. M., & Scholes, R. J. (1976). The nature of comprehension errors in Broca's, Conduction and Wernicke's aphasics. *Cortex, 12,* 258–265.

Horgan, D. (1981). Rate of language acquisition and noun emphasis. *Journal of Psycholinguistic Research, 10,* 629–640.

Jackson, H. J. (1931). *Selected writings of John Hughlings Jackson.* Ed. James Taylor. London: Hodder & Stoughton.

Kean, M. L. (1979). Agrammatism: A phonological deficit? *Cognition, 7,* 69–83.

Kempler, D. (1988). Lexical and pantomime abilities in Alzheimer's disease. *Aphasiology, 2,* 147–159.

Kolk, H., & Heeschen, C. (1985). Agrammatism versus paragrammatism: A shift of behavioral control. Paper presented at the Academy of Aphasia 23rd Annual Meeting, Pittsburgh, October.

Lapointe, S. (1985). A theory of verb form use in the speech of agrammatic aphasics. *Brain and Language, 24,* 100–155.

Lenneberg, E. (1967). *Biological foundations of language.* New York: Wiley & Sons.

Linebarger, M., Schwartz, M., & Saffran, E. (1983). Sensitivity to grammatical structure in so-called agrammatic aphasics. *Cognition, 13,* 361–392.

Luria, A. (1966). *Higher cortical functions in man.* New York: Basic Books.

Marchman, V., Miller, R., & Bates, E. (1989). Prespeech and babble in children with focal brain injury. *Project in Cognitive and Neural Development* (Tech. Report No. 89-01). La Jolla, CA: University of California, San Diego.

Marie, P. (1906). Revision de la question de l'aphasie: La troisieme convolution frontale gauche ne joue aucun role special dans la fonction du langage. *Semaine Medicale, 21,* 241–247. Reprinted in M. F. Cole & M. Cole (Eds.), [1971], *Pierre Marie's papers on speech disorder.* New York: Hafner.

Menn, L., & Obler, L. (in press). *Agrammatic aphasia: Cross-language narrative source book.* Amsterdam: John Benjamin.

Miceli, G., Silveri, M. C., Romani, C., & Caramazza, A. (1989). Variation in the pattern of omissions and substitutions of grammatical morphemes in the spontaneous speech of so-called agrammatic patients. *Brain and Language, 36,* 447–492.

Nelson, K. (1973). Structure and strategy in learning to talk. *Monograph of the Society for Research in Child Development, 38*(1&2, Serial No. 49).

Norman, D., & Shallice, T. (1980). Attention to action: Willed and automatic control of behavior. In R. Davidson, G. Schwartz, and D. Shapiro (Eds.), *Consciousness and self-regulation: Advances in research, vol. 4.* New York: Plenum.

Peters, A. (1977). Language learning strategies: Does the whole equal the sum of the parts? *Language, 53,* 560–573.

Peters, A. (1983). *The units of language acquisition.* Cambridge: Cambridge University Press.

Posner, M., & Snyder, C. (1975). Attention and cognitive control. In R. Solso (Ed.), *Information processing and cognition.* Hillsdale, NJ: Erlbaum.

Reznick, S., & Goldsmith, S. (1989). Assessing early language: A multiple form word production checklist. *Journal of Child Language, 16,* 91–100.

Riva, D., & Cazzaniga, L. (1986). Late effects of unilateral brain lesions before and after the first year of life. *Neuropsychologia, 24,* 423–428.

Riva, D., Cazzaniga, L., Pantaleoni, C., Milani, N., & Fedrizzi, E. (1986). *Journal of Pediatric Neurosciences, 2,* 239–250.

Rizzi, L. (1985). Two notes on the linguistic interpretation of Broca's Aphasia. In M. L. Kean (Ed.), *Agrammatism.* New York: Academic.

Shankweiler, D., Craine, S., Gorrell, P. , & Tuller, N. (1989). Reception of language in Broca's aphasia. *Language and Cognitive Processes, 4,* 1–33.

Shiffrin, R. M., & Schneider, W. (1977). Controlled and automatic human information processing: II. Perceptual learning, automatic attending, and a general theory. *Psychological Review, 84,* 127–190.

Smith, S., & Bates, E. (1987). Accessibility of case and gender contrasts for agent-object assignment in Broca's aphasics and fluent anomics. *Brain and Language, 30,* 8–32.

Swinney, D., Zurif, E., & Nicol, J. (in press). The effects of focal brain damage on sentence processing: An examination of the neurological organization of a mental module. *Journal of Cognitive Neuroscience.*

Talay, A., & Slobin, D. (1988). Grammatical impairment in Turkish. Symposium on Aphasia in Non–Indo-European Language, Academy of Aphasia, Montreal, October.

Thal, D., & Bates, E. (1988a). Language and gesture in late talkers. *Journal of Speech and Hearing Research, 31,* 115–123.

Thal, D., & Bates, E. (1988b). Relationships between language and cognition: Evidence from linguistically precocious children. Paper presented to the Annual Convention of the American Speech-Language-Hearing Association, Boston, November.

Thal, D., & Bates, E. (in press). Continuity and variation in early language development. In J. Colombo & J. Sagan (Eds.), *Individual differences in infancy: Reliability, stability, and prediction*. Hillsdale, NJ: Erlbaum.

Thal, D., Marchman, V., Stiles, J., Trauner, D., Nass, X., & Bates, E. (1989). Early language in children with focal brain injury. *Project in Cognitive and Neural Development* (Tech. Rep. No. 89-02). La Jolla, CA: University of California, San Diego.

Tyler, L. (1985). Real-time comprehension processes in agrammatism: A case study. *Brain and Language, 26,* 259–275.

Vargha-Khadem, F., O'Gorman, A., & Watters, G. (1985). Aphasia and handedness in relation to hemispheric side, age at injury and severity of cerebral lesion during childhood. *Brain, 108,* 677–696.

Vihman, M. (1981). Phonology and the development of the lexicon: Evidence from children's errors. *Journal of Child Language, 8,* 239–264.

Vihman, M., & Carpenter, K. (1984). *Linguistic advance and cognitive style in language acquisition*. Manuscript, Stanford University Department of Linguistics.

Von Stockert, T., & Bader, L. (1976). Some relations of grammar and lexicon in aphasia. *Cortex, 12,* 49–60.

Wernicke, C. (1874). Der aphasische Symptomenkomplex. Breslau: Cohn & Weigart. (Translated in *Boston Studies in Philosophy of Science, 4,* 34–97).

Woods, B., & Teuber, H. (1978). Changing patterns of childhood aphasia. *Annals of Neurology, 3,* 273–280.

Wulfeck, B. (1988). Grammaticality judgments and sentence comprehension in agrammatic aphasia. *Journal of Speech and Hearing Research, 31,* 72–81.

Zurif, E., & Caramazza, A. (1976). Psycholinguistic studies in aphasia: Studies in syntax and semantics. In H. Whitaker and H. A. Whitaker (Eds.), *Studies in neurolinguistics, vol. 1*. New York: Academic.

Zurif, E., Gardner, H., & Brownell, H. (in press). The case against the case against group studies. *Brain and Cognition.*

Zurif, E., & Grodzinsky, Y. (1983). Sensitivity to grammatical structure in agrammatic aphasics: A reply to Linebarge, Schwartz and Saffran. *Cognition, 15,* 207–221.

CHAPTER 8

Evidence from Syntax for Language Impairment

PAUL FLETCHER

INTRODUCTION

As reported at earlier symposia in this series, the group at Reading has been engaged recently in detailed studies of the syntax profiles of groups of normal English-speaking children from three to seven years of age. The purpose of this work (see, for example, Fletcher & Garman, 1988a, b; Fletcher, Garman, Johnson, Schelleter, & Stodel, 1986) in the beginning was to provide reference profiles against which the language of school-age language-impaired children could be measured and evaluated. The starting point for the study was syntax, or at least a particular description of it as instantiated in LARSP (Language Assessment Remediation and Screening Procedure; see Crystal, Fletcher & Garman, 1989), and the perspective was a normal developmental one. In his address to the AFASIC Congress in England in 1987, Jon Miller reminded the audience of the problems of this approach, in particular the tendency of studies of language impairment couched in terms of categories of normal development to ignore idiosyncratic features of the language-impaired (LI) data that may be important. In addition, Miller pointed out a tendency among researchers

This chapter is based on a paper presented at the 10th Annual Symposium on Research in Child Language Disorders, University of Wisconsin–Madison, June 1, 1989.

into specific language impairment (SLI) to assume that the language-impaired constitute a homogeneous group. He asked researchers to pay serious consideration, particularly among older language-impaired children to the identification of subgroups, defined by distinct language performance. This chapter represents an initial exploration of this task, using data from reference profiles and from a group of fifteen school-age SLI children who were included in this study. This chapter will examine some recurring features of the language-impaired data, and consider their implications for the interpretation of impairment within a dynamic model of language performance. The categories identified are then, in conjunction with some normal developmental categories, applied to the sample of SLI children to determine whether coherent subgroups emerge.

THE STUDY

There are aspects of three phases of the study that are relevant to the general task of this chapter. Those phases are data collection, transcription, and analysis, each to be dealt with in turn.

DATA COLLECTION

From a sample of 160 children at four different locations in England, data collection centered on the elicitation of a spontaneous speech sample from the child, in a conversation with a female adult previously unknown to the child, in a quiet area of the child's nursery or school. This setting and choice of interlocutor was a deliberate attempt to mimic the typical initial encounter between a speech therapist and a child who is being assessed. We were well aware of the type of bias built into this particular type of language sample. A comparison for example between interrogative frequencies in our children's data and those that appear in samples collected in the home in the Bristol survey (see Fletcher & Garman, 1988b, p. 315, compared to Wells, 1985, Table A17) shows considerable discrepancies, with a much lower incidence in our samples. Other sampling effects appear within the data, according to the elicitation procedure used. The elicitation procedure for the 45-minute conversations included a segment in which adult and child chatted around a game consisting of either a house interior or a farmyard, and an appropriate set of stickers to be located at suitable points on these pictures. In another segment there were no specific props, but the adult talked to the child about school and home experiences, and about significant past and future events in his or her life. It turns out, for example, that modal auxiliaries (as in "the clock *could* go here") are more frequent in the sticker game segment than in the more general conversation. On the other hand, the general conversation, steered as it was to topics which allow past and future reference, encouraged a higher frequency of temporal adverbials, specifying the tense choices that were made (e.g., *"on Friday I went to see Ghostbuster"*). Neither of these outcomes is particularly surprising, but researchers need to be alert to these and other potential sampling differences both in selecting stretches of transcript for analysis, and in selecting syntactic categories to apply to the data.

TRANSCRIPTION

The decisions required to implement transcription in a systematic fashion in a computer database is addressed in detail elsewhere (Johnson, 1986; Fletcher & Garman, 1988b). Conversations are transcribed orthographically, so far as is feasible, and include all false starts, repetitions and repairs. (This aspect of the data will be discussed below.) All child utterances are segmented into units for grammatical analysis. Two general points about this procedure can be made briefly. First, in our view it is not possible to rely on the prosodic system of English to identify units for grammatical analysis. For a replicable procedure we rely on the identification of clausal units in the data. The outcome of the clausally based segmentation is that each child utterance is divided into communication units consisting of *either* one main clause plus any subordinate clause or nonclausal structure attached to or embedded in it, *or* two linked main clauses meeting certain conditions on their linkage. Clearly any statement made about the frequency of occurrence of syntactic or other categories in the data is relative to the definition of analytical units, which must affect comparability with other studies.

ANALYSIS

The *analysis* initially effected on this data reflected our experience with LARSP and involved the application of an extensive set of clause, phrase, and inflectional categories to the data to derive frequency-based reference profiles for each of the age groups we were interested in. An example of this, for clause types in the free conversation of five-year-olds, appears as Figure 8.1. While it is certainly an advance to have soundly based quantitative profiles, LARSP presents certain problems for the identification of indices of normal development, and for characterizing differences between normal and SLI children. First, the sheer size of the profile—over two hundred separate categories—obscures developmental trends. Second, as the profile was initially designed for a preschool-age group, its application to a database from children up to 7 years of age may miss developmental change between 5 and 7 because the relevant categories are not included. And finally, in restricting the categories of comparison to only those found useful in characterizing normal development, significant features of the

		Minor	Responses		Vocatives	Other	Problems	Word
		Major	Comm. V'	Quest. 'Q'	Statement 'V' (Clause) / 'N'	Other (Phrase)	Problems (Phrase)	Word
Stage I (0:9–1:6)								
Stage II (1:6–2:0)	Conn.		VA	2.27 QA	SV 3.25 / SO / SC / Neg X — AX 1.38 / VO 1.13 / VC / Other	DN / Adj N / NN / PrN	VV / V part / Int X / Other	-ing / pl
Stage III (2:0–2:6)		X + S:NP · X + V:VP · X + C:NP · X + O:NP · X + A:AP	VXY / let XY / do XY	QXY 0.25 / VS(X) 1.38	SVC 4.25 / SVO 8.88 / SVA 4.63 / Neg XY — VCA / VOA 0.25 / VO O / Other	D Adj N / Adj Adj N / PrDN / $Pron^P_O$	Cop / Aux^M_O / Other	-ed / -en / 3s
Stage IV (2:6–3:0)		XY + S:NP · XY + V:VP · XY + C:NP · XY + O:NP · XY + A:AP	+S / NXY+	QVS 0.25 / QXY+ 0.13 / N S(X+) 0.13 / tag 0.13	SVOA 3.5 / SVCA 0.63 / SVO O / SVOC 0.13 — AAXY 1.75 / Other 0.88	NP Pr NP / Pr D Adj N / cX / XcX	Neg V / Neg X / 2 Aux / Other	gen
								n't / .cop / .aux
Stage V (3:0–3:6)	and	Coord.	Coord.	Coord.	Coord. — 1 0.75 1 + 0.13	Postmod. clause 1 / 0.38	1 + / 1 0.38	-est
	c	Other	Other	Other 0.13	Subord. A S 0.25 C — 1 1.13 1 +	Postmod. phrase 1 +		-er
	s		0.13		0.25 O 2.13			-ly
	Other				Comparative			

Fig 8-1. Partial LARSP profile (clauses only) for 5-year-olds (n = 8; mean frequencies per 40 analysable units). From "Larsping In Numbers" by P. Fletcher and M. Garman, 1988. Reprinted with perission by BJDC (British Journal of Disorder of Communication).

data from SLI children may be missed (cf. Miller, 1987, p. 102). It was in an attempt to meet this objection that we came to a reappraisal of our framework for analysis and interpretation.

FROM PRODUCT TO PROCESS

As a corrective to the potential normal developmental bias of the LARSP analysis framework, a small sample of school-age SLI children was included in the database. These subjects were from residential schools for the language-impaired and from language units in England and Scotland. The fifteen children in the sample ranged in age from 6 ; 2 to 9 ; 11 years; four of them were girls. On a number of different syntactic measures, it proved difficult to distinguish these children from the normal five-year-olds in terms of their expressive language. This in itself is nonnormal, considering the ages of the SLI children. But this is an unsatisfying conclusion—indeed, it seems only to be a starting point (see, again, Miller, 1987). Are there features of the language-impaired data that are being missed, when our perspective is limited to what is sufficient for an account of normal development? Perusal of the SLI data threw up three areas not covered by the normal categories: mazes, formulation problems, and grammatical errors.*

MAZES

This term has become to be used for the false starts, repetitions, and repairs that are to be found in spontaneous speech, and which have long been noted in SLI children (Miller, 1987). Some examples of these from our transcripts appear in Table 8-1. What would be the implications of including these features of the data in the analysis? Self-repairs occur in adult spontaneous speech and are part of what Garrett (1982) has referred to as "the naturally displayed evidence of the language production system." A systematic approach to mazes would involve a serious attempt to identify their place in such a system, which in turn of course means considering at least in outline what the lineaments of such a system are, and then reviewing the place within the system of the other analysis categories.

In a study of the spontaneous self-repairs made by normal adult speakers who had been asked to describe certain visual patterns, Levelt (1983) outlines two functions that the monitor, the final component of a language production mechanism, fulfills: it checks whether what was said corre-

---

*This is not to say of course that these features do not appear in the normal data, only that our identification of them as of interest comes from an examination of the SLI data.

Table 8-1. Mazes in the SLI sample

DAV	(but there) it's something strange
DAM	(do some) does some cows eat hay
JUL	(and the children are out on the) the children are on the roof
PET	why don't you (put) give us some hard ones
SEA	(but I gid) but I did get something
LLO	because (they get) I get scared
SHE	(this bed) this one have to go in there
AMY	(because it) when we press it hard it not work
ZAR	and we can put (it) the chair here
CHR	and (our cousin) our two cousins live in America
DAI	and then there's (stripes or) dark blue stripes over that
CHH	that's (a, you know, a, [[another[[) an oven
LEE	(I think she) I think he's smoking
AND	that's (why) why I don't throw snowballs
ALI	(but I've) I've got windows

sponds to what was intended, and it assesses standards of production. The message check leads to the speaker changing the message in midstream, or in response to the realization that the message may be ambiguous in context, to lexical change or to syntactic plus lexical change. The check on standards of production may lead to the correction of phonological error, or to some purely syntactic reorganization. Mazes are then seen, in adult corpora, to be of various types, and to reflect the speaker's on-line monitoring of a production process with different levels. Exactly what these levels might be will be discussed below. For the moment, after recognizing the existence and potential bases of mazes, the discussion will look more closely at their nature and distribution in the SLI data, and make comparisons with the normals*:

1. The group means for frequency of occurrence of mazes do not show a significant difference as between the normal (LN) and impaired (LI) children. Means, standard deviations, and ranges for this and other analysis categories are reported in Table 8-2. It will be noted that the standard deviation for the LN group is large. This is mainly the effect of one outlier, whose maze proportion of .28 was more than twice the value of anyone else in the group (and considerably higher than the top end of the LI range).

---

*As indicated above, on a number of syntactic measures reported elsewhere, the group of SLI children was not distinct from a group of 5-year-old normal children. The normal-SLI comparisons in this chapter therefore involve a group of 5-year-olds (n = 12). Normals are referred to as LN, and impaired individuals as LI.

2. The structure of a repair can be considered, following Levelt (1983), to involve an original utterance (OU), which contains the trouble spot or *reparandum*; this is then followed, either immediately or after a delay or a span of retracing, by the repair. Figure 8-2 provides schematic examples, for two of the utterances from Table 8-1. While the incidence of repairs may not differ between LI and LN, there do seem to be qualitative differences:

a. Both groups are more inclined to make repairs at the beginnings of utterances, but the LI group are more likely to provide repetitions in initial position than reformulations;
b. The delay and retracing phases of the repair are on average longer for the LI group;
c. The LN groups reparanda are equally split between single lexical items and longer constituents, whereas the LI group repair a higher proportion of constituents of phrase length or longer. Among the latter are a group of repairs which result in the more precise specification of NPs (see the examples in Table 8-1 from ZAR, CHR, DAI).
d. Like the LN group, the LI group show considerable variability in their use of mazes, as a glance at the ranges in Table 8-2 will show. Levelt remarks in relation to his normal adult data that many mistakes—in his data roughly half—are never repaired (Levelt, 1983, p. 54). The LI group as a whole lets many more mistakes than this past, but there is a great deal of individual variability.

Fig. 8-2. The structure of repair.

```
                      OU                        R
1.        ---------------------   -----------------
          because    they    get    I    get    scared
                     ----    ---    -
                     Rm      D      A


                  OU                          R
          ------------   --------------------------------
2.        but    I    gid    but    I    did    get    something
                     ---    -------    ---
                     Rm      S         A

OU        original utterance
R         repair
Rm        reparandum (trouble spot)
D         delay
A         alteration
S         span of retracing
```

Source: Adapted from Levelt, 1983

Table 8-2. Means, standard deviations, and ranges for analysis categories

		LN	LI
Maze[a]	Mean	0.09	0.09
	Sd	0.07	0.05
	Range	0.01–0.28	0.03–0.19
Formulation[a]	Mean	0.03	0.13
	Sd	0.02	0.06
	Range	0.00–0.06	0.06–0.28
Complex[b]	Mean	5.5	5.6
	Sd	2.94	3.42
	Range	1–10	1–10
Phrase structure[c]	Mean	0.29	0.24
	Sd	0.09	0.08
	Range	0.13–0.43	0.08–0.39
Verb expansion[c]	Mean	0.41	0.30
	Sd	0.13	0.11
	Range	0.17–0.61	0.18–0.56
Grammatical error[a]	Mean	0.01	0.10
	Sd	0.01	0.09
	Range	0.00–0.03	0.03–0.36

[a]Proportion per 100 A-units
[b]Frequency per 40 A-units
[c]Proportion per 40 A-units

What can be concluded from this brief review of maze behavior? First, that a lot more detailed data analysis needs to be done before any firm conclusions are drawn about similarities or differences between the LN and LI groups. This in itself would constitute a minor research project. But there is enough here to at least hypothesize that LI children are actively monitoring their own speech. They are able to detect mismatches with their original message in terms of inappropriate lexical choice. They can identify syntactic problems, recognize lack of specificity and modify, and detect phonological error. They may, however, be less able to detect problems than their normal (syntactic) peers, and they may take a little longer to effect a repair when they have noticed it.

Acknowledging, via maze analysis, the existence of a monitor seems to commit us, at the very least, to a production system with a message construction level, and a formulating level that draws on the messages constructed and generates phonetic strings. This view of language production as proceeding from "conceptual intention to utterance" led to an insightful case study of a school-age language-impaired child by Chiat and Hirson (1987; see also Fletcher, 1987). They were able to attribute a major part of the child's expressive problems, bewilderingly heterogeneous if assessed syntactically, to phonological difficulties at the very end of the production process. They place responsibility for the child's output problems on "phonological constraints, which limit the processing of detail within a rhythmic structure." A dynamic view of language production, with a series of levels or components delineated on the route to the phonetic string, affords the prospect of a typology of disorders related to the production process. This is in line with some recent work in aphasia (see Lesser, 1987), and in accord with the spirit of the research paradigm for normal language development espoused by Chapman (1988). But are there other features of the LI data, in addition to mazes, which further support the dynamic view of the language production process?

FORMULATION PROBLEMS

This category represents, in the first instance, a recognition by the analyst that something, as yet unspecified, has gone wrong in the formulation of the utterance, somewhere between message ("conceptual intention") and the phonetic string. What makes them different, at least at first sight, from the maze category, is that no attempt is discernible on the speaker's part to repair the problem or problems. The problem with the utterance is intuitively more serious than the omission of a grammatical element such as a determiner, an auxiliary, or an inflection. Formulation problems are almost exclusively the province of the LI group; they do not appear to be a significant feature of the language output of normal five-year-olds. (Table 8.2 reveals that the distributions of scores on this category are quite distinct for LI and LN groups. The range for the LN group is 0.00–0.06, while that for the LI group is 0.06–0.28). Within the LI group, however, there is considerable variability in the incidence of formulation problems. For the moment, the author will consider the LI group as a whole, what major types of formulation problem emerge, and if it is possible to relate them to a language production model. In sketching out some features of the production model elaborated by Garrett (e.g., 1988), and favored by Levelt (1983), we do not intend to claim that it is uncontroversial (see e.g., Stemberger, 1985). But at the rather crude level of linkage of this discussion, the Garrett model will serve as a useful exemplar.

The Garrett model posits two serially ordered syntactic processors, the first referred to as "functional," at which the semantic properties and syntactic relations of the lexical items corresponding to the main features of the message are specified. The subsequent, positional level processor assigns ordered syntactic structures and segmental and prosodic structures for lexical items. The reasoning for the specific organization assigned to this production model depends on the nature of speech errors from corpora of adult speech. It would be interesting if rather different data from the LI children could be located within the model also. There are three distinct types of error that occur in the LI corpus that may be argued to be related to the model (the three types, with a set of examples for each, appear in Table 8-3).

1. *Syntactic relations.* This type of error suggests a difficulty in the initial specification of syntactic relations between the abstract lexical items in clause constituents—in Garrett's terms, at the *functional* level. So for example in 1a, "my mum was take me a picture," "me" appears to have been assigned the inappropriate thematic role of benefactive, instead of being the complement *within* the object NP of "a picture." A benefactive NP with "take" can appear either before the object NP, or after it with a preposition—cf., "Molly took George breakfast/Molly took breakfast to George." In the LI child's example, the error can plausibly be assigned to the wrong thematic role application. In example 1b, "Scotland don't," the

Table 8-3. Some examples of formulation errors

1. SYNTACTIC RELATIONS
    a. my mum was take me a picture
    b. Scotland don't
    c. one is in the fishfinger
    d. one is in the tomato
    e. here they got eyes to me
    f. he puts webs
    g. we went in Weymouth seaside

2. BLENDS
    a. where shall we put it here
    b. are there any tables are here
    c. that's how long
    d. that's how big
    e. to see if I need any trouble with my speaking
    f. what's that is
    g. and one's gone off too

3. LEXICAL SELECTION
    a. he give the milk out
    b. we went up in the mountains and saw some of the donkeys
    c. she's sitting on a table getting some milk
    d. that is in the telly
    e. and cook over there
    f. do writing a picture
    g. for the wind to go round

child is trying to tell his interlocutor, whose claim is that settees (chesterfields/couches) always have pillows (cushions) on them, that such isn't the case in Scotland. On a reasonable interpretation of the likely message, "Scotland" should be a locative adverbial, with an agent role specified and eventually surfacing as the subject of "don't." One reason for the sentence that is produced would be the absence of any agent role at F-level. In its absence, the only candidate for sentence subject at positional level is "Scotland." Example 1c, "one is in the fishfinger," comes from a child trying to describe a picture in which there are plates with food of various types. "Fishfinger" is inappropriately located as a head noun within a PP specifying location, when it is the item to be located.

2. *Blends.* Unlike the syntactic relation errors which (so far as I am aware) are not attested in the adult speech error corpora, adults do make mistakes similar to those listed under the second subheading in Table 8-3. Most of these examples seem to represent competition between different syntactic frames for the same message. Thus 2a, "where shall we put it here" shows elements of both "where shall we put it" and "shall we put it here; that's how long" (example 2c) seems to reflect both "that's how long it is" and "it's that long." Other examples perhaps show the effects of two competing messages: 2e, "to see if I need any trouble with my speaking," mixes "if I need any help" and "if I have any trouble."

3. *Lexical selection.* Lexical choice errors on the part of the LI children are category-specific and usually semantically related to the item they are presumed to be in place of. So in 3c, "she's sitting on a table getting some milk," "table" is selected instead of "chair." In 2f, "writing" is accessed instead of either "painting" or "drawing a picture." In some examples the inappropriacy of the lexical choice is only apparent in context. In 3b the child is talking about a visit made to the New Forest, a wooded area of southern England that is not particularly hilly (so why "mountains"?) and where there is a famous breed of ponies (hence "donkeys"). Lexical selection errors, in terms of the production model, arise at the positional level when specific word forms are being retrieved for the abstract lexemes represented at F-level. The errors seen in the output of the LI children are similar to those attested in normal adult output (though in the LI data they are presumably more frequent).

GRAMMATICAL ERROR

The final category identified in the LI data identifies omissions of determiners, auxiliaries, and copula verbs, as well as agreement errors, overgeneralized inflections or the omission of morphological endings. On a few occasions the omission of a lexical verb was counted as a grammatical error. The figures in Table 8-2 reveal that grammatical error is another category like formulation, on which the LI and LN children seem to represent distinct populations, with means of .01 and .10 respectively, and ranges that are .00–.03 for the LN, and .03–.36 for the LI group. (It should however be pointed out that 13 of the 15 individuals in the LI group have error proportions of .13 or less, with the other two to some extent outliers at .26 and .36). The figures for error exclude omissions of subjects, and of subjects plus auxiliaries. Missing subjects were initially identified (as in "went to the pictures") as errors, but an examination of data across the age range, and of some normal adult data, revealed that the ellipsis of subjects (and on some occasions of subjects plus auxiliaries) was normal practice in certain linguistic contexts, and the LI group behaved no differently to the other groups in this respect.

The features of the LI data included under the heading of Grammatical Error seem very similar to those with which everyone is familiar from the acquisition literature for English, though they would be expected only in much younger children. In trying to explain why a set of elements as grammatically disparate as determiners, auxiliaries, and various inflectional endings should be vulnerable to omission by members of the LI group, one can perhaps, like Chiat and Hirson (1987), rely on the final stage of the production process. For an admittedly much wider range of errors than those identified under this heading, they point to phonological mapping as the source of their subject's problems. For the set of unstressed syllables and brief phonetic elements that realize the majority of the categories of omission under the Error heading, the problem can perhaps be located more plausibly at the final stage of the route from message to articulatory event.

If the interpretation of the three salient categories of the LI data described here is even partially correct, they must be included in any characterization of language impairment attempted. In what has been said so far, syntax, as it is normally construed, has had little part. And yet mazes, formulation problems, and errors all seem to reflect, albeit in different ways, difficulties with the deployment of a syntactic repertoire in real-time speech production. To fill out this process-oriented view of the LI children's language production ability, categories are required that will gauge attainment levels in key syntactic areas.

SYNTACTIC CATEGORIES

The major aim of this chapter is to begin to address the issue of a linguistic typology of LI children. Since there is a small sample, and three process-related categories needed for subtyping are already identified, it was possible to select only a small number of syntactic areas in the analysis. These are listed in Table 8-2 as Complex, Phrase Structure, and Verb Expansion.*

*All the examples that appear in the following sections to illustrate the syntactic categories are taken from transcripts of the LI group.

Complex

It is generally agreed that one of the major dimensions of grammatical development from four years on is in the area of complex sentence construction (see, e.g., Bowerman, 1979). This category covers a rather disparate set of constructions: verb complements ("I think the house going to be there"); subordination, with various kinds of semantic links between clauses ("when we press it hard it not work, I had to put the light on because she kept asking me"); postmodifying (relative) clauses ("the meals what I don't like"); and certain types of coordination ("I got a sister but she's a nuisance"). Means, standard deviations and ranges are similar for LN and LI groups in this category.

Phrase Structure

Children with a language age of five years or so have mastered the main features of the internal structure of phrases (though LI children may still have some problems with verb phrases—see below). So any measure of this facet of their syntactic ability that relied on frequency of, for example, noun phrases would almost certainly fail to discriminate among children. The measure adopted here to assess phrase structure ability is the proportion of simple clauses in the sample which have more than one phrasal expansion. Some examples ("expanded" phrases underlined):

why is <u>your house</u> <u>a mess</u>
<u>some people</u> <u>have put</u> them on
it's a <u>little girl</u> <u>with her mummy</u>
dad saw <u>a tractor</u> <u>in Wallingford</u>
I <u>can't do</u> it <u>really well</u>

There may well be better ways of measuring the internal complexity of simple clauses. This one has the merit of being easy to apply and seems to reflect in a straightforward way the informational content the child is able to deploy, in his part of a conversational interaction, with his available syntactic resources.

Verb Expansion

This measure, of verb premodification (by auxiliary or catenative verbs), was included because it has regularly been identified as an area of difficulty for language-impaired children by researchers (see, e.g., Fletcher & Peters, 1984; Leonard, Sabbadini, Leonard & Volterra, 1987). The means for this category are significantly different between the two groups, though the ranges overlap considerably.

TOWARD A TYPOLOGY OF
SPECIFIC LANGUAGE IMPAIRMENT

The literature on the typology is extensive (see, e.g., Aram & Nation, 1975; Crystal, 1986; Wilson & Risucci, 1986; Wolfus, Moscovitch, & Kinsbourne, 1980; Wren, 1980). The majority of studies, however, have either relied on standardized (speech and) language tests or used a mixture of these tests and psychological measures. Those that do apply detailed syntactic measures (Crystal, 1986; Wren, 1980) use multivariate techniques on quite small numbers of subjects (around 30), measured on a large number of variables (the LARSP set for Wren, and the LARSP set plus semantic and nonfluency variables for Crystal). We are in agreement with the general approach followed by Wren and Crystal, believing that if a language-impaired population exists as "a relatively discrete class of neurologically based disorders" (Wilson & Risucci, 1986, p. 289), it should be possible to define them in terms of their *language* behavior. However we concur with Wilson and Risucci in preferring a hypothesis-testing approach to classification systems rather than the shotgun method. In adopting a specific process-oriented approach to the characterization of the expressive language of a group of LI children, through the categories selected, the theoretical framework of a production model, within which various possibilities exist for behavioral subgroupings, becomes possible. The validation of a typology arising out of this theoretical framework will depend in part on its success at classifying a majority of the subjects (internal validation), and in part on its "predictive, descriptive and clinical validity" (external validation, p. 289). A prime goal of subgrouping would be to identify children with different types of problems so that remediation could be targeted more effectively. The success of a classification will depend in part on its fit with clinicians' inferential diagnoses, and the extent to which remediation based on it turns out to be effective.

On the dimensions outlined, what subgroups of this small group of children emerge? As the categories turn out to be relatively independent of one another (there is not a single significant inter-correlation for the six categories), the performance of each child on each of them was examined; the standard deviation for each category was used to designate a child as either –, indicating a score at or below –1SD; or +, indicating a score at or around the mean; or ++, indicating a score at or around +1SD. Patterns of these symbols are then used to subgroup the children. Table 8-4 shows the patterns, suggested subgroups, and other information about the children. The table is organized in columns as follows (where relevant, an abbreviation in parentheses, as used in the table, follows the description for a particular column below):

Table 8-4. Identifiable sub-classes in the LI group

N	Age	Sex	Com-prenension	Maze	Formu-lation	Complex	Phrase Structure	Verb Expansion	Error
1. JUL	9;1	M	-32	-	-	+	++	++	-
2. PET	7;9	M	-26	-	-	+	+	++	-
3. LEE	8;7	M	-26	+	++	-	-	-	+
4. LLO	7;6	M	-32	+	++	-	-	-	+
5. CHR	8;7	M	+4	++R	+	++	++	+	-
6. CHH	7;11	M	NK	+R	+	++	+	+	-
7. DAVI	7;7	M	NK	+R	+	+	++	+	-
8. DAM	7;0	M	-12	++R	+	-	+	+	-
9. ALI	6;2	M	NK	+	+	-	++	+	-
10. SHE	7;10	F	-24	-	-	-	+	+	++
11. AMY	7;3	F	-1	-	-	++	+	-	++
12. SEA	9;11	M	-24	++R	+	++	+	-	-
13. ZAR	8;3	F	-15	++	++	+	+	+	++
14. DAV	8;1	F	-33	-	++	+	+	-	-
15. AND	9;8	M	-36	-	+	+	+	+	+

Sample number for child

Child's I.D.

Child's sex

Child's age in year and months at the time of recording

Child's Comprehension: deficit in months at or near to time of recording, on either Reynell Developmental Language Scales (Receptive) or Test for Reception of Grammar; NK indicates no available score (COMP).

Maze: a minus here represents a very low maze score; a plus represents a score at about the average for the group; ++ indicates a high maze score; (R) following the symbol indicates that the child had a preponderance of repairs that were reformulations rather than repetitions (MAZE).

Formulation: a minus here represents a very low proportion of formulation problems; a plus reflects a score at about the mean for the group; ++ indicates that this individual has a high number of formulation problems (FORM).

Complex, Phrase Structure, Verb Expansion: the next three columns classify children on their syntactic repertoire scores. In all cases, a minus represents a low score, plus a score at or about the mean for the group, and ++ a very high score, relative to the mean for the group (PLEX, PS, VE).

Grammatical Error: in the final column of Table 8-4, a minus represents very little grammatical error, a plus, an average number of errors, and ++ a high incidence (ERR).

SUBGROUPS

Four groups, covering nine out of the fifteen individuals in the LI sample, emerge clearly out of the procedure illustrated in Table 8-4. The features of these groups will be considered in turn:

Group A

This group consists of two children, JUL and PET, who have low levels of mazes, formulation problems, and grammatical error, and average or good syntax. Whatever their language problems are, they do not appear to be in the syntactic repertoire or its deployment, either at higher levels of the production process or in phonological mapping. It may be that, relative to their language age, their expressive syntactic system is functioning as well as can be expected, and perhaps comprehension (which clearly shows a deficit relative to chronological age) needs to be the focus of remediation.

Group B

Here again we find two children, LEE and LLO, who coincidentally show the same comprehension deficits (in absolute terms) as JUL and PET, but whose expressive pattern is quite different—in fact the inverse, point for point, of the previous pattern. Here serious formulation problems can be seen, as well as a restricted syntactic repertoire across the three areas being measured, and (if the interpretation of the significance of grammatical error is correct) phonological mapping problems.

Group C

The next subset has three members, CHR, CHH, and DAVI. The most salient discriminating characteristic of this trio is their high-level deployment problem as evidenced by formulation errors and a high or very high level of mazes, among which there is a majority of reformulating mazes—repairs in which a change in lexis or structure is made, rather than a stretch of utterance simply being repeated. The syntactic repertoire of these three is at or well above average for all three syntactic categories, and there is very little grammatical error.

Group D

This subgroup of two, DAM and ALI, is similar in a number of respects to the previous group; the only obvious difference is that there is a complex sentence "deficit" in C2. Otherwise availability of syntactic structure, formulation problems, and low grammatical error all match quite well.

At this point in Table 8-4, all those individuals who share complete profiles across the categories have been classified into one subgroup or another. The results so far are quite encouraging, in that 60% of the subjects have been grouped, and the characteristics of the groups can be interpreted in terms of the model from which the analysis categories derive. How do the remaining six subjects fare?

Group E

It might be possible to argue for one further group, consisting of SHE and AMY. They show differences in their syntactic abilities, with SHE low on complex sentences, and AMY on verb expansion, but their production process profiles are similar, with limited high-level problems, but serious grammatical error difficulties.

Some of the remaining four subjects can be seen to resemble already established groups in their profiles. SEA, for example, only differs from the members of Group C in his low verb expansion score. ZAR appears to have the high-level deployment problems of Group C and a high grammatical error score, suggesting difficulties at all stages of the production process. This very fact, however, suggests that she may be the only representative here of a distinct group. The last two subjects, DAV and ANDR, can neither be readily assimilated or compared to existing groups, nor present alternative easily interpretable patterns.

ENVOI

This chapter, of course, raises many more questions than it answers. We require a finer-grained analysis of errors, and More thought needs to be given to the relationship between output errors and the levels of the production model, and no doubt to the production model itself. The categories chosen to estimate level of syntactic ability may need rethinking. The problem of analysis is a multivariate one, and requires a suitable statistical design, to replace the reliance on descriptive statistics as the basis for Table 8.4. And we need much more sophisticated ways of approaching comprehension ability, to relate it to the expressive problems described here. The author remains convinced that a "serious and careful appraisal of a quantity of faithfully transcribed speech is . . . the best source of information about a language-impaired child" (Fletcher, 1987, p. 71). But a dynamic perspective is needed on the child's speech production as a reminder that the output transcribed is the product of a complex of interacting subsystems operating in real time. The data presented here is part of an argument about evidence for language impairment, not so much from syntax, but from syntax deployed in the language-production process.

Acknowledgments
Research reported here was supported by MRC grant 68306114N, and NATO Collaborative Research Grant RG84/0135 (with Jon Miller and Robin Chapman).

Our thanks and appreciation are due to the staff and pupils of the following centers who contributed to the project: John Horniman School, Dawn House School, Rosehill School and the Children's Unit, Astley Ainslie Hospital.

I am grateful to my colleagues Susan Edwards and Michael Garman for their comments on an earlier version of this paper.

REFERENCES

Aram, D., & Nation, J. (1975). Patterns of language behavior in children with developmental language disorders. *Journal of Speech and Hearing Research, 18,* 229–241.

Bowerman, M. (1979). The acquisition of complex sentences. In P. Fletcher and M. Garman (Eds.), *Language acquisition: Studies in first language development* (pp. 285–305). Cambridge: Cambridge University Press.

Chapman, R. (1988). Child talk. Unpublished manuscript, University of Wisconsin–Madison.

Chiat, S., & Hirson, A. (1987). From conceptual intention to utterance: A study of impaired language output in a child with developmental dysphasia. *British Journal of Disorders of Communication, 22,* 37–64.

Crystal, D. (1986). The diagnosis of language disorders in children. Final Report on MRC Grant No. G 8306096 NA.

Crystal, D., Fletcher, P., & Garman, M. (1989). *The grammatical analysis of language disability: A procedure for assessment and remediation,* 2d ed. London: Cole and Whurr.

Fletcher, P. (1987). The basis of language impairment in children: A comment on Chiat and Hirson. *British Journal of Disorders of Communication, 22,* 65–72.

Fletcher, P., & Garman, M. (1988a). Normal language development and language impairment: Syntax and beyond. *Clinical Linguistics and Phonetics, 2,* 97–113.

Fletcher, P., & Garman, M. (1988b). LARSPing by numbers. *British Journal of Disorders of Communication, 23,* 309–321.

Fletcher, P., & Peters, J. (1984). Characterising language impairment in children: An exploratory study. *Language Testing, 1,* 33–49.

Fletcher, P., Garman, M., Johnson, M., Schelleter, C., & Stodel, J. (1986). Characterising language impairment in terms of normal language development: advantages and limitations. *Proceedings from the Seventh Wisconsin Symposium on Research in Child Language Disorders.* Madison: University of Wisconsin–Madison.

Garrett, M. (1982). Production of speech: Observations from normal and pathological language use. In A. W. Ellis (Ed.), *Normality and pathology in cognitive functions.* New York: Academic.

Garrett, M. (1988). Processes in language production. In F. Newmeyer (Ed.), *Linguistics: The Cambridge survey, vol. III* (pp. 69–96). Cambridge: Cambridge University Press.

Johnson, M. (1986). A computer-based approach to the analysis of child language. Unpublished Ph.D. thesis, University of Reading.

Leonard, L., Sabbadini, L., Leonard, J., & Volterra, V. (1987). Specific language impairment in children: A cross-linguistic study. *Brain and Language, 32,* 233–252.

Lesser, R. (1987). Cognitive neuropsychological influences on aphasia therapy. *Aphasiology, 1,* 189–200.

Levelt, W. (1983). Monitoring and self-repair in speech. *Cognition, 14,* 41–104.

Miller, J. (1987). A grammatical characterisation of language disorder. *Proceedings of the First International Symposium on Specific Speech and Language Disorders in Children* (pp. 100–113). London: AFASIC.

Stemberger, J. (1985). An interactive activation model of language production. In A. W. Ellis (Ed.), *Progress in the psychology of language, vol. I* (pp. 143–186). Hillsdale, NJ: Erlbaum.

Wells, G. (1985). *Language development in the pre-school years.* Cambridge: Cambridge University Press.

Wilson, B., & Risucci, D. (1986). A model for clinical-quantitative classification. Generation I: Application to language-disordered preschool children. *Brain and Language, 27,* 281–309.

Wolfus, B., Moscovitch, M., & Kinsbourne, M. (1980). Subgroups of developmental language impairment. *Brain and Language, 10,* 152–171.

Wren, C. (1980). Identifying patterns of language disorder. *Proceedings from the First Wisconsin Symposium on Research in Child Language Disorders* (pp. 113–124). Madison: University of Wisconsin–Madison.

CHAPTER 9

On the Nature of the Impairment in Language-Impaired Children

SUSAN CURTISS AND PAULA TALLAL

The most obvious "impairment" in language-impaired (LI) children is their "impairment" in language acquisition. They talk later than normal. Their acquisition rate is slower than normal. But what is actually wrong with them, that is, what is the nature of the impairment? As research on this population has progressed, LI children have been found not only to demonstrate language-learning difficulties, but also to have a number of nonlinguistic impairments, including deficits in specific aspects of information processing, cognition, and memory. How are these nonlinguistic deficits related to the language-acquisition problems of LI children? Are the nonlinguistic deficits the primary disabilities, which are then reflected in difficulties with language acquisition, or are the difficulties with language acquisition primary impairments, which are distinct from other, nonlinguistic deficits? This chapter will report on some of the answers to these questions that are emerging from a large-scale longitudinal study, "Evaluating the Outcomes of Children with Preschool Language Impairments."*

*The research reported herein was supported by NIH contract #NIH NO1 NS92322.

This chapter is divided into three parts. The first is concerned with the relationship between nonlinguistic processing abilities and linguistic performance. This section will report on two findings from the study; the first concerns the relationship between nonlinguistic sequencing and handling crucially sequenced information in linguistic structures; the second reports on the effects of syntactic redundancy on linguistic processing. The second section deals with the question of deviance versus delay in the acquisition of linguistic form. The third section attempts to integrate these different sets of findings into a coherent picture.

The subject populations upon whom this study is based and the methods used to test them are outlined below.

SUBJECTS AND PROCEDURES

SUBJECTS

The subjects fell into three major groups: (1) 67 children diagnosed as having a preschool language impairment, (2) 57 normally developing, age-matched peers, and (3) 32 normally developing language-matched peers. All three groups of children were participating in a large-scale longitudinal study of the linguistic, cognitive, neuroperceptual, academic, and social/emotional outcomes of children with preschool language impairments at 4 years of age (see Tallal, Curtiss & Kaplan, 1988; & Ziegler, Curtiss & Tallal, 1989, for further details of the study and study population).

The language-impaired subjects met the following criteria:

1. A nonverbal performance IQ of 85 or better on the Leiter International Performance Scale;
2. A mean "language age" (computed by averaging together expressive and receptive standardized test scores) at least one year below both performance mental age (MA) and chronological age (CA). The following standardized expressive and receptive language tests were used: the Sequenced Inventory of Communicative Development (SICD) (Hedrick, Prather, & Tobin, 1979); the Token Test (DiSimoni, 1978); the Northwest Syntax Screening Test (Lee, 1971); the Carrow Elicited Language Inventory (CELI) (Carrow, 1974); and the Arizona Articulation Proficiency Scale (AAPS) (Fudala, 1980);
3. Normal hearing acuity, no motor handicaps, and no oral structural or motor impairments affecting nonspeech movements of the articulators;
4. An Anglo language background without significant dialectal or language differences from Standard American English in the home environment;

5. Demonstrated language skills to or greater than those expected at one year of age in normal development;
6. No obvious signs of infantile autism or emotional difficulties.

The age-matched controls were matched to the LI children as a group on the basis of IQ, chronological age, socioeconomic, geographic, and schooling characteristics. They had to meet all of the criteria used to select the LI children regarding perceptual, motor, and neurological integrity, and home linguistic environment. They met the following additional criteria:

1. A mean language age not more than six months below performance MA or CA;
2. A speech articulation age not more than six months below CA;
3. No emotional or neurological problems.

The language-age matched controls were matched to the LI children on the basis of standardized language test scores, IQ, and SES. These children all performed within normal limits for their CA on standardized tests of cognitive and language development, and met all of the same criteria as the age-matched normals regarding emotional, linguistic, perceptual, motor, and neurological considerations.

There were, in addition, a number of LI and normal children who participated only in specific aspects of the study, whose data were included in the relevant sections

PROCEDURES

Language

Both receptive and elicited expressive production tests from the CYCLE (Curtiss & Yamada, 1988) were used. Each CYCLE-R (receptive) test consists of five items. The CYCLE-R tests consist largely of sentence-picture matching items, with foils that allow for a variety of error analyses in most cases. A passing score on each test is 4 out of 5 correct.

Each CYCLE-E (elicited production) test consists of a pair of items that utilize a sentence-completion format in which picture and prosodic cues, in combination with the sentence frame presented, constrain the possible logically and grammatically appropriate responses. A passing score on these tests is 2 out of 2 "correct."*

Each CYCLE test is assigned to a level, corresponding to the age at which 80% of the normative sample passed the test. Thus items assigned to level

---

*"Correct" is interpreted as a well-formed version of the structure being targeted or an appropriate, although syntactically irrelevant, response.

2 are earlier acquired than those items at levels 3, 4, 5, and so on. In addition, items from the CYCLE-P (phonological measures) testing discrimination of consonant and vowel oppositions were also administered.

The LI and age-matched normal children were tested yearly; the "language-matched" normals were tested at 6-month intervals. A difference in sampling intervals for the two populations was built into the design in an attempt to equalize acquisition rates for the two groups. After a child had achieved a passing score on a test 2 data points in a row, he or she was automatically assigned a passing score on that test from that point on.

Nonverbal. The LI and age-matched normals were given subtests of the repetition test at years 1, 3, and 5 (Tallal & Piercy, 1973a, b). In the repetition test two different stimuli are used in combination. Subject's responses are made by pressing either of two identical, clear panels that are mounted, one above the other, on a metal response box. The stimuli consist of two different complex tones, computer-generated so as to approximate the acoustic characteristics of steady-state vowels but with a spectral distribution not reproducible by the human vocal tract. In the experiment reported herein, stimulus 1 was a 75 msec duration complex tone with a fundamental frequency (F0) of 100 Hz and stimulus 2 was a 75 msec duration complex tone with a F0 of 305 Hz.

Every child was first "pretested" with the *Association* subtest of the repetition test, to establish that they could demonstrate the prerequisite perceptual skills necessary to perform the other tasks in the test series. In this "pretest," stimulus 1 and 2 are presented one at a time, in random order. Subjects are trained to press the bottom panel on the response box each time stimulus 1 was presented and the top panel each time stimulus 2 was presented. The two stimuli were presented, one at a time, in random order, with immediate corrections of errors until a criterion of 12 correct responses in a series of 16 consecutive stimuli was reached. This strict criterion was employed as it was imperative to ensure that each of the subjects could discriminate between the two stimuli and had fully established the correct association to each, before proceeding to the more complex tasks utilizing combinations of the two. The number of trials to criterion and number of correct responses were recorded. Testing was discontinued after 24 trials if a subject failed to reach criterion.

In the next subtest, the *temporal order* subtest, subjects were trained to respond to stimulus 1 and 2 presented sequentially, with a 500 msec interstimulus interval (ISI). Four possible stimulus patterns (1=1, 2=2, 2=1, 1=2) were presented in random order. The subjects were required to wait until both stimuli were presented before pressing the correct response panels in the same order as the stimuli were presented. The experimenter demonstrated the method four times to each child, and then administered 12 test trials. The score was the total number of correct responses.

In the *serial memory* subtest, the same two stimulus elements were used and the procedure was the same, except that the ISI was held constant at 500 msec and the number of elements in the stimulus patterns ranged from 3 to 7. The stimulus arrangements were random. A single score for this subtest was obtained consisting of the total number of stimulus elements responded to correctly out of 81 (3 X 3s + 3 X 4s + 3 X 5s + 3 X 6s + 3 X 7s).

THE RELATIONSHIP BETWEEN NONLINGUISTIC PROCESSING IMPAIRMENTS AND LINGUISTIC PERFORMANCE

SEQUENCING IN LANGUAGE-IMPAIRED CHILDREN

Reports of sequencing deficits in LI children date at least as far back as the Lowe and Campell (1965) study in which LI children required significantly longer intervals between auditory signals than age-matched peers in order to make accurate judgments concerning order of presentation. Numerous other studies have since investigated sequencing abilities in LI children, examining sequencing of both visual and auditory information, using tasks that require a fine degree of temporal order resolution as well as tasks involving material presented more slowly and for longer durations (e.g., Aten & Davis, 1968; Furth, 1964; Furth & Pufall, 1966; Frumkin & Rapin, 1980; Kirk, McCarthy & Kirk, 1968; McCroskey & Thompson, 1973; Poppen, Stark, Eisenson, Forrest & Wertheim, 1969; Rosenthal, 1972; Stark, 1967; Tallal, 1976; Tallal & Piercy, 1973a, b, 1974, 1975). Despite many differences in task and stimulus characteristics, all of these studies report that LI children demonstrate sequencing difficulties relative to normals.

The fact that LI children consistently evidence deficits in sequencing raises interesting questions regarding the impact such deficits might have on language learning. Since, in spoken language, most linguistic information is presented sequentially,* impairments in sequencing might impact globally on language acquisition (e.g., degrading the input or, more accurately, degrading the "intake"—what LI children perceive as the input) in a general fashion. Such deficits might also have a more specific impact on acquisition, for example, affecting the acquisition of linguistic structures in which the sequence of linguistic elements plays a crucial grammatico/semantic role. It was this latter relationship that was explored.

---

*In "fusional" languages, where individual morphemes encode several pieces of information (e.g., some combination of person, number, gender, and tense), or in languages where different "tiers" carry different pieces of grammatical information (e.g., some tone languages), aspects of grammatical information are transmitted in the signal simultaneously, and are thus exceptions to the predominant sequential character of linguistic transmission in spoken language.

To investigate the relationship between nonlinguistic sequencing impairments and language acquisition the impact of a sequencing deficit at the level of syntax was examined. Only at the level of syntax was it possible to compare performance on structures embodying crucial sequential cues with performance on structures that do not involve such cues. At the level of phonology and morphology, no such comparisons could be made.

Performance on linguistic structures in which word order provides the crucial cues for correct semantic interpretation was examined and compared with performance on an opposing set of structures in which key grammatical formatives, not word order, provide the essential interpretive cues. To this end items from the CYCLE were organized into two separate clusters: a [+sequentially cued] (+sc) cluster in which word order uniquely signalled grammatical and thematic role and a [-sequentially-cued] (-sc) cluster in which key formatives cued roles and relations. The [+sc] cluster was comprised of the receptive and expressive *active voice word order* tests, which involve semantically reversible SVO sentences (e.g., "The girl is pushing the boy" versus "The boy is pushing the girl"), in which word order provides the only cue to the relationship between the NPs and the verb. The [-sc] cluster included the *attributive/stative* test, a receptive test involving a single subject-predicate clause expressing an attribute or stative relationship between subject and predicate (e.g., "The ball is big" versus "The ball is little" or "The man is big"), and the *negation in simple sentences* test, an expressive test in which a predicate must be negated (e.g., "Here the boy *is* pulling the wagon but here the boy _____ [is *not* pulling the wagon"]).

These two clusters were fashioned so as to be equivalent in level of mastery and to involve structures at the early end of the developmental spectrum of language acquisition so that both groups were dealing with structures they could process at least in part (both clusters were comprised of structures for which 80% of the children in the normative population had demonstrated mastery by age 3). (For more details on this and other aspects of this experimental study, see Curtiss, Katz, & Tallal, forthcoming.)

Performance of LI children was compared with their age-matched counterparts on these clusters. A 2 X 2 X 3 repeated measures ANOVA using groups, clusters, and years (1–3) was performed.* There was a significant group effect, $p < .0001$, wherein the age-matched normals performed significantly better than the LI group throughout; a significant year effect, $p < .0001$, wherein performance for both groups improved significantly across the 3 years; and a significant cluster effect, $p < .0001$, reflecting better performance on the [-sc] cluster throughout. There was also a cluster by group effect, $p < .0005$, reflecting the fact that the LIs performed significantly worse on the [+sc] cluster than on the [-sc] cluster, whereas perform-

---

*Only 3 years were used, as performance had reached a ceiling by year 4.

ance on the two clusters was not significantly different for the normals (as substantiated by a posthoc test), and a year by group interaction, $p < .0001$, reflecting a sharper slope of change for the LI group. The three-way interaction, however, was not significant.

In the next analysis the relationship between performance on nonlinguistic sequencing tasks and performance on these linguistic clusters was directly examined. The same population of LI and normal children was used. Correlations between performance on each of the two linguistic clusters and performance on a nonlinguistic sequencing cluster comprised of the three subtests of the repetition test described above were calculated. Since most of the LI children had failed to pass the pretest for the nonverbal sequencing cluster at year 1 of the study (when they were 4 years of age), nonverbal performance at year 3 (at 6 years of age), the second nonverbal data point, was used to test the relationship between nonverbal sequencing and linguistic performance.

Table 9-1 presents a list of the correlations obtained. None of the correlations between nonverbal sequencing and linguistic performance was significant for the normal children. Performance on nonverbal sequencing and performance on the [+sc] cluster, both at years 2 and 3, were significantly correlated for the LI children.

These results suggest that a nonlinguistic sequencing impairment may impact directly on the processing of linguistic structures in which the sequential order of linguistic elements uniquely signals grammatico/ semantic information. The impact appears to be one of making such structures more difficult for LI children to process than for children without such impairments. Such an impairment does not appear to result in the construction of aberrant (impossible or ungrammatical) representations of such structures, however. In fact, the premastery errors made by LI children mirror those made by normal children in both comprehension and production. This was true not only with the structure tested in the [+sc]

Table 9-1. Correlations between nonverbal sequencing and linguistic sequencing

	[+sc] with nonverbal	*[−sc with nonverbal]*
YEAR 2 LANGUAGE / YEAR 3 NONVERBAL		
Language-impaired	.4938*	.2367
Normal	.1799	.2718
YEAR 3 LANGUAGE / YEAR 3 NONVERBAL		
Language impaired	.3914*	.1024
Normal	.2723	.0598

*Significant at $p < .005$.

cluster, but also with a number of structures requiring crucially sequenced constituents.

As a specific example, examine the error patterns displayed by the LI and normal children for the active voice word order items. On the CYCLE-R test, each test sentence is accompanied by a set of four pictures—the correct answer and three decoys, each of which represents a particular error type. Using the item, "The girl is pushing the boy" as an example, the decoys/error types are as follows:

1. A reversal of thematic roles ("The boy is pushing the girl");
2. Both NPs pictured as agents ("The boy and girl are pushing");
3. A decoy in which either only the first or second half of the sentence is represented correctly ("The girl is pushing the clown" or "The clown is pushing the boy").

Figures 9-1, 9-2, and 9-3 illustrate the percent of each error type made by the LI and two normal groups of children for those years in which the three groups were making errors. For all groups, the most frequent error by far is a reversal of NP roles, and the breakdown of errors is nearly identical across groups.

In production, as well, LI children make the same kinds of errors on SVO structures as do normal children. Table 9-2 presents a breakdown of error frequency and type for those data points at which any errors were made. LI children make neither different nor a greater number of constituent order errors in producing SVO structures than language-matched normal children.

Fig. 9-1. Active voice (year 1).

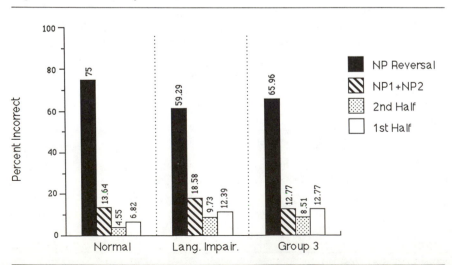

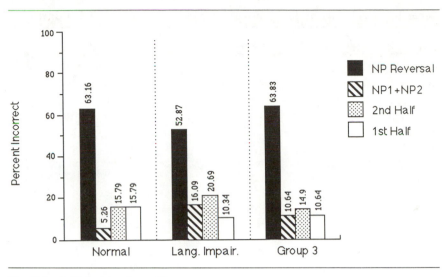

Fig. 9-2. Active voice (year 2).

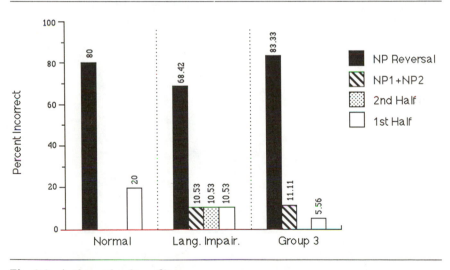

Fig. 9-3. Active voice (year 3).

The same pattern of nearly identical error types and frequency for LI and normal children have been found across many structures which involve the ordering of grammatical constituents (e.g., Prep NP, AUX Neg, AUX VP, Complementizer clause, etc). Thus, the deficiencies in sequencing that affect the processing of structures embodying crucially sequenced cues do not show up as violations of grammatical principles or as developmentally aberrant misanalyses. (For more details on patterns of errors made by LI and normal children, see Curtiss & Tallal, forthcoming, a.)

Table 9-2. Breakdown of SVO word order errors in LI and normal children

	LIs		Age-matched		Language-matched	
DPI						
n	94		63		34	
SV errors	11	(8.86%)	2	(2.3%)	5	(11.6%)
SV correct	117		84		38	
VO errors	8	(5.2%)	2	(1.8%)	3	(5.5%)
VO correct	145		110		52	

Error types
1. NP reversal
2. VS order (Here kicking the girl.)
                          V   S

	LIs		Age-matched		Language-matched	
DP2						
n	89		59		34	
SV errors	2	(1.8%)	0		3	(5.9%)
SV correct	109		88		48	
VO errors	0		0		2	(3.7%)
VO correct	159		109		52	

Error types
LIs: 1 NP reversal
            1 VS order
Language-matched: 2 NP reversals
                      1 VS order

	LIs		Age-matched	Language-matched
DP3				
n	43		9	37
SV errors	3[a]	(4%)	0	0
SV correct	72		17	71
VO errors	0		0	0
VO correct	81	17	73	

Error types:
[a]Only errors were of the type: "The dog is chasing the dog," where it is not clear whether the subject or object is incorrect. These may have been speech errors, rather than true constituent order errors.

THE EFFECT OF SYNTACTIC REDUNDANCY ON LINGUISTIC PROCESSING

Linguistic structure contains many redundant features, all of which are assumed to aid linguistic processing, at least for the adult. The effect of syntactic redundancy on linguistic processing in children has been little studied, however. As syntactic redundancy systematically increases sentence length, in some instances its effect may be to impose an increased processing *burden* on language-learners, whose short-term memories are not fully mature. LI children, in particular, may be burdened by the added length resulting from double or triple marking of syntactic information, since they have been found to evidence short-term memory deficits even in relation to other children (Ceci, Ringstrom & Lea, 1981; Doehring, 1960; Furth, 1964; Kirchner & Klatzky, 1985; Stanton, 1976; Tallal, 1975).

To test the effect of syntactic redundancy on LI children as compared to normal children, comprehension of sentences that differed in degree of redundancy, but which were structurally identical at the level of D-structure and encoded identical or nearly identical semantic information, were examined. These sentences were divided into two groups. One set of sentences, the *redundant* set, contained redundant marking of the linguistic information; in the other set, the *nonredundant* set, these redundant cues were absent. The redundant set consisted of two types of sentences: those containing double marking of number and those containing an overt (surface) marking of a subject relative clause (in the form of complementizer plus *be*). The *nonredundant* set consisted of the same two sentence types, but with no redundant marking of number in the first case, and with no overt marking of the relative clause in the second. Examples of each type are presented in Table 9-3 below.

Table 9-3. Examples of redundant and nonredundant sentences

Redundant	*Nonredundant*
Point to the picture of three hats.	Point to the picture of the hats.
The girl who is smiling is pushing the boy.	The girl smiling is pushing the boy.
The girl who is pushing the boy is smiling.	The girl pushing the boy is smiling.

A first analysis, illustrated in Figure 9-4, compared the LI with age-matched normals. A repeated measures analysis of variance (ANOVA) using groups, clusters (redundant and nonredundant), and years (1–5) was performed. There was a significant group effect reflecting that the age-matched normals performed significantly better than the LI group throughout (p < .0001), and a significant year effect indicating that performance for both groups improved significantly across the five years of the study (p < .0001). There was no cluster effect, but a cluster by group interaction, p < .0001, indicating that the LI children consistently performed better on the nonredundant cluster, whereas the age-matched normals consistently performed better on the redundant set, much as would be expected for adults. Thus, the pattern of performance across the two clusters was different for the two groups even though performance *level* across the clusters was not significantly different within each group.

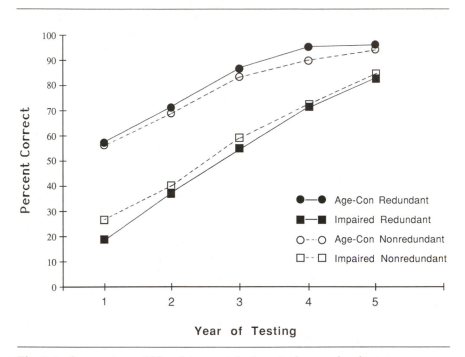

Fig. 9-4. Comparison of LI and age-matched controls on redundant structures over five data points.

In a second analysis, illustrated in Figure 9-5, we compared LI children with the language-matched controls. A repeated-measures ANOVA was again performed, using groups, clusters, and comparable data points; that is, years 1, 2, and 3 for the LIs and data points 1, 3, 5 for the language-matched normals (who were tested every 6 months). Again, there was a significant "year" effect, indicating that performance for both groups improved significantly across the three data points ($p < .0001$). There was also a significant cluster effect ($p < .0004$); performance on the nonredundant cluster was better overall, in contrast to the results with the age-matched normals. There was no significant cluster by group or three-way interaction, however. This analysis, therefore, suggested that LI and younger normal children prefer nonredundant shorter strings. A third analysis, comparing LI and their language-matched counterparts in more detail, however, revealed an interesting difference between the two groups, a difference only hinted at by the graphic representation of the data in Figure 9-5.

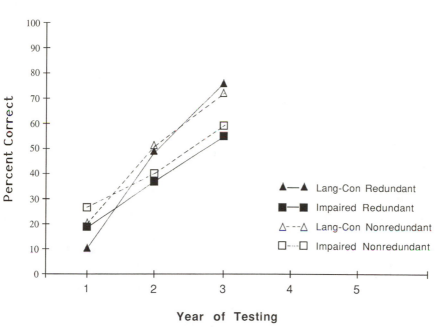

Fig. 9-5. Comparison of LI and language-matched controls on redundant and nonredundant structures over three data points.

In the third analysis, a repeated measures ANOVA was again performed, using groups, clusters, and all five data points for both groups. Again there was no group or cluster X group effect, and again there was a cluster effect, with performance on the nonredundant items better overall. However, this time, when all five data points were considered, there was a significant three-way interaction (p < .03). Upon inspection of the data, illustrated in Figure 9-6, it is apparent that while the LI children consistently preferred the nonredundant, shorter sentences, the language-matched children preferred the nonredundant sentences only at data points 1–3, but preferred the redundant sentences at data points 4 and 5. That is, they switched processing preference, and began performing like the age-matched normals after data point 3.

As can be seen, after data point 3, the language-matched controls perform like the age-matched controls. They prefer the redundant, albeit longer, sentences. In contrast, the LI children continue to demonstrate the same pattern of performance throughout, performing like much younger,

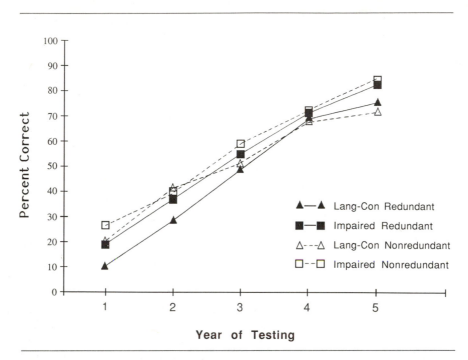

Fig. 9-6. Comparison of LI and language-matched controls on redundant and nonredundant structures over five data points.

normal children through all 5 years of the study. This result supports the hypothesis of a maturational lag for LI children. While there is a clear switch from a preference for shorter, nonredundant sentences at the youngest age to longer, redundant sentences by about age 4 in normal children, no such change in processing "strategy" for the LI children can be observed. (For more details on the results of this study see Curtiss & Tallal, forthcoming, b.)

DEVIANCE VERSUS DELAY

One of the central questions regarding LI children is whether they manifest delayed but normal patterns of acquisition or deviant acquisition patterns. This question has important implications for a theory of language acquisition in general, because a finding of deviance in LI children's language acquisition may illuminate the consequences of alterations or impairments of the relevant mechanisms or the consequences of utilizing alternate mechanisms for language acquisition. It is also an important issue both theoretically and practically in understanding the nature of language acquisition in the language-impaired child.

In this study to date, the focus has been on whether or not LI children display deviant grammar acquisition, in particular, in whether or not LI children manifest deviance at the representational level. What would constitute such deviance? Since the process of mastering a first language involves constructing (or "selecting") a grammar; that is, building linguistic representations and increasing the knowledge base or changing it in principled ways (i.e., moving from "stage" to "stage"), deviance at this level might be predicted to result in structure-specific difficulties, that is, difficulties with grammatical structures that embody particular formal properties, in rules and representations unattested in the grammars of linguistically normal children, or in clear deviations from the normal relationship obtained between one aspect of grammar and another. A number of studies have addressed this question, directly or indirectly, yet the issue is by no means resolved.

Since the studies reporting delayed but normal development have focused on one piece of the grammar at a time (e.g., Cousins, 1979; Freedman & Carpenter, 1976; Ingram, 1972; Leonard, Bolders & Miller, 1976; Menyuk, 1964) and the studies suggesting deviance report asynchronies between acquisition of one piece of the grammar and another (e.g., Johnston & Kamhi, 1984; Johnston & Schery, 1976; Steckol, 1976), it would seem important to examine patterns of acquisition across components in order to uncover deviance. To further investigate the delay versus deviance question, therefore, the acquisition of a set of linguistic structures and the relationship obtaining between one structure and another was examined, *within the same population of normal and LI children.* The order in which these linguistic structures are mastered was investigated looking at comprehension as well as production. Included in the set were structures of morphology, syntax, and semantics, some of which are mastered in close proximity to one another in normal acquisition, and some of which are mastered at distinctly different points in normal acquisition. Deviance in building the knowledge base as well as in moving from "stage" to "stage" would be revealed in this investigation as difficulties with specific structures relative to the normal children and atypical patterns of acquisition order for structures within and across components.

The subjects consisted of 28 of the larger group of LI children who comprised three defined clinical subtypes: (1) those evidencing greater expressive than receptive language problems; (2) those evidencing predominantly receptive difficulties; and (3) those manifesting both expressive and receptive impairments. These three subtypes were equally represented in the group of 28 LI children (9, 9, and 10, respectively). On induction into the study, the LI children ranged in age from 4 ; 0 to 4 ; 9 with a mean age of 4 ; 4.

The normal controls used in this study consisted of the 32 normally developing children matched to the LI children at entry to the study on the basis of language age as determined by performance on the same set of standardized language tests. The normal controls ranged in age from 2 ; 1 to 3 ; 8, with a mean age of 2 ; 9 years at the beginning of the study.

The data were analyzed in two ways. An analysis was made of the data point at which subjects attained mastery of a given linguistic structure. In addition, an analysis was completed of the consistency with which subjects' acquisition of structures matched an increasing, sequential progression. The list of structures tested are presented in Table 9-4.

POINT OF ATTAINMENT

First, an analysis was made comparing the percent of subjects (N and LI) passing each test, as a function of the data point at which mastery was reached (hereafter referred to as "point of attainment"). The chief finding

Table 9-4. Linguistic structures tested in the delay versus deviance study

Receptive		Expressive	
#	Name of test	#	Name of test
1	Negation in simple sentences	16	Negation in simple sentences
2	Object pronouns: him, her	17	SV (simple declaratives)
3	Locative preps: in front, in back	18	Regular past tense
4	Subject (SS) relative clauses	19	Future conditionals
5	Noun singular/plural	20	Possessive morpheme
6	Progressive aspect: /-ing/	21	Negation in embedded clause
7	Aux Be singular	22	Verb singular (3rd person)
8	Regular past tense	23	Case marking prep: with
9	Aux Be plural	24	Regular past participle
10	Subject pronouns: she, he, they	25	Counterfactual conditionals
11	Possessive morpheme	26	Subject (SO) relatives with relativized object
12	Subject (SS) relative clauses ending in a N-V sequence	27	Case marking prep: by
13	Object (OS) relative clauses	28	Passive (with specified agent)
14	Verb plurals	29	Passive aux and past participle
15	Object relatives with relatived objects (OO)		

is that the overall distributions of point of attainment are highly similar between the two groups, for both receptive and expressive tests. That is, there seem to be few cases where the distribution of point of attainment for normal children is not closely matched by that of the LI subjects. For example, 74% of the control subjects and 85% of the LI subjects passed receptive test #1 (negation in simple sentences) at the first data point. Similarly, 20% of the control subjects and 10% of the LI subjects passed test #1 at the second data point. Thus, by data point 2, 95% of both groups had passed this test.

To investigate group differences statistically, two series of chi-square tests were calculated. The first series examined the percent of subjects' point of attainment for each test, while the second series examined the percent of subjects' mean point of attainment for each level. Each chi-square test compared the distribution of point of attainment for normal and LI groups. For the analyses examining mean point of attainment values, a mean score of <=1.0 was ranked as level 1, <=2.0 as level 2, . . . to 5.0 and "above."

Table 9-5 shows the results of the individual test analyses, listing the value of X2, df, and probability for each comparison. Also shown are the components of the grammar (morphology, syntax, and semantics) to which the tests correspond. With the exception of test #7 (aux be singular, p < .005) there were no significant differences as a function of group either on an item-by-item basis or with reference to specific components of grammar.

DEVIATION FROM LINEAR SEQUENCE

The degree to which each group deviated from the linear sequence of acquisition expected from the CYCLE levels was also examined. For this analysis, the number of times the expected linear progression through levels was violated was computed for each subject. Each deviation from the expected sequence was counted such that one violation was scored each time an item from a higher level showed a point of attainment less (earlier) than a preceding level. A deviant acquisition pattern would presumably show a greater number of sequence violations than the norm.

A deviant pattern was not observed for the LI scores. When the number of violations is examined as a function of group and test type (R, E), largely similar means and variations were observed for both groups in both test types. To test this statistically, a two-way ANOVA was conducted, examining both group and test factors. The results show no significant main effects for group or test variables, and no group by test interaction.

These results argue for delay without deviance. The patterns displayed by both groups was remarkably similar across five different points in time,

Table 9-5. Point of attainment comparisons for individual tests

Receptive

MORPHOLOGY

Test	#	df*	X2	sig level
Noun singular/plural	5	5	2.469	.7811
Auxiliary be singular	7	5	17.278	.004
be + ing	6	5	7.843	.1651
Auxiliary be plural	9	5	2.872	.7197
Regular past tense	8	5	4.905	.4276
Possessive	11	5	1.364	.9282
Verb plural	14	5	7.627	.178

SYNTAX

Test	#	df*	X2	sig level
Subject (SS) relatives	4	5	.944	.967
Subject relatives NV	12	5	7.531	.1841
Object (OS) relatives	13	4	8.106	.0878
Object (OO) relatives	15	4	1.09	.7192

SEMANTICS

Test	#	df*	X2	sig level
Negative in simple sentence 1	4	3	.742	.4421
Him/her 2	3	2	.924	.4035
Front/back	3	4	4.750	.3140
She/he/they	10	5	4.389	.4948

Expressive

MORPHOLOGY

Test	#	df*	X2	sig level
Regular past tense	18	5	2.926	.7114
Possessive	20	5	8.275	.1417
Verb singular	22	5	5.528	.3549
Regular past participle	24	1	.273	.6015
Passive past participle	29	2	.941	.6248

SYNTAX

Test	#	df*	X2	sig level
Negative in simple sentence	16	3	.728	.8665
Simple declaratives	17	5	5.968	.3094
Negative in embedded sentence	21	5	9.138	.1037
Relativized object	26	5	5.651	.3417
Counterfactual	25	5	9.177	.1022
Passive	28	4	6.316	.1768
Future conditionals	19	5	1.561	.9059

SEMANTICS

Test	#	df*	X2	sig level
With	23	5	5.757	.3306
By	27	3	1.541	.6729

*Number of comparable data points between the two groups.

charting a major period of active language acquisition (5 years for the LI children; 2½ years for the younger, normal children).

SUMMARY AND DISCUSSION

Patterns of language acquisition in LI children, competence and performance, were examined in an attempt to better understand the nature of the language-learning difficulties these children display. In the first study discussed, the potential impact of a sequencing defect on handling syntactic material in which the sequential order of constituents plays a crucial role was examined. What was found was that LI children evidence more difficulty with such material than with otherwise equivalent structures, unlike developmentally normal children, who do not show such differences. What is more, their difficulty with "sequentially cued" syntactic structures is significantly correlated with their performance on nonverbal sequential tasks. Despite their difficulties, however, they make the same kinds of errors in both comprehension and production of such structures.

In the second study discussed, the impact of syntactic (and semantic) redundancy on sentence processing in LI and normal children was examined. Here the findings showed that the age-matched normals preferred the redundantly marked sentences throughout (i.e., from ages 4–8, while the LI children preferred the nonredundant sentences throughout). The language-matched children, however, presented the most informative picture—they preferred the nonredundant sentences at the early data points (before the age of 4 for the most part) and then switched to a preference for the redundant sentences after that point, suggesting that during the course of normal language development, a maturational change in the processor occurs such that the positive effect of syntactic redundancy outweighs the negative effect of increased length.

The third study examined longitudinal patterns in the acquisition of specific morphological and syntactic structures by comparing the order in which items were acquired relative to other items both within the same grammatical component and across components. The patterns displayed by the two groups were strikingly similar with respect to point of mastery for each of the structures examined relative to other structures as well as the actual sequence of acquisition displayed.

What do these results suggest regarding the nature of the language-learning impairments of LI children? The first two studies indicate that the nonlinguistic sequencing and short-term verbal memory impairments of LI children have rather specific consequences for linguistic processing. The nonverbal sequencing impairments appear to adversely affect the processing of crucially sequenced syntactic material (i.e., where order of constituent units determines grammatical role) but not otherwise parallel syntactic material. Short-term verbal memory impairments appear to increase the impact of sentence length on sentence processing. It seems, then, that the nonverbal impairments of LI children may affect linguistic processing efficiency and strategy.

The first and third studies presented above suggest that these impairments do not, in contrast, appear to affect the kinds of linguistic representations LI children compute; that is, at the representational level, LI children look quite normal. Even for those structures whose processing was compromised, the kinds of comprehension misinterpretations and production errors made in this study were nearly identical across groups, as was the order of acquisition. LI children appear to be constructing the same grammars, in the same way, as normal children.

The mechanisms by which knowledge of grammar develops and is represented may well be intact in LI children, therefore. However, the essential and continual contribution of certain nongrammatical abilities to normal and mature linguistic processing is highlighted by children with developmental language impairments. In some respects LI children may simply have immature processors which appear to be "stuck" at an early developmental state (cf., the redundancy results), giving rise to deficient processing compared to normal children. In other respects, perhaps, LI children may actually have impaired processors. In either event, the result is less performance for the same amount of representational knowledge.

The picture emerging from this study, therefore, is one which suggests that LI children demonstrate impaired linguistic processing in the face of normal language-learning mechanisms. The fact that they appear to construct grammars with the same content and in the same developmental manner as do linguistically normal children seems rather surprising, given all of the deficits and difficulties LI children have been shown to have and the fact that they have always been referred to as "language impaired." These findings suggest that they may be better referred to as "processing impaired"—children who exhibit a multiplicity of processing deficits, many of which conspire to make the comprehension and production of language an arduous affair.

REFERENCES

Aten, J., & Davis, J. (1968). Disturbances in the perception of auditory sequence in children with minimal cerebral dysfunction. *Journal of Speech and Hearing Research, 11*, 236–245.

Carrow, E. (1974). *Carrow Elicited Language Inventory (CELI)*. Boston: Teaching Resources.

Ceci, S., Ringstrom, M., & Lea, S. (1981). Do language-learning disabled children

(L/LDs) have impaired memories? In search of underlying processes. *Journal of Learning Disabilities, 14,* 159–162.

Cousins, A. (1979). Grammatical morpheme development in an aphasic child: A longitudinal study. Paper presented at the Boston University Conference on Language Development.

Curtiss, S., Katz, W., & Tallal, P. (forthcoming).

Curtiss S., & Tallal, P. (forthcoming, a). Language Impaired children: An impairment of competence or performance?

Curtiss, S., & Tallal, P. (forthcoming, b). The effect of syntactic redundancy on sentence processing in language-impaired and normal children. Submitted for publication.

Curtiss, S., & Yamada, J. (1988). *The Curtiss-Yamada Comprehensive Language Evaluation (CYCLE).* Unpublished test.

DiSimoni, F. (1978). *The Token Test for Children.* Boston: Teaching Resources.

Doehring, D. (1960). Visual spatial memory in aphasic children. *Journal of Speech and Hearing Research, 3,* 138–149.

Freedman, P., & Carpenter, R. (1976). Semantic relations used by normal and language impaired children at stage I. *Journal of Speech and Hearing Research, 19,* 784–795.

Frumkin, B., & Rapin, I. (1980). Perception of vowels and consonant-vowels of varying duration in language-impaired children. *Neuropsychologia, 18,* 443–454.

Fudala, J. B. (1980). *The Arizona Articulation Proficiency Scale (AAPS),* rev. Los Angeles: Western Psychological Services.

Furth, H. (1964). Sequence learning in aphasic and deaf children. *Journal of Speech and Hearing Disorders, 29,* 171–177.

Furth, H., & Pufall, P. (1966). Visual and auditory sequence learning in hearing-impaired children. *Journal of Speech and Hearing Research, 9,* 441–449.

Hedrick, D., Prather, E., & Tobin, A. (1979). *Sequenced Inventory of Communication Development (SICD).* Seattle: University of Washington Press.

Ingram, D. (1972). The acquisition of the English verbal auxiliary in normal and linguistically deviant children. *Papers and Reports in Child Language Development, 4,* 79–92.

Johnston, J., & Kamhi, A. (1984). Syntactic and semantic aspects of the utterances of language-impaired children: The same can be less. *Merrill-Palmer Quarterly, 30,* 65–85.

Johnston, J., & Schery, T. (1976). The use of grammatical morphemes by children with communication disorders. In D. Morehead and A. Morehead (Eds.), *Normal and deviant child language.* Baltimore: University Park Press.

Kirchner, D., & Klatzky, R. (1985). Verbal rehearsal and memory in language disordered children. *Journal of Speech and Hearing Research, 28,* 556–565.

Kirk, S., McCarthy, J., & Kirk, W. (1968). *The Illinois Test of Psycholinguistic Abilities (ITPA),* rev. ed. Urbana: University of Illinois Press.

Lee, L. (1971). *Northwest Syntax Screening Test (NSST).* Evanston, IL: Northwestern University Press.

Leonard, L., Bolders, J., & Miller, J. (1976). An examination of the semantic relations reflected in the language usage of normal and language disordered children. *Journal of Speech and Hearing Research, 19,* 371–392.

Lowe, A., & Campbell, R. (1965). Temporal discrimination in aphasiod and normal children. *Journal of Speech and Hearing Research, 8,* 313–314.

McCroskey, R., & Thompson, N. (1973). Comprehension of rate controlled speech by children with specific learning disabilities. *Journal of Learning Disabilities, 6,* 621–627.

Menyuk, P. (1964). Comparison of grammar of children with functionally deviant and normal speech. *Journal of Speech and Hearing Research, 7*, 264–270.

Poppen, R., Stark, J., Eisenson, J., Forrest, T., & Wertheim, G. (1969). Visual sequencing performance of aphasic children. *Journal of Speech and Hearing Disorders, 26*, 83–86.

Rosenthal, W. (1972). Auditory and linguistic interaction in developmental aphasia: Evidence from two studies of auditory processing. *Papers and Reports in Child Language Development, 4*, 19–34.

Stanton, A. (1976). Qualitative assessment of comprehension and imitation in language-delayed pre-school children in comparison with normal children of the same age. *British Journal of Disorders of Communication, 11*, 63–71.

Stark, J. (1967). A comparison of the performance of aphasic children on three sequencing tests. *Journal of Communication Disorders, 1*, 31–34.

Steckol, K. (1976). The use of grammatical morphemes by normal and language impaired children. Paper presented at the American Speech and Hearing Association convention.

Tallal, P. (1975). Perceptual and linguistic factors in the language impairment of developmental dysphasics: an experimental investigation with the Token Test. *Cortex, 11*, 196–205.

Tallal, P. (1976). Rapid auditory processing in normal and disordered language development. *Journal of Speech and Hearing Research, 19*, 561–571.

Tallal, P., Curtiss, S., & Kaplan, R. (1988). The San Diego longitudinal study: Evaluating the outcomes of preschool impairment in language development. In S. Gerber and G. Mencher (Eds.), *International Perspectives in Communication Disorders*. Washington, DC: Gallaudet University Press.

Tallal, P., & Piercy, M. (1973a). Defects of non-verbal auditory perception in children with developmental aphasia. *Nature, 241*, 468–469.

Tallal, P., & Piercy, M. (1973b). Developmental aphasia: Impaired rate of nonverbal processing as a function of sensory modality. *Neuropsychologia, 11*, 389–398.

Tallal, P., & Piercy, M. (1974). Developmental aphasia: Rate of auditory processing and selective impairment of consonant perception. *Neuropsychologia, 12*, 83–94.

Tallal, P., & Piercy, M. (1975). Perceptual and linguistic factors in the language impairment of developmental dysphasics: An experimental investigation with the Token Test. *Cortex, 11*, 196–205.

Ziegler, M., Curtiss, S., & Tallal, P. (1989). Selecting LI children for research studies. (Submitted).

CHAPTER 10

Quantifying Productive Language Disorders

JON F. MILLER

This chapter is an initial attempt to quantify productive language performance by identifying and establishing the validity of several general measures of language taken from free speech samples. The study was motivated
by the review chapter by Miller in this volume (see chapter 1), which
documents several shortcomings in the published research on child language disorders. One of the more serious problems discussed was the lack
of language-matched control groups in studies investigating children over
5 years of age. While some studies have matched subjects on language test
scores, there is a serious need for general measures of productive language
development in older children that can serve the same function as mean
length of utterance (MLU) has for children under 5 years of age. Language
production is the most seriously impaired process among language-disordered children. Production seems to be affected at a number of linguistic
levels, vocabulary, syntax, semantic, and pragmatic, suggesting that a
single general measure of production will be inadequate. Johnston (1988)

This chapter is based on a paper presented at the Wisconsin Symposium for Research on Child
Language Disorders, University of Wisconsin–Madison, June 1, 1989. Preparation of this
paper was supported in part by research grants No's, R01-NS2551717, NIDCD, NIH, Judith
Johnston and Jon Miller, Principle Investigators, and R01-HD22393, NICHD, NIH, Jon Miller,
Principle Investigator.

argues that some research questions, such as mapping discourse skills across speaking contexts, require documenting the status of syntactic development in both experimental and control groups. Other problems, such as documenting patterns of language performance among various disordered populations (i.e., syndromes associated with mental retardation), would require several different measures of language production quantifying different language characteristics. The problem of determining what criteria to use in matching subjects is significant. It is obvious that the criteria used in matching subjects is critical for the proper interpretation of the experimental data. Johnston (1988) suggests the use of language comprehension measures for matching experimental and control groups would certainly improve many studies. The fact remains, however, that if it is necessary to match subjects on language production criteria, only MLU can be used and then only for children under 5.

The solution to this dilemma is to create some measures of language production that measure different features of language performance. In addition to measuring different aspects of language performance, they must be developmentally sensitive. Developmental sensitivity means highly correlated with chronological age. If such measures can be identified and validated, they will help researchers deal with two other major problems in conducting research on language disorders in children: (1) how to developmentally organize subject groups to investigate various types of "error patterns" in language production (Miller, 1987); (2) general measures of language performance will provide an organizational structure for "normative" data bases of free speech samples for children older than five. Free speech sample data organized around general developmentally sensitive variables will allow documentation of developmental change in individual variables as well as the synchrony of progress among variables.

The goal of this chapter is to identify and validate several general measures of productive language performance. Several candidates have emerged from an ongoing project investigating productive language development in normal children. They focus on vocabulary diversity, a composite measure of speaking rate, sentence formulation, and speech motor proficiency, and MLU as an index of syntax using different segmentation criteria.

GENERAL MEASURES
OF LANGUAGE DEVELOPMENT

Assumption: If a variable measures an aspect of language and is correlated with advancing age, then it probably is sensitive to developmental changes in language performance. This assumption underlies most research on language development and this study is no different. The assumption is important to keep in mind while exploring variables which may predict age and measure a general aspect of language performance. This chapter will begin with MLU as the most widely accepted general measure of language development in young children.

Mean length of utterance in morphemes is considered to be a general measure of syntactic development. It was originally used by Roger Brown and his students to define stage-like advances in syntactic development, arguing that grammatical complexity must increase as utterance increased. MLU also provided a convenient way of summarizing performance over a large number of utterances both within and between subjects. Research on syntactic development has used MLU as a general index to (1) clearly document the period of development under study improving comparison and generalization of the findings, (2) summarize the data from a number of studies (Miller, 1981), and (3) document language-matched control groups to effectively study language change when delayed relative to age expectations (Morehead and Ingram, 1973). Theoretically, MLU is useful only through the period of simple sentence development, MLUs of four to five morphemes. The stability of MLU and its high correlation with age was originally demonstrated by Miller & Chapman (1981) for normal children and recently for normal and disordered children by Klee, Schaffer, May, Membrino & Mougey (1989). The link between MLU and structural complexity is broken with the onset of complex syntax allowing children to produce increasingly complex utterances without necessarily producing longer utterances. Despite this, Loban (1976) found mean length of utterance in C-units to systematically increase through the school years, grades K–12. Loban's segmentation criteria was essentially grammatical and was a modified version of the T-unit used by Hunt (1965) to study written language. A C-unit defines an utterance essentially as "each independent grammatical predication" checked by intonation, stress, and pause patterns. This criteria provides a systematic mechanism for dealing with conjoined utterances. Pause and intonation criteria reliably segment most utterances with the exception of those that are conjoined. This is particularly true with narrative samples as children get older. The Loban segmentation criteria make it possible to explore how MLU correlates with age in older children and how MLU relates to other general measures of language change. This exploration assumes that MLU-C-units is an index of something related to syntactic development.

Two additional measures are proposed for exploration: (1) the number of different words (NDW) produced in a sample of standard length (measured in utterances) as a measure of general semantic progress or semantic diversity and (2) the total number of words (TNW) produced in a sample of standard length (measured in time) as an index of general language facility. The TNW index reflects a number of factors including speaking rate, length of utterance, speech motor maturation (Kent, 1976, 1984), utterance formulation ability, and word-retrieval efficiency. One might expect some differences in TNW relative to speaking contexts where comprehension effectiveness and language-use variables such as gaining and holding the floor may be more evident in conversation than narration.

METHOD

In order to explore these variables, language samples from 192 children 3–13 years of age were analyzed using SALT (Miller & Chapman, 1982–87). Table 10-1 provides a description of the sample, age, sex, and SES stratification. The data are from an ongoing project to develop a reference database for SALT interpretation (Miller, 1986). The language samples were taken by an adult examiner interacting with each child individually in a school setting. Two speaking contexts, one conversation and one narration, were audiotape-recorded for each child. The conversational condition introduced the same topics to the child for discussion, school activities, family activities, friends, and holidays. In the narrative condition the child was asked to (1) tell a favorite story. If that failed, they were asked to (2) tell about a television program. If that failed, they were asked to tell a nursery story suggested by the examiner (e.g., The Three Bears), and if that failed, then (4) a picture book of a nursery story was introduced and reviewed with the child, then the child was asked to retell it. Ninety-eight percent of the subjects produced narratives using conditions 1 or 2.

Segmentation criteria followed Miller (1981) with the addition of

Table 10-1. RDB subjects[a]

	Age		Sex		
Age Group	M	R	M	F	Number
3-year-olds	3.1	2.8–3.4	13	14	27
4-year-olds	4.1	3.9–4.3	18	12	30
5-year-olds	5.5	5.2–5.8	14	13	27
7-year-olds	7.1	6.7–7.8	12	15	27
9-year-olds	9.1	8.8–9.4	10	17	27
11-year-olds	11.1	10.8–11.3	14	13	27
13-year-olds	13.1	12.8–13.3	14	13	27

[a]Subjects were 192 children from Madison, Wisconsin, 6 groups of 27 children, 3–13 years of age. All children were drawn from preschools in Madison or the Madison metropolitan public school system. Subjects were sampled from the diverse socio-economic areas represented in Madison, Wisconsin. The subject population is a random sample reflecting the diverse SES of Madison.

Loban's criteria for dealing with conjoined sentences. Two versions of each transcript were constructed using different length criteria. First, each transcript was cut at 100 complete and intelligible utterances. A second set of transcripts was cut at 12 minutes in duration. These two versions allow direct comparison between subjects for both frequency and rate variables. Two variables were analyzed on the 100 C&I utterance transcripts using SALT1, MLU in morphemes, and NDW. A third variable, NDW, was calculated with SALT1 on 12 minute, C&I utterance versions of the transcripts. Mean length of utterance and NDW required the same number of utterances to establish equivalency between subjects.

The results of the SALT1 analysis were sent to a data base for storage where the data could be formatted for statistical analysis. It was predicted that (1) each of these three variables would increase in frequency with increasing age, and (2) each of the variables would be significantly correlated with age in the conversation and narrative samples. The magnitude of each correlation with age would determine the potential usefulness of these variables for predicting productive language status in normal and disordered children.

ANALYSIS

The following analyses were run on the data using SPSSX on a VAXstation 2000 connected to the Waisman Center VAX Cluster.

1. Regression analyses, using each variable to predict age.
2. Multiple regression analyses for the conversational sample variables and the narrative samples independently where the three variables were added one at a time into the prediction equation to examine its influence on the composite equation.
3. Two multiple correlation analyses, one for the conversation and one for the narrative variables to document the relationship among each of the variables.

RESULTS

Tables 10-2 and 10-3 list the correlations and coefficient of determination (r^2) for the conversation and narrative samples. All three variables increase linearly with age and each is significantly correlated with age. The magnitude of the coefficients of determination are very high, particularly for the narrative sampling condition, indicating that each is capable of predicting age accounting for 49% to 78% of the variance. In order to explore the relationship among the variables and the degree to which they overlap

Table 10-2. Predicting age: Conversational samples

	r	r²
Mean length of utterance	.70	.49
Number of different words	.75	.57
Total number of words	.77	.59
Combined	.82	.68

Table 10.3. Predicting age: Narrative samples

	r	r²
Mean length of utterance	.80	.65
Number of different words	.80	.65
Total number of words	.86	.73
Combined	.88	.78

each other in predicting age, multiple regression analyses were run. Two multiple regression analyses were run, one for the conversational samples and one for the narrative samples, using age as the dependent variable. The results show an increase in the amount of variance accounted for by each variable individually when added in the following order, MLU, NDW, TNW. See Table 10-4 for the comprehension data and Table 10-5 for the narrative data. These data show that each variable contributes something independent to the prediction of age indicating that each variable is assessing something independent relative to productive language. If the order of variable entry into the prediction equation is reversed, we find that TDW and TNW account for all of the variance, MLU contributes nothing new. There appears to be considerable overlap between one or both of these variables and MLU. The pattern of the results of the analyses thus far is

Table 10-4. Multiple regression analysis of conversational samples

DEPENDENT VARIABLE:	CHRONOLOGICAL AGE		
Variables	r±2	*BETA*	*Change in r²*
Mean length of utterance (100 utterance samples)	.49	−.45736	—
Number of different words (100 utterance samples)	.57	.78643	.08*
Total number of words (12-minute samples)	.68	.52700	.11*

* = significant change, p = <.001

Table 10-5. Multiple regression analysis of narrative samples

Dependent Variable:	Chronological Age		
Variables	r^2	*BETA*	*Change in r^2*
Mean length of utterance (100 utterance samples)	.65	–.01197	—
Number of different words (100 utterance samples)	.68	.33638	.03*
Total number of words (12-minute samples)	.78	.58635	.10*

* = significant change, p = <.001

consistent for both the conversation and narrative data, although the magnitude of r^2 is higher for all of the narrative data.

In order to document the relationship between each of the variables in both speaking conditions, two multiple correlation analyses were calculated. The correlation matrix for the conversation and narrative data (Tables 10-6 and 10-7) indicate that each variable is significantly correlated with each other and age. The magnitude of these correlations ranges from r = .70 to .94 in conversation to r = .77 to .88. The ranking of these correlations is informative about their relative association. MLU and NDW have the highest correlations in both sampling conditions, conversation r = .94 and narration r = .89. The correlation between MLU and TNW in conversation is .77 and .84 in narration. The order of magnitude of the correlations between MLU and NDW and TNW is the same for both conversation and narration though the interval between them is quite different. In conversation, MLU has the highest correlation with NDW at .94 and the lowest with TNW at .77. In narration the correlation for MLU and NDW is .89 and TNW is .84. The correlation between NDW and TNW is consistent for both conversational and narrative samples at r = .76 in conversation and .77 in narration. There is a great deal more variation in the size of the correlations

Table 10-6. Correlation matrix conversational samples

	Chrono-logical Age	*Mean Length of Utterance*	*Number of Dif-ferent Words*	*Total Number of Words*
CA	—			
Mean length of utterance	.70	—		
Number of different words	.75	.94	—	
Total number of words	.77	.77	.76	—

Table 10-7. Correlation matrix narrative samples

	Chrono- logical Age	Mean Length of Utterance	Number of Dif- ferent Words	Total Number of Words
CA	—			
Mean length of utterance	.80	—		
Number of different words	.80	.89	—	
Total number of words	.86	.84	.77	

among all variables in conversation versus the narrative sampling condition. It appears that MLU and NDW overlap a great deal in what they measure with correlations of .89 and .94 compared to MLU and TNW with correlations of .77 and .84. While all of the correlations are extremely high, it is important to note that each variable measures something slightly different.

DISCUSSION

As predicted, each of these variables assess something slightly different about productive language, although clearly there is overlap among the measures. The multiple regression analysis reveals that NDW and TNW each add significantly to prediction equation for age. With all three variables added in the equation, MLU does not contribute to the prediction of age beyond the variance accounted for by TNW and NDW. NDW and TNW account for all of the variance in predicting age. This pattern is consistent in conversation and narration. It appears that MLU and NDW may be measuring some of the same characteristics of productive language performance. This is somewhat puzzling since age and MLU correlate highly with each other and NDW is the same for both conversation and narrative samples, MLU is significantly longer in the narrative samples. Apparently these variables change together across age.

INTERPRETATION

1. Each variable, MLU, NDW, and TNW, is significantly correlated with age. While each can be argued to assess something independent about productive language, a composite measure of NDW and TNW is the best predictor of age in both the conversation and narrative

sampling conditions.
2. Scaling the variables relative to their power in predicting age results in the following for conversation: r^2 = .49 MLU, .57 NDW, .59 TNW and for narration, r^2 = .65 MLU, .65 NDW, .73 TNW. The magnitude of the variance accounted for the correlations is uniformly higher in the narrative condition, suggesting that this condition is the best reflection of developmental change in general language skills through this period of development.
3. The consistency of each variable in predicting age in the narrative condition suggests that each may be informative about the general development of different aspects of language production.

The problem of differentiating different types of language disorders requires general developmental measures to document overall productive language performance. Such measures might be considered comparable to assumptions of adult competence used in characterizing loss of language function in adults due to brain injury or disease processes. That is, general measures such as NDW, TNW, and MLU provide an index of language performance prior to adult competence. These measures will provide the means to describe the relationship among linguistic levels at different points in development defined by semantic diversity (NDW), syntax (MLU), overall verbal productivity (TNW), or in combination. This strategy will provide the opportunity to document different patterns of development where progress in language development is slower than expected for chronological age. Explanations for lower than expected MLU might include specific structural description, as well as documentation of speech motor performance. Fewer different words than expected may be attributable to smaller vocabulary or retrieval problems. Fewer total words per unit time may be attributable to context, opportunity to talk, social-affective variables, or formulation deficits. Each of these conditions has a variety of potential explanations from lack of experience to storage deficits. Understanding the patterns of productive language will determine if there is a single cause or more than one causal construct. If different patterns of productive deficits exist then they might be most evident where nonverbal cognitive skill and language comprehension are asynchronous relative to each other and language production skills. The general measures of productive language development provide us with the tools to document different types of productive language disorders relative to language comprehension and nonverbal cognitive skills.

The three variables proposed in this chapter allow explanation of development or disordered performance to focus on specific aspects of language, semantic diversity, syntax or overall productivity rather than age. The details of language development can then be defined by relationship among variables documenting specific aspects of language performance relative to general development. These measures will provide opportunity to document different patterns of language disorders, if they exist, by quantifying "error" patterns in language production relative to developmental level of language performance.

A great deal of work remains to be done to validate the use of these measures to identify children with language disorders. The robust correlations of each of these measures of general language performance with age suggests they may play a leading role in developing the next generation of research studies investigating the character and explanation of language disorders in children.

REFERENCES

Hunt, K. (1965). *Grammatical structures written at three grade levels* (Res. Rep. No. 3). Urbana, IL: National Council of Teachers of English.

Johnston, J. (1988). Specific language disorders in the child. In N. Lass, L. McReynolds, J. Northern, & D. Yoder (Eds.), *The handbook of speech pathology*. Philadelphia: W. B. Saunders.

Kent, R. (1976). Anatomical and neuromuscular maturation of the speech mechanism: Evidence from acoustic studies. *Journal of Speech and Hearing Research, 19*, 421–445.

Kent, R. (1984). Psychobiology of speech development: Coemergence of language and a movement system. *American Journal of Physiology, 246*, 888–894.

Klee, T., Schaffer, M., May, S., Membrino, I., & Mougey, K. (1989). A comparison of the age-MLU relation in normal and specifically language impaired preschool children. *Journal of Speech and Hearing Disorders, 54*, 226–233.

Loban, W. (1976). *Language development: Kindergarten through grade twelve.* (Res. Rep. No. 18). Urbana, IL: National Council of Teachers of English.

Miller, J. (1981). *Assessing language production in children*. Baltimore: University Park Press.

Miller, J. (1986). SALT Reference Database. Unpublished paper, Language Analysis Laboratory, Waisman Center, University of Wisconsin–Madison.

Miller, J. (1987). A grammatical characterization of language disorder. In A. Martin, P. Fletcher, P. Grunewell, & D. Hall (Eds.), *First international symposium: Specific speech and language disorders in children* (pp. 100–114). London: AFASIC.

Miller, J., & Chapman, R. (1981). The relation between age and mean length of utterance in morphemes. *Journal of Speech and Hearing Research, 24*, 154–161.

Miller, J., & Chapman, R. (1982; 1983; 1984; 1985; 1986; & 1987). *SALT: Systematic Analysis of Language Transcripts (SALT)*: A computer program designed to analyze free speech samples—Apple II Version. Language Analysis Laboratory, Waisman Center, University of Wisconsin–Madison.

Morehead, D., & Ingram, D. (1973). The development of base syntax in normal and linguistically deviant children. *Journal of Speech and Hearing Research, 16*, 330–352.

SECTION   IV

Directions for Future Research

In this section, you will find a unique collection of 15 first person accounts of future directions for research on language disorders in children. The goal of this section was to characterize the changing foci of language disorders research from the broadest possible perspective. The authors included in this section have made significant contributions to the research literature through their work investigating specific populations, processes, language levels or methodology. The perspectives these investigators have for future research issues collectively define what we hope to learn about language disorders in the next ten years. Each chapter is a personal account by the author reflecting their own view of the future. Themes were not shared among contributors in advance. You will note, however, a number of commonalities among the chapters even where populations and developmental periods addressed are quite diverse. The need for careful description of populations and longitudinal research are prominent examples of these common themes. We should appreciate the diversity and uniqueness of each chapter as well as the similarities. Both consensus and diverse points of view will provoke new insight and understanding of the nature of language disorders and advance our ultimate goal of developing effective prevention and intervention methodologies.

Section IV is organized in general by functional topics but you will note several chapters defy the categorization employed. Perhaps this is a commentary about the field of language disorders. Our characterizations of disordered performance are part medical model, part process model, part etiological and part linguistic. After reading the chapters in this section I feel confident that the field will one day, emerge with a unique taxonomy contributing to both developmental theory and explanation of disordered language performance.

It is a privilege for me to share with you the vision for future research articulated by each of these authors. I believe you will find this section a unique mind expanding, consciousness raising, and perspective shaping cognitive experience.

PART A

Research Sources

CHAPTER 11

Research in Specific Language Impairment: A Federal Perspective

JUDITH A. COOPER

The prevention, understanding, and treatment of language disorders in children is frequently, as we assume it should be, an outgrowth of research investigations. Carefully designed investigations allow a scientific field to move forward; their absence encourages the field to stagnate in past achievements, in outdated or misguided philosophies and approaches. Research which challenges and at the same time expands current knowledge is the life-blood of a discipline.

The funding of research is a critical issue to scientists, as well as to administrators. Researchers in child-language disorders may look to their own departments, universities, private agencies, or to the federal government for this support. The purpose of this chapter is to discuss research support for child-language disorders, in particular, Specific Language Impairment (SLI), from the perspective of one federal funding agency, the National Institutes of Health (NIH). This chapter will focus on past funding and support trends in SLI, characteristics of supported research, and potential directions for research in SLI. Factors that have contributed to past and current levels of support should be of interest to those who are interested in seeking or seeing an increase in research support for SLI.

A few introductory comments are needed, to put the comments of this chapter into perspective. Historically, the NIH has encouraged and supported language research in several of its institutes. The majority of support for research into SLI has come from the Division of Communicative Disorders, of the National Institute of Neurological and Communicative Disorders and Stroke (NINCDS). This Division served as the focal point within the federal government for research in this disorder, from 1975 until October 1988, when the Division became a component of the National Institute on Deafness and Other Communication Disorders (NIDCD). Information presented in this chapter is based on data generated during the Division's "life" in NINCDS, as well as its beginnings in NIDCD.

RESEARCH SUPPORT IN SPECIFIC LANGUAGE IMPAIRMENT: FUNDING AND SUPPORT TRENDS

NIH INTEREST IN SLI

The question is often raised of NIH interest in a particular area of language research. In general, NIH "interest" in any topic originates with the research community, which identifies questions and issues ready to be addressed. Thus, the currently supported studies in SLI represent areas of concern or interest to language investigators, areas that scientists deemed worthy of investigation and for which strong, competitive proposals were developed.

A slight exception to this philosophy is the issuance of "program announcements," a vehicle whereby Institutes within the NIH identify areas in which more research would be welcomed, for reasons such as seemingly little activity in the area, minimal submissions to or support by the NIH in the area, or developments that necessitate prompt attention. In recent years, announcements related to child language disorders have been issued and have focused on such areas as the genetic basis of these disorders, language learning, and treatment. The issuance of these announcements has been associated with an increased number of applications, as well as increased funding, in these areas.

It is important to distinguish between Institute *interest* in a topic, and Institute *support* of a topic. Institute interest almost certainly extends beyond the research areas supported to include specific impaired groups, deficit profiles, and questions not currently under investigation. There may be interest, but an absence of current support because of either lack of or the noncompetitive quality of the grant applications.

FUNDING TRENDS IN SPECIFIC LANGUAGE IMPAIRMENT

Specific dollar support is *not* set aside or budgeted for SLI. What is spent on research is directly determined primarily by two factors: the number of high quality applications submitted, and the overall Institute budget.

Over the past ten years, the number of funded projects in SLI has slowly increased. As indicated in Figure 11-1, the first part of the last decade saw no more than one funded project per year, but this has increased recently. NIDCD FY88 support of research in SLI involved 12 grants, or 3% of all grants awarded for that year. Research dollars for FY88 totaled slightly over $1 million.

The fact that support has continued relatively unchanged over the past decade is due largely to the fact that there has been only a small increase in applications submitted during this period. As indicated in Figure 11-2, the

Fig. 11-1. Number of research projects in specific language impairment (1979–1988) funded by the National Institute of Neurological and Communicative Disorders and Stroke.

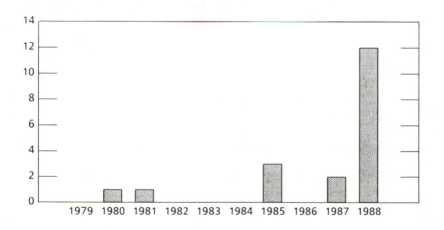

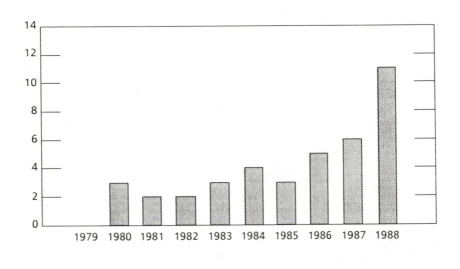

Fig. 11-2. Number of grant submissions in special language impairment (1979–1988) assigned to National Institute of Neurological and Communicative Disorders and Stroke.

number of applications submitted to the NIH that focused on some aspect of SLI has recently seen an upward swing. In the first part of the last 10 years, four or fewer applications in SLI were submitted each year. However, recent trends suggest that investigators are now looking in increasing numbers to the NIH for support. For example, in FY88, 11 applications in SLI were submitted. This increase is quite modest, when put into the context of other areas of speech, language, and hearing (e.g., the number of applications in speech and voice disorders average approximately 45 per year, and applications in more basic science areas well over 100 per year). Thus, with the relatively few number of submissions yearly, it is not surprising that the research support for SLI has not notably increased.

Why aren't more investigators whose research focuses on SLI looking to the NIH for funding? Several factors might be contributing to investigators seeking funding elsewhere.

- **Misconceptions about favoritism.** Many researchers perceive favoritism in the NIH and funding process. They believe the chances of someone "new" entering the system are quite remote and that once an investigator is funded, subsequent research inevitably will be accepted and funded. Often accompanying this belief is the perception that some institutions or individuals are judged by a different measure and have an edge over others who are less well known. Three bits of information are offered to refute these misperceptions: (1) Currently, the NIH offers a FIRST (First Independent Research Support and Transition) award for those newly independent investigators without extensive research experience or NIH-funded research. Clearly recipients of these awards are new to the "system," bringing with them fresh ideas and approaches. In addition, FIRST awards are funded at a higher rate than regular research grants. (2) In considering research grants in SLI supported in FY88, over 80% of the investigators are in some phase of their initial grant, suggestive that most have relatively young grants, and are in general new to NIH funding. (3) Investigators above and below 35 years tend to be funded at the same rate at the NIH, suggesting more senior investigators do *not* have a distinct advantage in the review process.

- **Competition**. The highly competitive nature of the review process may discourage some from submitting applications. Preparation of an application is quite time consuming and intellectually strenuous. This factor, in combination with investigator awareness of the rigorous review process and limited available funds, may discourage the young or even established investigator. Many applicants who fail to be funded initially do not re-enter the system. It is disappointing not to receive an award after months of preparation and waiting. Many, however, attempt to incorporate the written suggestions and criticisms of the review group in a revised application, thereby improving greatly their chances of funding.

- **Unfamiliarity with the system**. A naïveté regarding types of available awards, procedures for developing a strong proposal, and how one may approach program staff for advice often dissuade a potential applicant from applying.

- **Limited number of investigators**. One must certainly consider the possibility that the "critical mass" of investigators in SLI is relatively small compared to other disciplines, thereby placing somewhat of an automatic "cap" on the potential number of grant applications. The number of new investigators entering research is directly influenced by the availability of mentors and training sites that can provide a strong research foundation. The number of currently supported NIH training facilities in SLI is minimal. Increasing the number of research training facilities is critical to expanding the cadre of investigators. Without such facilities, the number of investigators with sufficient background to develop competitive grant proposals will remain limited.

CHARACTERISTICS OF SUPPORTED RESEARCH IN SPECIFIC LANGUAGE IMPAIRMENT

The research projects in SLI that are supported by NIDCD were judged to be outstanding by the initial review group responsible for their evaluation. These review groups considered such criteria as the scientific merit, the qualifications of the investigator, and the proposed design and data analysis in evaluating the merit of the research proposed. In considering the comments of the Initial Review Group regarding these applications, several factors appear to characterize them all:

- Research that has both theoretical and clinical significance
- Design appropriate for the questions proposed
- Well-detailed methodology
- Research that builds on the investigator's previous work

What commonalities can be identified in currently supported research in SLI? During FY88, 12 studies in SLI were supported. The areas of investigation, or the "themes" of research, included phonology, treatment, characteristics, and etiology. The specific foci of these projects, presented in Table 11-1, suggest that no one particular area of investigation is in danger of being saturated by federal support. Researchers are posing, and gaining acceptance for, a wide variety of questions related to SLI.

Regarding characteristics of the supported investigators in SLI, all 12 have a doctoral degree*. All but one of these investigators received their doctoral training in speech pathology/communication disorders/speech and hearing sciences and are currently associated with a university department in those disciplines.

---

*Although possession of a terminal degree is not a criterion for submission or award of an NIDCD research grant, outstanding research expertise or potential (often reflected in publications in peer-reviewed journals) and prior experience in directing pilot or small-scale research projects, is critical. These types of research "qualifications" do not tend to be characteristic of individuals with less advanced degrees.

Table 11-1. Focus of FY 1988 research in child language disorders

Phonological knowledge and learning patterns
The study of the neurological basis of language
Cognitive factors in specific language impairment
Speech processing in childhood language disorders
Predicting the benefits of language treatment
Learnability of sound systems
Morphological deficits in specific language impairment
Early identification of risk for language disorder
Language impaired children's fast mapping of new words
Rule learning problems in language-impaired children
Studies in developmental phonological disorders
Predicate acquisition by language-disordered children

A NEW INSTITUTE AND NEW DIRECTIONS IN SPECIFIC LANGUAGE IMPAIRMENT

Within the stated mandate of NIDCD is the "conduct and support of research and training with respect to diseases affecting . . . speech and language," with investigations into "the etiology, pathology, detection, treatment and prevention" of such disorders. In January 1989, a task force comprised of scientists from across the United States met to establish a research plan for the new Institute. Research priorities for SLI were identified, and include the following*:

- The relationship of the speech perception and speech production mechanism to language

- Acquisition of reading and writing skills in language-impaired children

- Development of typologies or subgroups

- Investigation of the underlying processes that subserve language development and disorders

- Language learning and processing strategies in language-impaired children in different language environments

*National Strategic Research Plan: National Institute on Deafness and Other Communication Disorders. Bethesda, MD: National Institutes of Health, March 1989.

- The relationship of language impairment and psychosocial disorders in children

- Documentation of the precise etiology or neurological dysfunction that underlies these disorders, and the mechanism by which the dysfunction occurs

- New intervention strategies based upon current theoretical models

By identifying these priority areas, the new Institute and the NIH make a strong statement to the research community. Research on this population and in these areas is of high priority. Researchers are thereby encouraged to look to the NIH for support and encouragement of such investigations. Although the identification of the aforementioned areas is a necessary first step in addressing critical needs in SLI, it is obvious that most of the subsequent steps must be taken by the research community. It is the responsibility of this community to identify and develop the most appropriate studies to address these research needs.

SUMMARY AND CONCLUSIONS

In summary, the small group of investigators in language disorders who are currently supported by the NIDCD are characterized by doctoral training (most often in Speech and Hearing Sciences or Speech-Language Pathology), association with universities, and a tendency toward holding relatively "new" NIH grants. The foci of their investigations span phonological, treatment, etiologic, and characterization topics.

The number of applications submitted to NIH in SLI has remained stable and small in the last decade. This stability in submission and thus in funding is of concern, as the amount of dollars spent in language disorders are related to the number of applications submitted. The solution is not to simply deluge the NIH with a large number of applications in the area. The applications must be competitive, well developed, and strong. If researchers in SLI wish to see increased support for this area, the issues of increasing the number and improving the quality of the applications must be considered.

The future of research in SLI lies in the training of the next generation of investigators: in fostering an interest in the area of those disorders, in developing critical thinking skills and writing in doctoral students, and in providing the experiences essential to creating well-trained, competitive researchers. Postdoctoral training experiences, such as extended training in the laboratories of established researchers, must become more commonplace with those interested in pursuing research careers that target SLI.

The breadth and number of questions that remain unanswered or unaddressed in SLI suggest a need for close collaboration from researchers from a variety of disciplines, such as psychology, linguistics, genetics, and medicine. The study of disordered language is a complex undertaking, and the future success of understanding of this disorder may rest in researchers' ability to draw upon the expertise of professionals with diverse training. There is a critical need for more collaborative and multidisciplinary research endeavors.

The child language research community has a potentially powerful effect on federally supported language research. It is a challenge which must be met, for the purpose of solidifying and expanding understanding, diagnosis, and treatment of specific language impairment.

PART   B

Intervention

CHAPTER 12

Child Language Intervention: Research Issues on the Horizon

SUSAN ELLIS WEISMER

In many ways, intervention research has been the stepchild of the study of child language disorders. Yet, it seems to provide the ultimate challenge in terms of testing our theoretical constructs of language learning and the nature of language disorders. In reviewing the papers presented at the Wisconsin Symposium on Research in Child Language Disorders, I discovered that only five investigations dealing with remediation topics had been presented at the conference since it began in 1980. Admittedly, various practical and methodological concerns may dissuade investigators from undertaking intervention research (refer to the discussion of methodological issues in Chapter 13 in this volume). However, renewed interest and enthusiasm in pursuing this area seem to be signalled by the First National Conference on Treatment Efficacy (March 1989) sponsored by the American Speech-Language-Hearing Foundation. Theoretical, methodological, and ethical issues relating to remediation were addressed at the conference and data-based investigations were presented on various aspects of treatment efficacy research including the area of child language.

Over the past 10 years or so, intervention research has provided us with tentative answers to many questions concerning the impact of remediation. During the next decade we need to fill in the gaps in our information in certain areas, refine our questions, and expand our efforts to new lines of inquiry. The following discussion is intended to clarify these general comments by focusing on selected topics concerning the particular language domains and processes that have been targeted for treatment, the effectiveness of various intervention approaches and training procedures, interactions between child characteristics and intervention methods, and treatment of older children and adolescents. My primary interest has been with children who are identified as having specific language impairment or language-learning disabilities; therefore, much of the discussion will be aimed at these children. I will not address specific research issues pertaining to the treatment of children with hearing impairment, phonological disorders, or those who use augmentative communication systems.

LANGUAGE DOMAINS AND PROCESSES TARGETED FOR TREATMENT

With a few exceptions, studies have demonstrated that language intervention is effective in facilitating changes in language behavior and in affecting linguistic rule-learning (see reviews by Arnold, Myette & Casto, 1986; Leonard, 1981; Nye, Foster & Seaman, 1987). With respect to the domains of language functioning that have been examined, the majority of investigations to date have focused on training grammatical aspects of language (see review by Byrne Saricks, 1987). Although there are some studies directed at lexical training and the training of semantic roles (Connell, 1986a; Leonard et al., 1982), these areas of language functioning are still relatively underrepresented in treatment research. There are only a handful of intervention studies that have focused on pragmatic abilities (Conant, Budoff, Hecht & Morse, 1984; Olswang, Kriegsmann & Mastergeorge, 1982). The scarcity of pragmatic intervention research no doubt reflects the need for more elaborated theoretical frameworks and refined methodologies for measuring skills in this area.

Language comprehension processes have been a neglected area in intervention research. The vast majority of treatment studies have been solely concerned with productive language abilities (see review by Byrne Saricks, 1987). Perhaps it is time to re-evaluate the implicit assumption made by most interventionists that the most effective means of modifying children's linguistic knowledge is to ensure that they can produce the target form. Various investigators have explored the interaction between language processes by examining the impact of comprehension training on expressive language skills and/or the effects of productive language training on comprehension (Connell, 1986a; Cuvo & Riva, 1980; Ezell & Goldstein, 1989). This is a line of inquiry that future investigations might profitably pursue, as many issues remain unresolved. Similarly, there is a need for more research focusing on the complex interplay between various linguistic domains and the effect that intervention in one area of language functioning has on other areas (for example, the impact of phonological training on syntactic skills). Such information could provide insights into the nature of language-disordered children's linguistic knowledge and bear on the issue of efficiency of training.

INTERVENTION
APPROACHES AND TRAINING PROCEDURES

A variety of intervention approaches have been demonstrated to improve language disordered children's performance, such as operant approaches, direct instruction, milieu training, and interactive approaches (see reviews by Cole & Dale, 1986; Connell, 1987; Warren & Kaiser, 1986). Likewise, a number of different training procedures have been found to be effective, including imitation (Connell, 1986b; Hegde, 1980; Rogers-Warren & Warren, 1980), modeling (Courtwright & Courtwright, 1976, 1979; Leonard, 1975; Wilcox & Leonard, 1978), and modeling plus an evoked production of the target (Culatta & Horn, 1982; Ellis Weismer & Murray-Branch, 1989; Leonard et al., 1982). Investigations demonstrating the effectiveness of treatment based on script theory (Constable, 1986) and discourse structuring techniques (Schwartz, Chapman, Terrell, Prelock & Rowan, 1985) also seem to offer interventionists promising alternative methods of language training.

At this time, the bulk of experimental evidence does not clearly support the use of one approach or training procedure over another. Findings from the few studies that have directly compared intervention methods have not been particularly illuminating. Most of these investigations have contrasted treatment methods based on distinct theoretical frameworks. I have discussed the problems that arise in interpreting the results of such investigations elsewhere (see Ellis Weismer & Murray-Branch, 1989). Briefly, it is difficult to determine which dimensions of the training situation affected performance when global treatment approaches or entire intervention programs are compared (e.g., Cole & Dale, 1986). On the other hand, studies comparing specific training procedures, such as imitation versus modeling, have often employed these procedures in ways that are not consistent with the overall intervention approach in which these techniques are typically embedded (e.g., Courtwright & Courtwright, 1976, 1979). Perhaps a more productive approach would be to pursue the question of the "most effective" training method from within one's own theoretical framework. For example, we might ask which of the various training procedures that are consonant with a given view of the language learning process and the nature of language disorders are most facilitating for particular linguistic features or specific children. What seems most important is not *which* theoretical model is adopted, but that a coherent conceptual framework is consistently employed to guide intervention efforts and related research questions.

An emerging area of inquiry in treatment research pertains to computer-based remediation procedures. Various researchers have recommended guidelines for microcomputer applications in language intervention (Larson & Steiner, 1985; Miller & Marriner, 1986). However, few studies have actually assessed the effectiveness of microcomputer programs. One study by O'Connor and Schery (1986) compared traditional language therapy to computer-aided intervention using the Program for Early Acquisition of Language (PEAL) (Meyers, 1985). Both programs were effective, but no significant difference between the treatments was found. More investigations of this type are needed to determine whether specific computer-based approaches offer unique motivational and learning benefits that justify their cost. Additionally, the use of computer-based programs utilizing synthesized speech should be carefully considered (see the discussion by Ellis Weismer, 1989, regarding the KEYTALK program by Meyers, 1988). A recent study by Massey (1988) indicates that we may need to be cautious about using synthesized speech as linguistic input with language-disordered children. A closer look at this issue is definitely warranted.

INTERACTION BETWEEN CHILD CHARACTERISTICS AND INTERVENTION METHODS

A number of studies have investigated the relationship between particular subject characteristics and language intervention efficacy (refer to Arnold et al., 1986: Nye et al., 1987). For example, the findings of Olswang and her colleagues (Olswang & Coggins, 1984; Olswang, Bain, Rosendahl, Oblak & Smith, 1986) indicate the importance of providing treatment at a point in time when the child demonstrates optimal readiness for learning. There is very little research, however, that has focused on child variables that may impact upon the *relative* effectiveness of various language treatment approaches. Response to different training methods may interact with certain characteristics of the child, such as cognitive or information processing skills, level of linguistic development, relationship between comprehension and production abilities, readiness to acquire the target form, learning history, or learning style. A few studies have explored some of these factors, including aptitude by treatment interactions (Cole & Dale, 1986; Friedman & Friedman, 1980) and linguistic facility by treatment interactions (Connell, 1987). This seems to be an especially important line of research to pursue since it could ultimately help us predict which intervention approaches or methods are more likely to be successful with particular children.

Another approach to the issue of interactions between intervention methods and child variables might be taken. We could consider the characteristics of the language-disordered children who are the focus of our programming efforts and then adapt training techniques in light of what we know about how they process information. By testing the effectiveness of these specially adapted approaches, we could draw inferences about the accuracy of our initial assumptions regarding child characteristics and gain information that would have direct clinical import.

There is evidence that children with specific language impairment may have attentional deficits and perceptional deficiencies that affect their ability to process brief, rapidly sequenced auditory (and visual) events (see review by Johnston, 1988b). The role that these presumed deficits may play in the language disorder is unclear. What is obvious is that language-disordered children have failed to identify the rules governing language by inducing the patterns in the linguistic signal in the normal way. Therefore, in order for intervention strategies to actually be therapeutic, they should include special considerations in terms of the linguistic input that is provided. Various modifications of the linguistic input have been suggested, including reduced rate of speech, increased pause length, exaggerated vocal stress, positioning of the target at the beginning or end of the utterance, and use of nonauditory cues (such as visual symbols or manual signing) paired with oral language input (see Ellis Weismer, 1988; Lahey, 1988). It is assumed that these modifications may facilitate segmentation of the speech signal and/or heighten the perceptual saliency of the target, thereby reducing processing demands and allowing the child to allocate more attention to the discovery of the linguistic rule.

Although several treatment studies have incorporated certain of these linguistic input modifications (Constable, 1986; Culatta and Horn, 1982), there are only a few investigations that have attempted to assess directly the impact of such modifications on language-disordered children's linguistic performance (Campbell & McNeil, 1985; Liles, Cooker, Kass & Carey, 1978; McCroskey & Thompson, 1973; Romski & Ruder, 1984). I am currently conducting a study exploring the effects of linguistic input modifications on the ability of preschoolers with specific language impairment to learn invented vocabulary and morphological markers. The variables being examined include vocal stress, rate of speech, and visual cues (i.e., gestures) accompanying spoken language. Hopefully, this line of research will lead to insights about the ways in which interventionists can optimize the match between language-disordered children's processing capabilities and the input they receive.

TREATMENT OF OLDER CHILDREN AND ADOLESCENTS

Thus far, most treatment research has centered on relatively young children. There is considerable evidence that a substantial number of language-disordered preschoolers go on to exhibit language problems (in both oral and written language skills) during the school years and because of the academic difficulties that these children encounter they are often identified as having languag-learning disabilities (see review by Johnston, 1988b). As we acquire more knowledge about normal linguistic developments in older children and adolescents (refer to Nippold, 1988) and expand our remediation efforts to individuals in the upper grades, intervention research in this area must keep pace. For instance, even though a number of studies have focused on treatment of early-developing forms such as the copula and auxiliary *be* (Connell, 1986b; Culatta & Horn, 1982; Hegde, 1980; Hegde, Noll, & Pecora, 1979), there is very little information available regarding remediation of more advanced syntactic features of language such as those detailed by Scott (1988). Another critical area for future research with older language-disordered children concerns the facilitation of metalinguistic skills such as the comprehension monitoring program reported by Dollaghan and Kaston (1986). Investigations exploring the impact that training in metalinguistic abilities may have on literacy (see Van Kleek & Schuele, 1987) could prove to be extremely useful. Finally, research is needed to examine the effectiveness of approaches that involve the teaching of strategies for learning (refer to Buttrill, Niizawa, Biemer, Takahashi & Hearn, 1989; Larson & McKinley, 1987) and contextually based intervention approaches (see Miller, 1989; Norris, 1989).

CONCLUDING COMMENTS

In this limited discussion, I have touched on selected issues in intervention research that are of particular interest to me. I would be remiss not to at least mention several important topics that have not been addressed. One of these areas concerns generalization of training effects. Differing views concerning the nature of generalization clearly impact upon how we define and measure it (see the thought-provoking exchange among Connell, 1988; Fey, 1988; Johnston, 1988a; Kamhi, 1988; & Warren, 1988). Another area that was not considered relates to indirect service delivery models. The effectiveness and cost-efficiency of parent programs and consultative roles for speech-language clinicians warrants further examination. Neither of these topics is easily investigated, but both have far-reaching implications.

Regardless of the specific treatment topics being addressed, some basic questions might be used to guide our investigations as we look forward to the challenges of language-intervention research in the next decade. These include (1) how will the study advance our information regarding the nature of language-disordered children's linguistic knowledge and communications skills?; (2) will the study help us understand the processes involved in learning language and provide insights about the differences that may exist between language-disordered and non-language-disordered children?; and (3) what clinical impact will the investigation have with respect to our programming efforts?

REFERENCES

Arnold, K., Myette, B., & Casto, G. (1986). Relationship of language intervention efficacy to certain subject characteristics in mentally retarded preschool children: A meta-analysis. *Education and Training of the Mentally Retarded, 21*, 108–116.

Buttrill, J., Niizawa, J., Biemer, C., Takahashi, C., & Hearn, S. (1989). Serving the language learning disabled adolescent: A strategies-based model. *Language, Speech, and Hearing Services in Schools, 20*, 185–204.

Byrne Saricks, M. (1987). Treatment of language disorders in children: A review of experimental studies. In H. Winitz (Ed.), *Human communication and its disorders* (pp. 167–201). Norwood, NJ: Ablex.

Campbell, T., & McNeil, M. (1985). Effects of presentation rate and divided attention on auditory comprehension in children with an acquired language disorder. *Journal of Speech and Hearing Research, 28*, 513–520.

Cole, K., & Dale, P. (1986). Direct language instruction and interactive language instruction with language delayed preschool children: A comparison study. *Journal of Speech and Hearing Research, 29*, 206–217.

Conant, S., Budoff, M., Hecht, B., & Morse, R. (1984). Language intervention: A pragmatic approach. *Journal of Autism and Development Disorders, 14*, 301–317.

Connell, P. (1986a). Acquisition of semantic role by language-disordered children: Differences between production and comprehension training. *Journal of Speech and Hearing Research, 29*, 366–374.

Connell, P. (1986b). Teaching subjecthood to language-disordered children. *Journal of Speech and Hearing Research, 29*, 481–492.

Connell, P. (1987). An effect of modeling and imitation teaching procedures on children with and without specific language impairment. *Journal of Speech and Hearing Research, 30*, 105–113.

Connell, P. (1988). Induction, generalization and deduction: Models for defining language generalization. *Language, Speech, and Hearing Services in Schools, 19*, 282–291.

Constable, C. (1986). The application of scripts in the organization of language intervention contexts. In K. Nelson (Ed.), *Event knowledge: Structure and function in development* (pp. 205–230). Hillsdale, NJ: Erlbaum.

Courtright, J., & Courtright, I. (1976). Imitative modelling as a theoretical base for instructing language disordered children. *Journal of Speech and Hearing Research, 19*, 655–663.

Courtright, J., & Courtright, I. (1979). Imitative modelling as a language intervention strategy: The effects of two mediating variables. *Journal of Speech and Hearing Research, 22,* 389–402.

Culatta, B., & Horn, D. (1982). A program for achieving generalization of grammatical rules to spontaneous discourse. *Journal of Speech and Hearing Research, 47,* 174–180.

Cuvo, A., & Riva, M. (1980). Generalization and transfer between comprehension and production: A comparison of retarded and nonretarded persons. *Journal of Applied Behavior Analysis, 13,* 315–331.

Dollaghan, C., & Kaston, N. (1986). A comprehension monitoring program for language-impaired children. *Journal of Speech and Hearing Research, 51,* 264–271.

Ellis Weismer, S. (1988). Specific language learning problems. In D. E. Yoder and R. D. Kent (Eds.), *Decision-making in speech-language pathology* (pp. 42–43), Philadelphia: B. C. Decker.

Ellis Weismer, S. (1989). Computer applications: KEYTALK review. *Child Language Teaching and Therapy, 5,* 221–228.

Ellis Weismer, S., & Murray-Branch, J. (1989). Modeling versus modeling plus evoked production training: A comparison of two language intervention methods. *Journal of Speech and Hearing Research, 54,* 269–281.

Ezell, H., & Goldstein, H. (1989). Effects of imitation on language comprehension and transfer to production in children with mental retardation. *Journal of Speech and Hearing Disorders, 54,* 49–56.

Fey, M. (1988). Generalization issues facing language interventionists: An introduction. *Language, Speech, and Hearing Services in Schools, 19,* 272–281.

Friedman, P., & Friedman, K. (1980). Accounting for individual differences when comparing the effectiveness of remedial language teaching methods. *Applied Psycholinguistics, 1,* 151–170.

Hegde, M. (1980). An experimental-clinical analysis of grammatical and behavioral distinctions between verbal auxiliary and copula. *Journal of Speech and Hearing Research, 23,* 864–877.

Hegde, M., Noll, M., & Pecora, R. (1979). A study of some factors affecting generalization of language training. *Journal of Speech and Hearing Disorders, 44,* 301–320.

Johnston, J. (1988a). Generalization: The nature of change. *Language, Speech, and Hearing Services in Schools, 19,* 314–329.

Johnston, J. (1988b). Specific language disorders in the child. In N. Lass, L. McReynolds, J. Northern, & D. Yoder (Eds.), *Handbook of speech-language pathology and audiology* (pp. 685–715). Philadelphia: B. C. Decker.

Kamhi, A. (1988). A reconceptualization of generalization and generalization problems. *Language, Speech, and Hearing Services in Schools, 19,* 304–313.

Lahey, M. (1988). *Language disorders and language development.* New York: Macmillan.

Larson, V., & McKinley, N. (1987). *Communication assessment and intervention strategies for adolescents.* Eau Claire, WI: Thinking Publications.

Larson, V., & Steiner, S. (1985). Language intervention using microcomputers. *Topics in Language Disorders, 6,* 41–55.

Leonard, L. (1975). Modeling as a clinical procedure in language training. *Language, Speech, and Hearing Services in Schools, 6,* 72–85.

Leonard, L. (1981). Facilitating linguistic skills in children with specific language impairment. *Applied Psycholinguistics, 2,* 89–118.

Leonard, L., Schwartz, R., Chapman, K., Rowan, L., Prelock, P., Terrell, B., Weiss, A., & Messick, C. (1982). Early lexical acquisition in children with specific language impairment. *Journal of Speech and Hearing Research, 25,* 554–564.

Liles, B., Cooker, H., Kass, M., & Carey, B. (1978). The effects of pause time on auditory comprehension of language disordered children. *Journal of Communication Disorders, 11*, 365–374.

Massey, H. (1988). Language-impaired childrens' comprehension of synthesized speech. *Language, Speech, and Hearing Services in Schools, 19*, 401–409.

McCroskey, R., & Thompson, N. (1973). Comprehension of rate controlled speech by children with specific learning disabilities. *Journal of Learning Disabilities, 6*, 621–628.

Meyers, L. (1985). *Programs for early acquisition of language* (Computer program). Los Angeles: PEAL Software.

Meyers, L. (1988). *KEYTALK* (Computer program). Calabasas, CA: PEAL Software.

Miller, J., & Marriner, N. (1986). Language intervention software: Myth or reality. *Child Language Teaching and Therapy, 2*, 85–95.

Miller, L. (1989). Classroom-based language intervention. *Language, Speech, and Hearing Services in Schools, 20*, 153–169.

Nippold, M. (Ed.) (1988). *Later language development: Ages nine through nineteen.* Austin, TX: PRO-ED.

Norris, J. (1989). Providing language remediation in the classroom: An integrated language-to-reading intervention method. *Language, Speech, and Hearing Services in Schools, 20*, 205–218.

Nye, C., Foster, S., & Seaman, D. (1987). Effectiveness of language intervention with the language/learning disabled. *Journal of Speech and Hearing Disorders, 52*, 348–357.

O'Connor, L., & Schery, T. (1986). A comparison of microcomputer-aided and traditional language therapy for developing communication skills in normal toddlers. *Journal of Speech and Hearing Disorders, 51*, 356–361.

Olswang, L., Bain, B., Rosendahl, P., Oblak, S., & Smith, A. (1986). Language learning: Moving performance from a context dependent to independent state. *Child Language Teaching and Therapy, 2*, 180–210.

Olswang, L., & Coggins, T. (1984). The effects of adult behaviors on increasing language delayed children's production of early relational meanings. *British Journal of Disorders of Communication, 19*, 15–34.

Olswang, L., Kriegsmann, E., & Mastergeorge, A. (1982). Facilitating functional requesting in pragmatically impaired children. *Language, Speech, and Hearing Services in Schools, 13*, 202–222.

Rogers-Warren, A., & Warren, S. (1980). Mands for verbalization: Facilitating the display of newly-taught language. *Behavior Modification, 4*, 361–382.

Romski, M., & Ruder, K. (1984). Effects of speech and speech and sign instruction on oral language learning and generalization of action + object combinations by Down's Syndrome children. *Journal of Speech and Hearing Disorders, 49*, 293–302.

Schwartz, R., Chapman, K., Terrell, B., Prelock, P., & Rowan, L. (1985). Facilitating word combination in language-impaired children in discourse structure. *Journal of Speech and Hearing Disorders, 50*, 31–39.

Scott, C. (1988). Spoken and written syntax. In M. Nippold (Ed.), *Later language development: Ages nine through nineteen* (pp. 49–95). Austin, TX: PRO-ED.

Van Kleek, A., & Schuele, C. (1987). Precursors to literacy: Normal development. *Topics in Language Disorders, 7*, 13–31.

Warren, S. (1988). A behavioral approach to language generalization. *Language, Speech, and Hearing Services in Schools, 19*, 292–303.

Warren, S., & Kaiser, A. (1986). Incidental language teaching: A critical review. *Journal of Speech and Hearing Disorders, 51*, 291–298.

Wilcox, M., & Leonard, L. (1978). Experimental acquisition of wh-questions in language-disordered children. *Journal of Speech and Hearing Research, 21*, 220–239.

CHAPTER 13

Needed: Intervention Research

DELORES KLUPPEL VETTER

Until investigation of intervention efficacy with language-disordered children becomes a research priority, potential clients and third-party providers of clinical services will severely call into question the bases of professional intervention (Vetter, 1985). It is not acceptable to the client (or the insurance company) to say, "Trust me. This therapy makes good sense from what I know about normal language development and language disorders. Come to see me for an hour twice a week. I charge $75 an hour. I am sure that in a couple of years, I will have helped you with your language disorder." There is a responsibility to children with language disorders and a responsibility to the public at large to know that what is being done is effective. There is a need to provide evidence to third-party providers that, in addition to the many investigations substantiating the diagnosis of language deficits, research has also documented successful intervention procedures for such deficits. Provision of services for children with language disorders should be based on sound data, should be humane, and should be offered in a cost-effective way to contribute to the quality of the child's life and to society as a whole.

WHY IS INTERVENTION RESEARCH NOT BEING DONE?

A variety of arguments are given by those concerned with language disorders regarding the lack of active investigation into the efficacy of intervention procedures. Such research is costly in terms of time, energy, and money. Fey (1986) and Larson and McKinley (1987) indicate that remediation of language disorders is a lengthy process regardless of whether the child is a preschooler or an adolescent. It is not surprising, then, that studies of intervention efficacy are usually not undertaken for dissertations, nor are they often pursued by academicians seeking tenure, since both of these cases have substantial pressures of time and money. A brief review of the work of academicians interested in child language indicates that by the time tenure has been achieved these researchers are likely to have developed programmatic investigations in one of two areas: the theory of normal language acquisition, or the nature and assessment of language disorders. After such programmatic research has been developed, investigators are less likely to change research focus toward intervention efficacy.

THEORY-DRIVEN INTERVENTION PROGRAMS

Because theories of language acquisition and information on the nature of language disorders are significant, and because more extensive data have been collected in these areas, researchers have, perhaps inadvertently, encouraged the notion of an etiology-based model for intervention. A tacit premise here is that if the nature of normal child language and child-language disorders are understood, the appropriate remediation will be obvious. Given the orientation that intervention has taken over the past twenty-five years, it is clear that as various theories, models, and descriptions of language development have appeared in the literature, the focus of intervention has followed. McLean (1983) provides a general historical summary of the content of language-training programs, but there are also specific instances that should be noted. After Chomsky's book on generative grammar was published (Chomsky, 1965), programs for teaching syntax were developed for use with language-disordered children (Miller & Yoder, 1972). When meaning and context were stressed (Bloom, 1970, 1973), these factors were incorporated into remediation procedures (Miller & Yoder, 1974). Accordingly, books describing the acquisition of pragmatics (Bates, 1976) and children's discourse (Ervin-Tripp & Mitchell-Kernan, 1977) exerted their influences on intervention procedures (Constable, 1983; Craig, 1983). This rapid incorporation of theory and data into intervention procedures indicates that many share Siegel and Spradlin's (1985) belief that "therapy is most useful when it organizes and integrates research-produced knowledge with knowledge drawn from other sources into a comprehensive therapeutic program that effects a positive change in the behavior of the client" (p. 227). Unfortunately Siegel and Spradlin, and others with similar beliefs, do not state that it is necessary to determine if a positive change occurs and, when it occurs, to determine that it is a result of the intervention procedures employed. Siegel (1987), in fact, categorizes investigations of therapy under "Wasteful Uses of Science " (p. 309) and continues to state that studies of intervention effectiveness are not proper questions for science.

The lack of research on intervention efficacy also is a function of the influence of publications questioning who is competent to do research and whether or not the efficacy of intervention should be studied. Speech-language clinicians are likely to have the most investment in the remediation of children with language disorders. When asked, clinicians give several reasons for not investigating intervention effectiveness, but the first is usually that they are not qualified to conduct research. This is unfortunate as the clinician is in a unique position to study the effectiveness of treatment. Often clinicians have a traditional, rigid idea of what constitutes research. Good research, however, relies more upon being able to frame a clear, answerable question with a known research hypothesis (Carver, 1978; Underwood, 1957) than on being able to conceptualize a design that yields a five-way interaction or to prepare a datafile for a computer to use in calculating multivariate statistics. Certainly university training programs must teach their graduate students how to think logically and to formulate questions that are both relevant to the clinical enterprise and answerable (Kent, 1983; Wiley, 1988). Speech-language pathologists, however, appear to have been more influenced by authors seriously questioning their competency to conduct clinical research (Jerger, 1963; Siegel & Spradlin, 1985). Unfortunately those publications in which the speech and language pathologist's knowledge and experience have been seen as providing unique qualifications for asking significant intervention questions have not been persuasive (Bloom & Fischer, 1982; McReynolds and Kearns, 1983; Ringel, 1972; Vetter, 1985). Another response given by speech-language pathologists is that they cannot conduct studies of intervention because they are concerned with the ethics of presenting exactly the same stimulus from child to child and expecting the same response, or they are concerned about withdrawal or reversal of treatment within a study. They appear to have conceptualized intervention research as requiring a remediation procedure that is represented by a most simplistic stimulus-response-reinforcement sequence. The variety and flexibility of designs available for conducting intervention research, whether single-subject or group studies, have not been seen as viable alternatives. In contrast, clinical psychologists have proposed procedures for treatment evaluation that are appropriate for the client populations they serve (Bloom & Fischer, 1982). Bedrosian's study (1981) with mentally retarded adults provides an example of complex procedures used in the remediation of certain pragmatic disorders.

INTERVENTION RESEARCH: METHODOLOGICAL ISSUES

In addition to the problem of motivating people to conduct investigations of intervention efficacy, the next decade must see responses being developed to methodological concerns. Levin (1985) has written comprehensively of methodological and statistical "bugs" often found in psychological research and in studies of children's learning in particular. Although all of Levin's "bugs" should be of concern to those conducting research, there are several whose resolution may be the most salient for future investigations of intervention efficacy.

HETEROGENEITY AND SAMPLE SIZE

Probably the most frequently stated concern about conducting research with language-disordered children is that the subjects are so heterogeneous that they can never be combined into a single group. This would not be a methodological concern if researchers used reasonable and explicit boundaries for the definition of the population they wish to study and if sample sizes were large. Most studies of child language are conducted on very small samples. The fact is, however, that if the number of subjects were large, language-disordered children should not necessarily be any more variable than are children who are selected for the control (normal) group. Nor should comparisons between two large groups, randomly selected from the same population of language-disordered children, necessarily yield heterogeneous variances. Researchers have tended to express a set of circular arguments where sample size is concerned. They initially state that language-disordered children are too heterogeneous for them to find sufficient numbers. Then they state that sample size is small because the group is heterogeneous. Confirmation of the belief in the heterogeneity of language-disordered children is derived from the notion that normal control subjects yield a single estimate of performance, the mean of the group. Available information, both from conferences and current literature, indicates that the relation between the mean and variance is irrelevant to some researchers, since the mean is discussed without reference to the variability of the distribution. This tends to reinforce the notion of the performance of children with normal language yielding a point distribution (rather than a distribution best described by a mean and variance). Consequently, normal performance is perceived as being substantially less variable than it is in reality.

SUBJECT MATCHING

One misdirected attempt to deal with the concern of heterogeneity has been to match subjects in the experimental group with normal controls on as many factors as possible: for example, gender, nonverbal intelligence test scores, and language age. Typically, this yields a normal control group that is chronologically younger and socially less experienced than the language-disordered children. In addition to whatever bias this selection process has contributed to the data, the researcher has likely violated two assumptions of parametric inferential statistics: random selection of subjects and a normal distribution (Eisenhart, 1947; Kirk, 1982). The nonnormal distribution might not pose a problem if the hypotheses could be tested through the use of nonparametric statistics (Siegel, 1956), but the violation of random sampling inherent in a matching process makes the interpretation of both parametric and nonparametric statistics questionable at best (Campbell & Stanley, 1963; Kirk, 1982). Thus, the use of matched subjects introduces a "bug" (Levin, 1985) and is not a solution to the problem of heterogeneity.

SINGLE-SUBJECT DESIGNS

Another suggestion for handling heterogeneity in small samples has been to use single-subject designs (Bloom & Fischer, 1982; McReynolds & Kearns, 1983; Vetter, 1985). Certainly single-subject designs, particularly multiple-baseline or multiple-target designs, lend themselves to the study of the unique case receiving treatment. In the final analysis, however, it will be necessary for those interested in remediating children's language disorders to demonstrate that the techniques and procedures they have employed are generalizable beyond the single case. Considerations for conducting single-subject or group design replications will have to be made by the researcher (Carver, 1978; Hersen & Barlow, 1976; Milliken & Johnson, 1984; Vetter, 1985).

PRACTICAL VERSUS STATISTICAL SIGNIFICANCE

Finally there is the issue of how intervention efficacy is determined. Or, stated differently, how does one measure change? And, how much change must there be before it can be concluded that the intervention procedure is effective? Speech-language pathologists involved in remediation of language disorders routinely determine when changes in behavior are relevant. Many researchers in education and psychology, however, have been unable or unwilling to specify the magnitude of the difference in effect size that is interesting, important, or clinically meaningful. Instead, they rely on the use of statistical tests of significance to determine when differences are important (Carver, 1978; Stevens, 1968). This particular use of tests of significance is not appropriate, and in fact, may lead to erroneous conclusions by researchers. When specific predictions are made and the hypotheses are tested, the power of the statistical test is invariably increased (Cohen, 1977). It is critical for those studying intervention efficacy, as well as those with other interests in child language, to give prior thought to effect size (Levin, 1985). Since tests of significance are frequently not used with single-subject designs, they might appear to be the method of choice for those unwilling to specify the magnitude required for a meaningful effect; however, those designs *also* require thought about effect size before the data are inspected (Bloom & Fischer, 1982; McReynolds & Kearns, 1983; Parsonson & Baer, 1978).

MISUSES OF STANDARDIZED TESTS

Often, the measure of intervention efficacy has been performance of language-disordered children on a standardized test. There are several methodological concerns associated with the use of this type of measure. Most standardized tests of language comprehension and production have not included children with language disorders in their standardization sample. In fact, the children appear to be supernormal. If the characteristics of the standardization sample are evaluated, the children frequently score 100 or above on an intelligence test, they have never had any special educational support, nor have they been treated for *otitis media*. When children with language disorders are given a test with this kind of standardization sample, it is not possible to know if the test will measure the same ability as it measured in the supernormal standardization sample. Is poor performance on the test a result of the language deficit, or is the test measuring some other characteristic of the language-disordered child? For example, it would be considered scandalous, and perhaps unethical, to test a child with a visual impairment using an oral language comprehension test with visual stimuli. Yet such tests frequently are administered to children with language disorders. The assumption is that the test results are valid even though we have no information about the child's test-taking skills or visual-processing abilities. It is essential that those constructing tests of language performance select appropriate standardization samples for the population for whom the test is intended. It is also imperative that those administering such tests use only those tests for whom their client could have been a member of the standardization sample (American Psychological Association, 1985).

Other concerns about the use of standardization tests in determining change due to intervention have been discussed by McCauley and Swisher (1984). Specifically, they have discussed potential misuses and misinterpretations of performance on norm-referenced standardized tests. Unfortunately some researchers have not heeded the information in that article, and in those cases, it often is not possible to differentiate treatment from subject effects based on norms.

EDUMETRICALLY SOUND MEASURES

One issue raised by McCauley and Swisher (1984) that must be emphasized is the need for criterion-referenced tests. Most currently available standardized tests of language comprehension or production have been constructed as norm-referenced tests. They have not been constructed for the purpose of evaluating remediation procedures, and they are not appropriate for such use. A better choice would be to use criterion-referenced tests. Unfortunately there are few, if any, criterion-referenced tests available to assess comprehension and production in children with language disorders. These tests, similar to achievement tests, would be constructed to reflect the array of knowledge and ability the child has in a specific domain, and they would sample widely at each level of difficulty or development. Performance on criterion-referenced tests, or other tests constructed to meet edumetric criteria (Carver, 1974), would provide information about an individual's level of functioning relative to the domain to be mastered, rather than to the average scores of others at given ages or grades. There is ample data available for the development of such tests. If investigations of intervention efficacy are carried out, tests meeting standards on the edumetric dimension will be valuable.

Bloom and Fischer (1982) suggest a number of other ways to measure change due to intervention, for example, quantification of clinical judgments, rating scales for use by judges, and self-rating scales. However, there has been little effort placed on the development of these other techniques for measuring change in behaviors related to language performance. Yet, these measures, in conjunction with performance on criterion-referenced tests, would provide cross-validation of the data obtained in any study of intervention efficacy.

WHAT MUST BE DONE

There are no unresolvable problems facing investigators interested in the efficacy of intervention applied to children with language disorders. On a number of occasions the argument has been presented urging research investigating clinical efficacy (Bloom & Fischer, 1982; McReynolds & Kearns, 1983; Vetter, 1985). The initial step toward acquiring data on intervention procedures requires a shift in primary focus of investigators and a change in attitude by speech-language clinicians toward conducting research. If efficacy data become a priority for professionals interested in children with language disorders, modulations in interests and attitudes will follow.

If allowed, most of the general methodological problems found in child-language research would plague studies of intervention procedures. These problems can largely be resolved through the use of appropriate experimental designs (Levin, 1985). Because of the potential overreliance on statistical tests, thought must be given to the instruments and measures used to document children's performance and to the development of hypotheses that predict the direction and magnitude of the expected change.

Numerous intervention procedures exist for use with language-disordered children. Speech-language clinicians have been intervening with children who present language disorders for many years. The time has come to establish the effectiveness of the intervention.

REFERENCES

American Psychological Association. (1985). *Standards for Educational and Psychological Tests*. Washington, DC.: Author.

Bates, E. (1976). *Language and context: The acquisition of pragmatics*. New York: Academic.

Bedrosian, J. (1981). A sociolinguistic approach for communication skills: Assessment and treatment methodology for mentally retarded adults. Unpublished doctoral dissertation, University of Wisconsin–Madison.

Bloom, L. (1980). *Language development: Form and function in emerging grammars*. Cambridge: MIT Press.

Bloom, L. (1973). *One word at a time: The use of single word utterances before syntax*. The Hague: Mouton.

Bloom, M., & Fischer, J. (1982). *Evaluating practice: Guidelines for the accountable professional*. Englewood Cliffs, NJ: Prentice-Hall.

Camp, D. T., & Stanley, J. C. (1963). *Experimental and quasi-experimental designs for research*. Boston: Houghton Mifflin.

Carver, R. P. (1974). Two dimensions of tests: Psychometric and edumetric. *American Psychologist, 29*, 512–518.

Carver, R. P. (1978). The case against statistical significance testing. *Harvard Educational Review, 48*, 378–399.

Chomsky, N. (1965). *Aspects of the theory of syntax*. Cambridge: MIT Press.

Cohen, J. (1977). *Statistical power analysis for the behavioral sciences* (2nd ed.). New York: Academic.

Constable, C. M. (1983). Creating communicative context. In H. Winitz (Ed.), *Treating language disorders: For clinicians by clinicians* (pp. 97–120). Baltimore: University Park Press.

Craig, H. K. (1983). Applications of pragmatic language models for intervention. In T. M. Gallagher & C. A. Prutting (Eds.), *Pragmatic assessment and intervention issues in language* (pp. 101–127). Austin, TX: PRO-ED.

Eisenhart, C. (1947). Assumptions underlying the analysis of variance. *Biometrics*, 3, 1–22.

Ervin-Tripp, S., & Mitchell-Kernan, C. (Eds.). (1977). *Child discourse*. New York: Academic.

Fey, M. E. (1986). *Language intervention with young children*. Austin, TX: PRO-ED.

Hersen, M., & Barlow, D. H. (1976). *Single-case experimental designs: Strategies for studying behavior change*. New York: Pergamon.

Jerger, J. (1963). Who is qualified to do research? Viewpoint. *Journal of Speech and Hearing Research*, 6, 301.

Kent, R. D. (1983). How can we improve the role of research and educate speech-language pathologists and audiologists to be competent users of research? In N. S. Rees & T. L. Snope (Eds.), *Proceedings of the 1983 National Conference on Undergraduate, Graduate, and Continuing Education* (pp. 76–86). St. Paul: American Speech-Language-Hearing Association.

Kirk, R. E. (1982). *Experimental design: Procedures for the behavioral sciences* (2nd ed.). Belmont, CA: Brooks/Cole.

Larson V. L., & McKinley, N. L. (1987). *Communication assessment and intervention strategies for adolescents*. Eau Claire, WI: Thinking Publications.

Levin, J. R. (1985). Some methodological and statistical "bugs" in research on children's learning. In M. Pressley & C. J. Brainard (Eds.), *Cognitive learning and memory in children* (pp. 205–233). New York: Springer-Verlag.

McCauley, R. J., & Swisher, L. (1984). Use and misuse of norm-referenced tests in clinical assessment: A hypothetical case. *Journal of Speech and Hearing Disorders*, 49, 338–348.

McLean, J. E. (1983). Historical perspectives on the content of child language problems. In J. Miller, D. E. Yoder, & R. Schiefelbusch (Eds.), *Contemporary issues in language intervention* (pp. 115–126). Rockville, MD: American Speech-Language-Hearing Association.

McReynolds, L .V., & Kearns, K. P. (1983). *Single-subject experimental designs in communicative disorders*. Baltimore: University Park Press.

Miller, J. F., & Yoder, D. E. (1972). A syntax teaching program. In J. E. McLean, D. E. Yoder, & R. L. Schiefelbusch (Eds.), *Language intervention with the retarded: Developing strategies* (pp. 191–211). Baltimore: University Park Press.

Miller, J. F., & Yoder, D. E. (1974). An ontogenetic language teaching strategy for retarded children. In R. L. Schiefelbusch & L. Lloyd (Eds.), *Language perspectives—acquisition, retardation, and intervention* (pp. 505–528). Baltimore: University Park Press.

Milliken, G. A., & Johnson, D. E. (1984). *Analysis of messy data: Volume 1. Designed experiments*. New York: Van Nostrand Reinhold.

Parsonson, B. D., & Baer, D. M. (1978). The analysis and presentation of graphic data. In T. R. Kratchowill (Ed.), *Single subject research: Strategies for evaluating change* (pp. 101–165). New York: Academic.

Ringel, R. (1972). The clinician and the researcher: An artificial dichotomy. *ASHA*, 14, 351–353.

Siegel, G. M. (1987). The limits of science in communication disorders. *Journal of Speech and Hearing Disorders*, 52, 306–312.

Siegel, G. M. & Spradlin, J. E. (1985). Therapy and research. *Journal of Speech and Hearing Disorders, 50,* 226–230.

Siegel, S. (1956). *Nonparametric statistics for the behavioral sciences.* New York: McGraw-Hill.

Stevens, S. S. (1968). Measurement, statistics, and the schemapiric view. *Science, 161,* 849–856.

Underwood, B. J. (1957). *Psychological Research.* New York: Appleton-Century-Crofts.

Vetter, D. K. (1985). Evaluation of clinical intervention: Accountability. *Seminars in Speech and Language, 6,* 55–65.

Wiley, T. (1988). Curricular arithmetic: How do we add and subtract. In *Proceedings of the Ninth Annual Conference on Graduate Education* (pp. 36–42). St. Louis: Council of Graduate Programs in Communication Sciences and Disorders.

PART   C

Speech Sound System

CHAPTER 14

Issues in Phonological Development and Disorders

CAROL STOEL-GAMMON

The field of phonological development and phonological disorders has advanced considerably in the past decade as the complex nature of phonological acquisition has become increasingly apparent. One of the major changes involves the use of phonological processes to describe children's error patterns. First introduced in order to account for normal development (Stampe, 1969), phonological process analysis is now widely used as a basis for assessment and treatment of children with phonological disorders (Hodson, 1986; Khan & Lewis, 1986; Shriberg & Kwiatkowski, 1980; Weiner, 1979). The advantage of phonological process analysis is that it focuses on sound classes and error patterns rather than on individual sounds, as was previously the case. While I use this type of analysis myself, and have advocated it for describing the phonological systems of both normally developing and phonologically disordered subjects (Stoel-Gammon & Dunn, 1985), process analysis provides only a partial description of a child's phonological system. It allows us to examine the mismatches between the adult target and the child's production in terms of syllabic structure and consonantal error patterns and is a reasonable place to *start* analyzing a child's system, but it is only that—a start. It must be supplemented with other types of analysis in order to obtain a more complete picture.

There are many areas in which we need additional information; I have chosen two of these to discuss in this chapter. The first area centers around the interface between phonology and lexicon, by exploring the possible interrelationships between these two facets of language. The second topic is the acquisition of vowels in normally developing and phonologically disordered subjects, and the relationship between vowels and other aspects of phonology. For each topic I will briefly review our current state of knowledge, pinpoint areas for future research, and discuss clinical implications.

THE PHONOLOGY-LEXICON INTERFACE

CURRENT STATE

It has been argued that in the earliest stages of meaningful speech, children acquire words as "unanalyzed wholes," and consequently, that phonological acquisition is word-based rather than phoneme-based (Ferguson & Farwell, 1975). This early period of development, often referred to as "the first 50 word stage" (Ingram, 1976), is distinct from the period that follows in that the phonology is less systematic and productions of a single phoneme may vary considerably across words. Most children with a lexicon under 50 words have a limited inventory of sounds, predominantly stops, nasals, and glides (Stoel-Gammon, 1985). Investigations of lexical selection and avoidance have shown that children make good use of their limited phonetic inventories by *selecting* for their productive vocabularies words that contain consonants from their inventories and *avoiding* words with consonants not in the inventory (Ferguson & Farwell, 1975; Schwartz & Leonard, 1982).

By the time children are 24 months old, their productive vocabulary is around 250 words (Nelson, 1973) and the average phonetic inventory includes 9–10 consonants in initial position, typically stops, nasals, fricatives, and glides, and 5–6 consonants in final position. Word and syllable shapes at this stage include both open (CV) and closed (CVC) syllables, which combine to form words with a variety of structures (e.g., CV, CVC, CVCV, CVCVC, and occasional initial and final consonant clusters) (Stoel-Gammon, 1987). Dyson (1988) has shown that between the ages of 2 and 3, the phonetic inventory continues to expand, incorporating more phones and a wider range of sound classes.

For the normally developing child, then, lexical and phonological acquisition move forward in synchrony; as the lexicon expands, so does the phonetic inventory needed to support the number of different words the child is trying to say. Among phonologically disordered subjects, however, the picture may be quite different.

FUTURE RESEARCH: QUESTIONS AND HYPOTHESES

The relationship between lexical and phonological development in phonologically disordered children has not been well documented, but it is my impression that these two aspects of development proceed at different rates for some children. I am particularly interested in the phonology-lexicon interface in those subjects who have a small repertoire of speech sounds, typically stops, nasals, and glides, with syllable types limited to CV and CVC. This pattern in not uncommon among children with functional articulation disorders (Dinnsen & Chin, 1988).

There are three "profiles" of interest among these subjects in terms of the relationship between lexical size and phonological development. The *first* profile, here called Type A, is one in which the two aspects are in phase with each other; that is, the phonetic repertoire is limited and the lexicon is small. The "disordered" aspect of development for Type A children is that both the sound inventory and lexicon size are well below age-level norms. The *second* profile, Type B, is characterized by a marked discrepancy between the child's phonology and the lexicon, with the lexicon being age-appropriate but the phonetic inventory very limited. Essentially, this is the case of a 4-year-old child with a 4-year-old vocabulary and the phonetic repertoire of a 21-month-old. The limited repertoire cannot adequately support the lexicon, and consequently, a large number of homonyms occur in the child's speech. For example, given a repertoire of stops, nasals, and glides, and the phonological processes of Velar Fronting (substitution of alveolars for target velars), Stopping (substitution of stops for target fricatives), and Cluster Reduction (reduction of consonant clusters to a single consonant), the child would produce the words *sack, track, tack, cat, clack, crack,* and *sat* as [tæt]. Obviously, the inability to differentiate among sets of words such as these would negatively impact intelligibility.

The *third* possible relationship between the lexicon and the phonology, Type C, is characterized by a normal-sized lexicon (as in Type B), but in this case, children would differentiate among potentially homonymous forms by marking contrasts in atypical ways. For example, [h] might be used as the substitute for target fricatives in order to effect a stop-fricative contrast, or suprasegmental features might indicate segmental information. Although the productions of both Type B and Type C children are clearly in error, the Type C child does a better job of distinguishing among words than the Type B child.

CLINICAL IMPLICATIONS

Increased understanding of the phonology-lexicon interface has several clinical implications. Returning to the "first 50 word stage," the major characteristic of the child's phonology during this stage is that the unit of acquisition is *whole words* rather than *segments*. Consequently, if a child is being assessed for a possible disorder, and that child has a productive lexicon of less than 50 words, I feel it is inappropriate to perform a phonological process analysis. Based on our knowledge of normal acquisition, one would not expect the child to evidence *systematic* segment-based error patterns of the sort captured by phonological processes. The child's productions should be analyzed to determine the inventory of sounds and syllable types, but an evaluation in terms of phonological processes is premature at this stage.

Using the same reasoning, I would hesitate to label a child with a lexicon of fewer than 50 words as *phonologically disordered* (providing there is evidence of some CV syllables with supraglottal consonants) or to advocate a program aimed exclusively at phonological remediation. Rather, intervention should be directed toward increasing the child's productive vocabulary. Given what we know about lexical selection and avoidance in the normally developing child, it would be wise to choose new words for the vocabulary that capitalize on the existing phonetic inventory in terms of sound types and syllable shapes. Thus, if the inventory includes open and closed syllables with stops, nasals, and glides, words conforming to this pattern would be obvious candidates for additions to the vocabulary. Once the child demonstrates a productive lexicon of more than 50 words, the phonological system can be evaluated and an appropriate intervention program implemented, if necessary.

For phonologically disordered children beyond the first 50 word stage, the most appropriate treatment program would depend, in part, on the nature of the phonology-lexicon interface. For children identified as a Type A (those with a small lexicon *and* a limited phonetic inventory for their chronological age), remediation should not be purely phonological, but should be aimed at increasing the lexicon as well as expanding the inventory of sounds and syllable structures. Type B children (those with an age-appropriate vocabulary, a small phonetic inventory, and many homonymous productions) should receive therapy aimed at expanding their phonetic inventory *and* at increasing their awareness of the effects of homonomy on intelligibility. A minimal pair approach would probably be the most effective in this case. Finally, children with a Type C profile (those with a large vocabulary, a small phonetic inventory, and the presence of atypical errors to make word contrasts) should also receive therapy to expand the inventory. In contrast to Type B children, however, the secondary focus for these subjects would not be on eliminating homonyms, but on suppressing the unusual error patterns that have been adopted.

Another implication of the phonology-lexicon interface concerns the terms "deviant" and "delayed," which often appear in descriptions of phonologically disordered subjects. Given the typology outlined above, I would argue that only Type A children can unequivocally be labeled as "delayed." These children are below age level for both lexical and phonological development. Type B children are more difficult to classify. Their phonetic repertoire is typical of a much younger child, suggesting that the term "delayed" is appropriate, but the mismatch between their sound repertoire and the size of their productive lexicon makes their *overall* system "deviant," since it differs substantially from the system of a normally developing child. Thus, on one level, phonological development, Type B children are *delayed*, but on another, the phonology-lexicon interface, they are *deviant*. The third group, Type C, would be presumably labeled as deviant by most clinicians because of the presence of atypical error patterns.

I should stress that the relationships between lexical and phonological development posited above are my impressions based on available literature and personal observations. They need to be supported, modified, or rejected by investigations that focus not on phonology alone, but on phonology as it relates to lexicon size. In carrying out future research in both the basic and applied areas of child language, we need to recognize that phonology is an integral part of the overall linguistic system.

VOWELS

CURRENT STATE

Historically, research in child phonology has focused on consonants. We now have a substantial body of knowledge regarding the emergence of consonantal phones, the order of acquisition of phonemes, the nature of error types, and similarities and differences between normally developing and phonologically disordered children. This information has been used clinically in the design and implementation of successful assessment and treatment programs. By comparison, our knowledge of vowels is woefully inadequate. Most researchers and clinicians tend to ignore vowels completely or discuss them only as an aside. Even the oft-cited norms of Templin (1957) are of no help when it comes to the acquisition of vowels. According to her findings, vowels were highly accurate in her 3-year-old subjects (mean percent correct: 93) and evidenced little improvement between 3 ; 0 and 8 ; 0 years.

One reason vowels are often ignored is that vowel errors tend to be less discrete than consonantal errors; they are, in some sense, less perceptible and seem to be more difficult to transcribe reliably. In addition, dialectal differences in the pronunciation of vowels may make us more tolerant of variations in the production of target vowels. In spite of these problems, researchers and clinicians must make a concerted effort to pay attention to vowels and to document their acquisition in young children.

Although normally developing children and some phonologically disordered subjects may acquire a complete and accurate vowel repertoire by the age of 3 ; 0–4 ; 0, as Templin's findings suggest, other phonologically disordered subjects do not. We know almost nothing about these disordered subjects. It seems that the literature on vowels in phonologically disordered subjects is limited to one published study (Hargrove, 1982) and a few unpublished conference presentations (Khan, 1988; Pollock & Swanson, 1986; Stoel-Gammon & Herrington, 1987). There is an obvious need for more research in this area, both on young normally developing children and on children with phonological disorders. In the section which follows, I will outline a series of questions regarding vowels, their developmental patterns, and their relationships to other aspects of phonology.

FUTURE RESEARCH: SOME SUGGESTIONS

1. *What is the relationship between the vowels of babbling and those of meaningful speech?* Studies of prelinguistic and early linguistic vocalizations show a clear continuity between the types of consonants that occur in premeaningful and early meaningful speech (see Locke, 1983, for a summary). Stops, nasals, and glides dominate in both types of vocalizations; moreover, these consonants are the ones that tend to be produced accurately first. For vowels, it seems that a different pattern holds. The most common vowels in prelinguistic utterances are lax front and central vowels (e.g., [ɪ, ɛ, æ, ʌ]); high front and high back vowels are rare (Irwin, 1948; Kent & Bauer, 1985). There appears to be little carryover from babbling to speech in terms of vowel types. Lax vowels do *not* occur more frequently than tense vowels and actually seem to be more difficult to target correctly; in particular, the tense phonemes /i/, /u/, and /o/ are acquired quite early, whereas /ɪ/ and /ɛ/ are late (Hare, 1983; Wellman, Case, Mengert & Bradbury, 1931). In sum, the continuity reported for consonants is apparently not found in the domain of vowels.

2. *What is the order of acquisition of vowel phonemes in the normally developing child?* This question is very straightforward, but we have no definitive answer. A brief survey of data from diary studies and cross-sectional investigations provides only a partial answer, or rather, several different answers. According to Wellman and colleagues (1931), single word samples collected from 206 children, 2 to 6 years old, provide the following ages of mastery: /i, a, u, o, ʌ ,ə / by 2 years; /ɛ / and /ɔ / are added by 3 years; and /ɪ, e, æ, ʊ / are mastered by 4 years; the r-colored vowels /ɚ/ are acquired later. This order is supported in part by the studies of younger children (Hare, 1983; Paschal, 1983), although differences are apparent, particularly in the order of mastery of /æ/, /ɛ/, /ɪ/ and /ɔ/ . In addition, Stoel-Gammon (1985) and Dyson (1988) reported that /ɚ/ emerged by 2;0 in a majority of their subjects. Olmsted's cross-sectional study of 100

subjects is of little help in determining the order of acquisition of vowels because of the presence of many reversals in accuracy levels between 18 months and 5 years (Olmsted, 1971). There are several possible explanations for the various findings: one is that they result from methodological differences in data collection (e.g., different target words; single word samples versus running speech) or in data reduction (different transcription and scoring systems); alternatively, it is possible that the acquisition of vowels is inherently more variable than the acquisition of consonants—perhaps there is no "typical" order of acquisition; rather each child follows his/her own developmental path. These possibilities need to be examined further.

3. *What is the nature of vowel errors?* The available literature suggests that certain error types are fairly common, specifically: /ɪ/ → [i]; /ʌ/ and /æ/ → [a]; /ɚ/ → [o] or [ʊ]; beyond this, however, there is little documentation of error types. A complete answer to this question would also provide information on the following related questions: Can vowel errors be grouped on the basis of distinctive features? What is the level of intrachild variation in vowel errors? What is the level of interchild variation?

4. *Do phonologically disordered subjects adhere to the same patterns of acquisition as normals?* Studies of consonants in phonologically disordered children have shown that, for the most part, order of acquisition and error types are similar to that documented for normally developing children. Once we learn more about normal patterns of vowel development, we need to determine if the same patterns occur in subjects with phonological disorders. We also need an estimate of the prevalence of vowel errors among disordered subjects.

5. *What is the appropriate frame work for describing vowel productions?* This question has two subparts—the first centers around the *features* used to classify vowels. While there is general agreement on the features associated with /i, ɪ, e, u, ʊ, o/, there is less consensus on the classification of other vowels. For example, some investigators consider /ʌ/ to be *mid* (on the front-back dimension) and *central* (on the high-low dimension); others classify it as *back* and *central*, and still others as *mid* and *low*. Similar problems exist with the classification of /æ ɔ, a / as *tense* or *lax*; some researchers call all three tense, others list them as lax. Until we can agree upon a feature classification for vowels, comparable to that for consonants, it will be difficult to compare vowel descriptions across studies and to classify vowel errors using a feature system.

The second issue deals with the terminology used to discuss vowel errors. Three terms appear commonly in the literature: substitution, neutralization, and distortion. It appears that researchers and clinicians often use these terms to describe the same phenomena. I would suggest that the term "distortion" be applied only when the realization of a target vowel is perceived as being *within* the phoneme boundaries for that vowel, but is distorted in some way; for example, a nasalized vowel in the context of oral consonants in English would be classified as a distortion. If, however, the child's production of a target vowel crosses a phoneme boundary, as in /ɪ / being produced as [i], the error type is no longer a distortion but a neutralization or a substitution; both terms imply a loss of contrast between the target vowel and the child's production and the two terms seem to be used interchangeably by many researchers. Ingram (1976), for example, writes of *substitution* errors for consonants, but *neutralization* errors for vowels. I feel that the term "substitution" is preferable to "neutralization" in describing unidirectional errors, as for example, when a child consistently produces [i] for /ɪ /. The term "neutralization" would be reserved for instances of bidirectional errors, as when a child produces [ɪ] for /i/ *and* [i] for /ɪ /;* the contrast between the two phonemes has been lost, but there is no single pattern of substitution.

6. *What relationships obtain between consonants and vowels in CV or VC sequences?* Obviously, two basic types of relationships are possible: (1) consonants can affect neighboring vowels, or (2) vowels can affect neighboring consonants. The effects of consonants on vowels are well documented for adult speech; we know, for example, that vowels are nasalized in the context of nasal consonants and are lengthened when they precede voiced consonants. We also know that children often produce a vowel correctly in the context of some consonants, but misarticulate it in others. In particular, vowels preceding liquids are often misarticulated, even when the liquid does not appear in the child's production (e.g., milk may be pronounced as [mok], even though /ɪ / is pronounced correctly in other words).

The influence of vowels on consonants in child speech has not received much attention. Stoel-Gammon (1983) summarized a small set of studies showing that labial consonants were substituted by alveolars in CV syllables with front vowels; thus, the word *baby* was produced as [didi], but *ball* was [ba]. A similar observation was made in a recent case study by Davis and MacNeilage (1988). We do not yet know how widespread these patterns are, but it is becoming increasingly clear that neither consonants nor vowels can be studied in isolation.

7. *What is the relationship between stress patterns and the acquisition of vowels?* Vowels form the nucleus of the spoken syllable and their articulation varies with changes in stress pattern. For instance, the phonemes /e/ and /o/ are produced as dipthongs in syllables of primary stress and monophthongs when they receive secondary stress. A number of researchers have noted that both normally developing and phonologically disordered children have difficulty producing syllables with tertiary (or reduced) stress (Allen & Hawkins, 1980; Davis & MacNeilage, 1988; Stoel-Gammon & Herrington, 1987). When in error, these syllables are either deleted or are articulated with secondary rather than tertiary stress. Given

that vowels tend to be produced accurately in stressed syllables, errors in the articulation of reduced vowels would appear to result from difficulties with the rhythmic patterning of syllable sequences in English. Thus, a full investigation of vowel acquisition must examine the interactions between the suprasegmental features of rhythm and stress and the segmental features of vowels.

CLINICAL IMPLICATIONS

Lack of knowledge of normal patterns of vowel development has adversely affected assessment and treatment programs for phonologically disordered children with vowel errors. Nearly all assessment batteries focus on consonants; vowels are evaluated with little concern regarding phonetic context and word structure. As Pollock (1987) has noted, an adequate assessment of vowels can be obtained only through a test that offers *multiple* opportunities for the production of each vowel and diphthong in a variety of contexts, including monosyllabic and multisyllabic forms, stressed and unstressed syllables, and with varied adjacent consonants. Current assessment batteries do not provide this framework. In fact, some widely used articulation tests fail to include target words with all the vowels of English; the Goldman-Fristoe Test of Articulation, for example, has no words with the vowels /ʊ/, /a /, or /ɔɪ / (Goldman & Fristoe, 1969). Pollock (1989) provides preliminary suggestions for the clinical assessment of vowels in children's speech.

Even when vowel errors are identified, clinicians have little guidance regarding target selection and appropriate treatment, because, once again, intervention programs have tended to focus on consonants. Since most subjects with multiple vowel error also have multiple consonant errors, the unstated assumption of many programs seems to be to treat the consonants first and maybe the vowels will improve without direct intervention. While this may be true for some subjects, I doubt it applies in all cases. At present, this assumption must be viewed skeptically until supported by clinical studies.

These questions should serve as a starting point for future research on vowels and on their interactions with other parts of the developing phonological system. It is my hope that during the next few years, we can accumulate a body of knowledge that will provide us with answers to these and related questions.

CONCLUSION

The purpose of this chapter has been to identify areas of future research in phonological development and disorders. There are many areas in need of study—I chose two in the hope of expanding our research and clinical programs beyond the narrow focus on consonants which is currently in vogue. The first topic, the phonology-lexicon interface, was selected in part to highlight the notion that phonology should not be studied in isolation; it is an integral part of language and its relationship to other aspects of the linguistic system must be considered. The second topic, vowels, represents an area in which there is a huge gap in our knowledge base. Vowels are as fundamental to speech as consonants, and yet we know little about their featural properties, their developmental patterns in young normal children, their role in phonological disorders, and appropriate methods of assessment and treatment. Research in this area is clearly necessary if we are to reach a complete understanding of the nature of phonological development and disorders.

ACKNOWLEDGMENT

Preparation of this chapter was supported, in part, by a grant from the National Institutes of Health (NS 26521-01). The author wishes to thank Judith Stone for her comments on an earlier draft.

REFERENCES

Allen, G., & Hawkins, S. (1980). Phonological rhythm: Definition and development. In G. Yeni-Komshian, J. F. Kavanagh, & C. A. Ferguson (Eds.), *Child Phonology: Vol. 1: Production* (pp. 227–256). New York: Academic.

Davis, B. L., & MacNeilage, P. F. (1988). *Phonetic relationships between adult targets and early child word productions.* Paper presented at the Symposium on Research in Child Language Disorders, Madison, Wis.

Dinnsen, D. A., & Chin, S. B. (1988). *Some phonological constraints on functional speech disorders.* Paper presented at the Annual Convention, American Speech-Language-Hearing Association, Boston.

Dyson, A. T. (1988). Phonetic inventories of 2- and 3-year-old children. *Journal of Speech and Hearing Disorders, 53,* 89–93.

Ferguson, C. A., & Farwell, C. (1975). Words and sounds in early language acquisition: English initial consonants in the first fifty words. *Language, 51,* 419–439.

Goldman, R., & Fristoe, M. (1969). *The Goldman-Fristoe Test of Articulation.* Circle Pines, MN: American Guidance Service.

Hare, G. (1983). Development at 2 years. In J. V. Irwin and S. P. Wong (Eds.), *Phonological development in children: 18–72 months* (pp. 55–88). Carbondale: Southern Illinois University Press.

Hargrove, P. M. (1982). Misarticulated vowels: A case study. *Language, Speech, and Hearing Services in Schools, 13,* 86–95.

Hodson, B. W. (1986). *The assessment of phonological processes* (rev. ed.). Danville, IL: Interstate Press.

Ingram, D. (1976). *Phonological disability in children.* New York: American Elsevier.

Irwin, O. C. (1948). Infant speech: Development of vowel sounds. *Journal of Speech and Hearing Disorders, 13,* 31–34.

Kent, R. D., & Bauer, H. F. (1985). Vocalizations of one-year-olds. *Journal of Child Language, 12,* 491–526.

Khan, M. L. (1988). *Vowel remediation: A case study.* Paper presented at the Annual Convention, American Speech-Language-Hearing Association, Boston.

Khan, M. L., & Lewis, N. P. (1986). *Khan-Lewis phonological analysis.* Circle Pines, MN: American Guidance Service.

Locke, J. (1983). *Phonological acquisition and change.* New York: Academic.

Nelson, K. (1973). Structure and strategy in learning to talk. *Monographs of the Society for Research in Child Development, 38.*

Olmsted, D. (1971). *Out of the mouth of babes.* Mouton: The Hague.

Paschall, L. (1983). Development at 18 months. In J. V. Irwin & S. P. Wong (Eds.), *Phonological development in children: 18 to 72 months.* Carbondale, IL: Southern Illinois University Press.

Pollock, K. E. (1987). *Vowel analysis using traditional articulation and phonological process test stimuli.* Poster session presented at the Annual Convention, American Speech-Language-Hearing Association, New Orleans.

Pollock, K. E. (1989). *Assessing vowel errors in children.* Miniseminar presented at the Annual Convention, American Speech-Language-Hearing Association, Boston.

Pollock K. E., & Swanson, L. A. (1986). *Analysis of vowel errors in a disordered child during training.* Paper presented at the Annual Convention, American Speech-Language-Hearing Association, Detroit.

Schwartz, R., & Leonard, L. B. (1982). Do children pick and choose? *Journal of Child Language, 9,* 319–336.

Shriberg, L., & Kwiatkowski, J. (1980). *Natural process analysis.* New York: Wiley and Sons.

Stampe, D. (1969). The acquisition of phonetic representation. *Papers from the Fifth Regional Meeting of the Chicago Linguistic Society* (pp. 433–444). Chicago: Chicago Linguistic Society.

Stoel-Gammon, C. (1983). Constraints on consonant-vowel sequences in early words. *Journal of Child Language, 10,* 455–457.

Stoel-Gammon, C. (1985). Phonetic inventories, 15–24 months: A longitudinal study. *Journal of Speech and Hearing Research, 28,* 505–512.

Stoel-Gammon, C. (1987). The phonological skills of two-year-olds. *Language, Speech, and Hearing Services in Schools, 18,* 323–329.

Stoel-Gammon, C. & Dunn, C. (1985). *Normal and disordered phonology in children,* Austin, TX: Pro-Ed.

Stoel-Gammon, C., & Herrington, P. (1987). *Vowel productions of normally developing and phonologically disordered children.* Paper presented at the Symposium on Research in Child Language Disorders, Madison, WI.

Templin, M. C. (1957). Certain language skills in children: Their development and interrelationships. *Institute of Child Welfare Monographs, 26.* Minneapolis: University of Minnesota Press.

Weiner, F. (1979). *Phonological process analysis.* Baltimore: University Park Press.

Wellman, B. L., Case, I.M., Mengert, I. B., & Bradbury, D. E. (1931). Speech sounds of young children. *University of Iowa Studies in Child Welfare, Vol. 2,* 5.

CHAPTER 15

Directions for Research in Developmental Phonological Disorders

LAWRENCE D. SHRIBERG

For the challenging goals of this book, this chapter offers some observations on theoretical, methodological, and clinical perspectives in developmental phonological disorders. First, a review of some historical and descriptive perspectives should provide a context from which to consider future research needs.

CHILDREN WITH DEVELOPMENTAL PHONOLOGICAL DISORDERS

HISTORICAL PERSPECTIVES

The nosological evolution from *articulation* disorders to the current *phonological* disorders has been recounted in many recent synthesis papers. Nearly universal acceptance of this change in focus (see Hoffman, Shuckers, & Daniloff, 1989 for a well-developed alternative position) appears to have been fueled by two independent forces, each of which has relevance in the current context of a perspective on research directions. In the clinical community, the Education of All Handicapped Children Act (1975) required speech-language pathologists to identify and provide services for younger children than previously had been advised in the speech pathology literature. Pressed to provide services for all children with exceptional educational needs, educators began to question whether precious clinical resources should be allocated to young children with "functional" articulatory involvement. At about the same time—and I nominate Ingram's (1976) scholarly textbook as the point of demarcation—articulatory aspects of speech performance began to be reconsidered from the perspective of linguistic systems. Across many speech disorders, including those associated with aphasia, hearing impairment, and mental retardation, a focus on organizational aspects of errors began to replace traditional emphasis on phonetic description. Using classificatory terms such as *phonological disorders, speech disorders of unknown origin,* and *speech delays* (note that the latter term is also used for children with late onset of speech, e.g., Paul, 1989), a considerable number of studies in the 1980s yielded descriptions of children with developmental phonological disorders.

CLINICAL PROFILE

Table 15-1 is a summary of 10 demographic, speech, and educational characteristics of several samples of children with developmental phonological disorders. These data were derived primarily from children in Madison, Wisconsin, with the usual caveats about external validity due to potential differences in subject groups, service delivery models, and research methods. The average or modal child referred for an evaluation of a speech disorder of unknown origin is male, aged 4 years, 2 months. Over two-thirds of the child's consonants are correctly articulated in continuous speech (70%), with consonant errors approximately equally divided among deletions (10%), substitutions (10%) and clinically notable distortions (10%). Typically, there is a substantial (10%) difference between the percentage of correct singleton consonants in continuous speech compared to correct consonant in clusters. Among clusters, those occurring in word-initial position are one-fourth as likely (15%) to be articulated correctly (no consonant deletion or substitution errors) as clusters occurring in word-final position (60%).

The profile in Table 15.1 also includes data tallied using the construct of *phonological process*, a cover term for errors aggregated by error-phoneme, error-type, and word-position. As shown, approximately 92% of speech-delayed children's substitution and deletion errors can be subsumed by one of eight *natural* phonological processes, with the remaining 8% of errors not "accounted for" by errors that presumably are either perceptually, cognitively, or motorically natural (see subsequent discussion). As

Table 15-1. A clinical profile of the "typical" child with a phonological disorder of unknown origin

Variable	Characteristic*
DEMOGRAPHIC	
1. Gender	Male
2. Age at referral	4;2
SPEECH AND PROSODY	
3. Percentage of consonants correct	70%
4. Distribution of consonant errors	10% deletions
	10% substitutions
	10% distortions
5. Correct singleton—correct cluster difference	10%
6. Correct word-initial cluster—word-final cluster ratio	1:4
7. Percentage of sound changes accounted for by eight natural phonological processes	92%
8. Intelligibility in continuous speech	80%
9. Probability of perceptible rhythm or voice involvement	25%
EDUCATIONAL STATUS	
10. Probable need for speech and/or other services through elementary grades	80%

*See text for description of each characteristic.

estimated by trained phonetic transcribers who were allowed to replay audiotapes as needed to gloss words, the average intelligibility of these children in continuous speech is 80%. Associated findings indicate that many (approximately 25%) of these children have perceptible deficits in either rhythm or voice characteristics of speech prosody. Finally, preliminary follow-up data indicate that among children referred during preschool years for moderate to severe phonological disorders of unknown origin, most (approximately 80%) continue to have exceptional educational needs through at least third grade.

Clearly, the paradigmatic shifts that presaged the "new look" in childhood speech disorders have been fruitful. The 10 entries in Table 15-1 provide a mandate for programmatic research in developmental phonologic disorders. Specifically, the profile attests to the service delivery needs of these children, with speech-language involvements having implications for academic, social, and, ultimately, vocational adjustment. The following section will conclude with some observations on these clinical perspectives.

THEORETICAL, METHODOLOGICAL, AND CLINICAL PERSPECTIVES

THEORETICAL PERSPECTIVES ON PHONOLOGICAL PROCESSES

One way to consider relevant theoretical issues for the 1990s is to examine the most widely debated construct of the past decade, the ubiquitous *phonological process*. With some license, my sense of the relevant literatures suggests five theoretical perspectives of the phonological process as a construct in theoretical systems.

The Phonological Process as a Descriptive Term

Historically, the earliest clinical implementation of Stampe's definition of the phonological process (Donnegan & Stampe, 1979; Stampe, 1973) exploited the descriptive adequacy of processes as cover terms for *all* sound changes. Among the several process-based assessment instruments to emerge in the early 1980s and throughout that decade, most have not developed explicit explanatory positions on the nature of delayed speech relative to the theory of natural phonology. Rather, with a few exclusionary constraints, children or adult's speech errors have been interpreted as *phonological simplifications* in contrast to the earlier notion of *articulatory errors*. The descriptive power of this approach and the simplicity of calculation have made process terms available and appealing for a variety of research questions. To date, this essentially atheoretical use of process terminology is the most prevalent of the alternatives here, both as independent and dependent variables in child phonology research and especially as clinical indices of severity of involvement.

The Phonological Process in Diagnostic Classification

A second perspective on Stampe's natural phonology was proposed by and appears to be advocated by only one research group (Shriberg, Kwiatkowski, Best, Hengst, & Terselic-Weber, 1986). The data in Table 15-1 have emerged from studies that Joan Kwaitkowski, many other colleagues, and I have undertaken in attempts to explain the causal antecedents of delayed speech of heretofore unknown origin. Our reading of Stampe was that natural phonology provides exactly the links between linguistic competence models and relevant psycholinguistic constructs in speech production models that are needed for diagnostic classification. Stampe's view that only *certain* sound changes are natural due to perceptual, cognitive, or production issues seemed to place the focus exactly on etiology. To use a statistical analogy, we are primarily interested in the analysis of the *residuals* from a natural process analysis. Accordingly, it is both the frequencies of natural processes that differ from reference statistics and those sound changes that are not "accounted for" by natural processes, that provide research leads to the perceptual, cognitive, and motoric involvements associated with diagnostic classification.* As shown in Table 15-1, this application of natural phonology indicates that approximately 92% of young children's speech sound errors can be described by eight putatively natural phonological processes, with the residuals having potential for diagnostic classification. Hypothesis testing studies based on this general framework will continue through the 1990s.

The Phonological Process and Underlying Representations

A third interpretation of the construct of phonological processes is reflected in the body of work by Dinnsen, Elbert, Gierut and colleagues (e.g., Elbert, Dinnsen & Weismer, 1984; Gierut, Elbert, & Dinnsen, 1987). The focus of this research program is to attempt to differentiate levels of phonological knowledge underlying sound change, with only certain sound changes qualifying as appropriate candidates for the term *phonological process*. From this perspective, phonological analyses that do not attempt to determine whether children have correctly represented the target phoneme underlyingly are considered incomplete. Assuming what appears to be a two-lexicon representation of a child's phonological knowledge, these researchers have proposed several typological systems to represent the status of underlying representations in a child's productive lexicon. Continuing work includes validity studies in prediction and intervention.

Nonlinear Phonologies

Whereas the previous three perspectives on phonological processes reflect developments within speech pathology, the remaining two perspectives reflect the potential impact of work elsewhere on speech pathology research. These paradigms generally do not invoke the construct of phonological processes in description or explanation of sound change. Thus, the

---

*For an example of the first type, a phonologically natural, but high frequency of occurrence of syllable deletion and final consonant deletion errors in a group of adults with mental retardation has been interpreted as evidence for continuing cognitive-linguistic constraints effecting sociolinguistic performance (Shriberg & Widder, forthcoming). For an example of the second type, a consistent, but relatively low frequency of occurrence of certain non-natural sound changes in some children has been associated with histories of recurrent otitis media with effusion (Shriberg, 1988).

fourth perspective in this list refers to contemporary developments in several nonlinear theories of phonology. Such proposals, including continuing developments in autosegmental and metrical phonology, portray underlying representations of sounds and words in ways that differ considerably from the taxonomic, generative, and natural phonologies that preceded them (e.g., Goldsmith, forthcoming). Most important in the present context are attempts of these theories to link segmental organization with suprasegmental tiers. Such analytic frameworks provide description at exactly the relevant levels that, to date, have not been attempted in such related areas as developmental apraxia of speech. Although no one theoretical proposal has emerged with immediate utility for applied research in speech pathology, we can expect to see continued efforts to understand how prosodic variables interact with other speech-language domains in normal and disordered communication.

Psycholinguistic Models

The fifth perspective on phonological processes is reflected in the information-processing approaches in the cognitive sciences literature, including several widely cited speech perception and production models (Bock, 1982; Garrett, 1975, 1980; Shattuck-Huffnagel, 1983) and the active area of connectionist models of speech-language acquisition and performance (e.g., Dell, 1986; MacWhinney, this volume, chapter 4). In comparison to the four previous perspectives, psycholinguistic models appeal to a wider range of cognitive and linguistic domains in attempts to identify and explicate the source of surface-level simplifications. Connectionist models of speech learning, in particular, do not invoke such linguistic abstractions as underlying representations and phonological processes. To date, most applications of these models have been in adult speech and language disorders and childhood language disorders. The many emerging psycholinguistic and neurolinguistic frameworks provide a rich source for a new generation of theory-corroborative studies in developmental phonological disorders.

Summary

In my judgment, the primary task of the 1990s will be to sort from among and within these five perspectives on developmental phonological disorders which is best able to provide a unified paradigm for the clinical goals of classification, prediction, intervention, and prevention. Whichever theoretical perspectives eventually emerge as the most highly valued, certain methodological needs remain to be addressed. Following are brief impressions of some major gaps.

METHODOLOGICAL PERSPECTIVES

Speech Sampling

Researchers continue to collect speech data in a variety of sampling contexts, involving such stimuli and procedural oppositions as imitative versus spontaneous, isolated versus embedded, citation versus continuous and narrative versus conversation. Such differences in sociolinguistic context and linguistic content make it difficult to compare data across studies. As methodological variables, there is a need for comprehensive studies of the effects of sampling context on phonetic, phonologic, and prosodic characteristics of normal and disordered speech. Differences associated with sampling variables are also of theoretical interest in their own right. For example, language productivity differences associated with narrative versus continuous speech samples are reported in the database described by Miller (see chapter 10); phonetic and phonologic differences associated with citation-form versus continuous speech samples are reported in the database described in Morrison and Shriberg (1989). Continued research of this type should consider multivariate description of sampling effects on language and speech variables within the same database.

Phonetic Transcription

A second general methodological need that clearly requires research attention is the use of phonetic transcription as the sole measurement modality for speech research. Current research in both normal and disordered speech-language continues to make extensive use of both narrow and broad phonetic transcription, but reliability and validity issues have influenced some workers to question the continued use of perceptual phonetics for certain questions. For example, several studies report that phonetic transcription may not be sensitive to oppositions in children's speech that are evident within acoustic analyses (cf., Leonard, 1985). The increasing availability of microprocessor technologies for acoustics-aided transcription should allow for efficient methods that yield valid and reliable data.

Assessment Instruments

The final entry here simply points to the need for a set of well-developed assessment procedures for a variety of research questions in child phonology. There is a clear need for psychometrically stable measures (cf., Shriberg, 1989) of such interrelated construct domains as *intelligibility, prosody, speech-motor function,* and *speech sound awareness.* Several test development projects currently underway may yield useful research instruments. Hopefully, the 1990s will see significant growth in the validity and reliability of the diverse perceptual, acoustic, and physiologic instruments needed in our speech-language research protocols.

CLINICAL PERSPECTIVES

The position expressed at several places within this discussion is that research directions in speech pathology should be dictated by the four clinical service needs of an allied health science: *classification, prediction, intervention,* and *prevention.* This final section notes a few perspectives in each area.

Diagnostic Classification

Interest in causality, so active in the classic studies of the 1940s and 1950s, seems recently to have returned to fashion following the behaviorist frameworks of the 1960s and the descriptive linguistic frameworks of the 1970s and early 1980s. Most notable in this regard are the epidemiological and familial-history studies that have begun to appear in several disorders literatures, including child language and phonology (e.g., Lewis, Ekelman & Aram, in press; Parlour & Broen, 1989; Tomblin, 1989). Note that many of the entries in Table 15-1 reflect questions that can be investigated using these methods. The gender ratio of 3:1 boys to girls with phonologic disorders is consistent with findings in other communicative disorders that indicate the possibility of a genetic basis for some forms of communicative disorders. With the currently available descriptive power of computerized speech-language analyses procedures, epidemiological designs will also be able to examine error patterns among siblings and other family members. In addition to their importance for diagnostic classification, such studies could eventually provide significant information for prediction, intervention, and prevention.

Prediction

Preliminary data from our own longitudinal samples indicate that certain children referred early for a speech delay of unknown origin normalize without formal intervention. Exactly which subject variables are associated with self-correction, or with a favorable prognosis when intervention is provided, remains a relatively unstudied area. Several recent follow-up studies indicate that intelligence, language comprehension, and language production factors are significant predictors of continued involvements. However, other than clinical-level observations about relative stimulability and consistency of error, linguistic analyses have not yielded a metric with adequate predictive validity. Once more, the expected proliferation of well-controlled databases should allow for many research designs toward a battery of effective predictor instruments.

Intervention

The extension of two research trends in intervention begun in the 1980s will be interesting to observe in the 1990s. The first major trend was the shift in management targets from emphasis on sound-level articulatory precision to procedures that attempt to increase the sociolinguistic value of intelligible speech. To date, no one well-controlled intervention study has clearly tested the superiority of these two perspectives. The second trend was the attempt to develop and test computer-assisted methods for the several phases of intervention in developmental speech disorders. The few available data indicate that complex subject factors seem to be more important to successful intervention than the mode of intervention. What is needed are clinical challenge studies in both areas, including speech recognition technologies that allow intervention programming based on signal processing paradigms (e.g., Waton, Reed, Kewley-Port & Maki, 1989).

Prevention

A sure mark of a mature research discipline is the development of preventative procedures. Primary, secondary, and tertiary forms of prevention (ASHA, 1987) in developmental speech-language disorders seem particularly likely targets for research in the last decade of this century. Most of the research in primary prevention will obviously occur in other areas of medicine and developmental neurobiology, informed by epidemiologic and other data from communicative disorders. Continuing prevention research on such world health problems as recurrent otitis media may ultimately have significant impact on the incidence of developmental speech-language problems, particularly among children in certain high-risk geographic and anthropologic groups.

REFERENCES

American Speech-Language-Hearing Association (1987). Prevention of communication disorders: A position statement. *ASHA, 29,* 51–52.

Bock, J. K. (1982). Toward a cognitive psychology of syntax: Information processing contributions to sentence formulation. *Psychological Review, 89,* 1–47.

Dell, G. (1986). A spreading-activation theory of retrieval in sentence production. *Psychological Review, 93,* 283–321.

Donnegan, P. J., & Stampe, D. (1979). The study of natural phonology. In D. A.

Dinnsen (Ed.), *Current approaches to phonological theory* (pp. 126–173). Blooming-ton: Indiana University Press.

Education of All Handicapped Children Act (PL 94–142). (1975). *Federal Register,* August 23.

Elbert, M., Dinnsen, D. A., & Weismer, G. (1984). Phonological theory and the misarticulating child. *ASHA Monographs,* No. 22. Rockville, MD: ASHA.

Garrett, M. (1975). The analysis of sentence production. In G. Bower (Ed.), *The psychology of learning and motivation: Vol. 9.* New York: Academic.

Garrett, M. (1980). Levels of processing in sentence production. In B. Butterworth (Ed.), *Language production: Vol. 1.* London: Academic.

Geirut, J. A., Elbert, M., & Dinnsen, D. A. (1987). A functional analysis of phonol-ogical knowledge and generalization learning in misarticulating children. *Jour-nal of Speech and Hearing Research, 30,* 462–479.

Goldsmith, J. (forthcoming). *Autosegmental and metrical phonology: A new synthesis.* Oxford: Basil Blackwell.

Hoffman, P. R., Shuckers, G. H., & Daniloff, R. G. (1989). *Children's phonetic disorders: Theory and treatment.* Boston: Little, Brown.

Ingram, D. (1976). *Phonological disability in children.* London: Edward Arnold.

Leonard, L. B. (1985). Unusual and subtle phonological behavior in the speech of phonologically disordered children. *Journal of Speech and Hearing Disorders, 50,* 4–13.

Lewis, B. A., Ekelman, B. L. & Aram, D. M. (in press). A familial study of severe articulation and phonology disorders. *Journal of Speech and Hearing Research.*

Morrison, J. A., & Shriberg, L. D. (1989). *Citing versus talking: Measurement validity in phonologic assessment.* Paper presented at the Annual Convention, American Speech-Language-Hearing Association, St. Louis.

Parlour, S. F., & Broen, P. A. (1989). *Familial risk for articulation disorder: A 25-year follow-up.* Paper presented at the Annual Meeting of the Behavior Genetics Association, Charlottesville, VA.

Paul, R. (1989). *Profiles of toddlers with delayed expressive language development.* Paper presented at the Biennial Meeting of the Society for Research in Child Develop-ment, Kansas City, MO.

Shattuck-Huffnagel, S. (1983). Sublexical units and suprasegmental structure in speech production planning. In P. MacNeilage (Ed.), *The production of speech.* New York: Springer-Verlag.

Shriberg, L. D. (1988). The otitis media-speech connection. *Journal of the National Student Speech-Language-Hearing Association, 15,* 56–67.

Shriberg, L. D. (1989). *Measurement validity.* Paper presented at the American Speech-Language-Hearing Foundation Conference on Treatment Efficacy, San Antonio.

Shriberg, L. D., Kwiatkowski, J., Best, S., Hengst, J., & Terselic-Weber, B. (1986). Characteristics of children with phonologic disorders of unknown origin. *Journal of Speech and Hearing Disorders, 51,* 140–161.

Shriberg and Widder (forthcoming). Speech and prosody characteristics of adults with mental retardation.

Stampe, D. (1973). *A dissertation on natural phonology.* Unpublished doctoral disser-tation, University of Chicago.

Tomblin, J. B. (1989). Familial concentration of developmental language impairment. *Journal of Speech and Hearing Disorders, 54,* 287–295.

Watson, C. S., Reed, D. J., Kewley-Port, D., & Maki, D. (1989). The Indiana speech training aid (ISTRA) I: Comparisons between human and computer-based evaluation of speech quality. *Journal of Speech and Hearing Research, 32,* 245–251.

CHAPTER 16

Similarities and Differences in Vocalizations of Deaf and Hearing Infants: Future Directions for Research

D. KIMBROUGH OLLER

The traditional belief that deaf and hearing infants produce the same kinds of speech-like sounds during the "babbling period" has recently been shown to be fundamentally flawed. In fact, the babbling vocalizations that provide the clearest indications of a developing speech capacity are clearly different in deaf and hearing infants during the first year of life and other differences may also be obtained. In order to delineate the differences and similarities, it is necessary to work within a carefully formulated framework of description. Until very recently no such framework was available, and perhaps for that reason it was possible to maintain a false characterization of babbling in deaf infants for many years.

The future of the study of vocal development in normal and handicapped infants depends both upon the elaboration of a rich framework and upon the acquisition of detailed longitudinal data. The purpose of this

Acknowledgment: The research reported here has been supported by NIH/NINCDS grant #1-R01-NS26121-01 to D. Kimbrough Oller.

chapter is to provide some indications of the importance of both the theoretical elaboration and the longitudinal empirical work.

THEORETICAL ACCOMPLISHMENTS
AND FUTURE NEEDS

The description of infant speech-like sounds was hampered through the first three-quarters of this century by a lack of agreement about how to characterize the notion "speech-like." Some authors (e.g., Irwin, 1947) presumed that all infant sounds other than vegetative utterances (cries, coughs, etc.) could be transcribed phonetically. This approach begged the question of how speech-like the sounds being transcribed were and consequently leveled potentially valuable differentiations among speech-like sounds occurring across the first year of life. Lynip (1951) attacked the transcription of infant sounds, pointing out that there did not exist and international alphabet for baby sounds and concluding that the only appropriate description of infant sounds was an instrumental acoustic one. Unfortunately, acoustic analysis of infant sounds in and of itself does not indicate the degree to which infant sounds resemble speech. Consequently, investigators following Lynip's recommendation provided acoustic characterizations that did no better than phonetic transcriptions in specifying the relationship of infant sounds and speech.

During the 1970s my colleagues and I at the University of Washington began to develop a new approach that we felt would help bridge the gap between those who advocated transcription and those who advocated acoustic analysis of infant sounds. We began by noting that transcription of infant sounds was most applicable when the sounds met certain criteria of syllabicity. Sounds occurring in the first half year of life commonly did not meet the criteria, while those occurring beyond six or seven months often did. We imposed rigid criteria in defining the term *canonical syllable* (Oller, Wieman, Doyle, & Ross, 1975): the syllable had to have at least one vowel and one consonant, and the formant transition from the consonant to the vowel had to be rapid and unbroken. Slow transitions produced what we termed *marginal syllables*.

When this definition was imposed during transcription of infant vocalizations, certain surprising facts became quickly obvious. The traditional belief (attributed to Jakobson, 1941) that babies babble all the sounds of all the world's languages with equal ease proved drastically incorrect. In fact, babies were seen to have very strong preferences in their canonical babbling for certain syllable types. The sounds preferred tended to be drawn from the same set that had for years been observed to be preferred by young children who were learning to speak meaningfully (see also Locke, 1984).

Perhaps even more interesting was the fact that, having differentiated baby utterances that included canonical syllables from those that did not, we were in a position to begin to study the ones that did not meet the canonical criteria from a new perspective. After moving to the University of Miami, I began to analyze "precanonical" sounds in the attempt to determine whether they might systematically manifest an emerging capacity for speech. This effort resulted in a stage model of infant vocal development (Oller, 1980) and a theoretical descriptive framework we called "metaphonology" (see esp. Oller, 1986). We recently revised the term to "infraphonology" because the purpose of the model is to provide an account of the infrastructure of the sound systems of natural languages. The model provides definitions of concrete phonetic units (segmentally specified syllables such as [pa], [dI], [qu], [eps], etc.), indeed the whole range of potential phonetic units in natural languages by specifying in acoustic terms how phonetic units are constructed. Having specified the rules of formation of syllables, any sound that is heard or analyzed acoustically can be judged in terms of the extent to which it meets the requirements of the rules. In other words, in an infraphonological framework, it is possible to judge the degree of speechiness of any sound and thus to characterize the vocalizations of a baby in terms of the extent to which those vocalizations resemble speech.

In the context of the model, it became possible to interpret sounds produced by infants at various ages. The patterns of sounds occurring had been described by our own group and by Stark (1980) with considerable agreement. In the first two months of life, infants were noted to produce a large number of nondistress sounds with "normal phonation," the pattern of vocal production that occurs most commonly in vowels of speech. Consequently, we began to refer to this period as the Phonation Stage. During the next two months (the Gooing Stage), infants were noted to produce normally phonated sounds in alternation with articulations occurring in the back of the mouth. Speech requires articulation in order to provide an acoustic landscape that is sufficiently differentiated to support a rich code of communication. During the next two months (Expansion Stage), many new vocal types appear to come under the infant's control: (1) vowel-like sounds that not only include normal phonation, but also rich formant structure; (2) squeals and growls, sounds that appear to indicate the infant's emerging control of pitch; (3) yells and whispers, sounds that indicate amplitude control; (4) "raspberries," articulations involving the lips; and (5) marginal babbles, sounds that include both vowel-like and consonant-like elements in presyllables. In the next few months infants enter the canonical stage, wherein they can produce consonants and vowels in fully well-formed syllables.

The infraphonological model affords an understanding of the significance of the changes in vocal control from stage to stage. Without the model, a canonical babble, a marginal babble, an isolated vowel, or a raspberry are an array of sounds produced by the infant, none of which is seen as more or less speech-like than the other. Within the model, a principled basis for differentiation is provided: marginal babbles are more speech-like than isolated vowels or raspberries because they include a combination of consonant-like and vowel-like articulations (canonical syllables always include at least one consonant and one vowel), and canonical syllables are more speech-like than marginal ones because the former include canonical syllable timing while the latter do not.

Another empirical outcome of detailing the model of infraphonology has been the discovery that vocalizations of deaf and hearing infants are fundamentally different during the first year of life. This finding flies in the face of traditional wisdom, but is unequivocal. Deaf infants enter the "canonical" stage of vocalization, during which canonical syllables are produced frequently and repetitively, substantially later than hearing infants do. In fact, it appears that there is no overlap in the distributions of ages of onset of canonical babbling in deaf and hearing infants (Kent, Osberger, Netsell, & Hustedde, 1987; Oller & Eilers, 1988) and a variety of additional differences appear to occur at later stages of development (see Stoel-Gammon & Otomo, 1986).

Infraphonology is potentially a very major theoretical endeavor that will encompass not only the definition of the canonical syllable, but also the specification of the limits natural languages impose upon segments, phonetic features, intonations, boundary markings, paralinguistic usage of loudness/pitch/duration, and the relationship of the natural value-bound signal system of our species (including cries, laughs, moans, shrieks, etc.) to the largely value-free (arbitrarily meaningful) system of speech. We have a long way to go in seeking to fill out the theory and each step may have potentially crucial benefits. For example, in the area of intonations, recent research by Papousek and Papousek (1988) and Fernald (1988) suggests that parents from a wide variety of language backgrounds (including Chinese, English, German, Italian, and others) communicate with their infants in the first half-year of life with a set of clearly definable intonation types, superimposed upon an apparently unlimited variety of phrases and sentences. For example, if the mother is consoling the child, there is a particular intonation that accompanies widely different sentences and phrases ("Oh, you look so sad," "Poor baby," etc.). It is not clear whether infants truly "understand" the intonations that parents use, but the attentiveness and responsiveness of infants in face-to-face conversations utilizing these patterns is suggestive of an innate awareness. An important goal for the future of infraphonology will be to try to account for "canonical" intonations, universal patterns that have relatively fixed values both in terms of meaning and boundary marking function. The emergence of canonical intonations and the elaborations of them could then be plausibly taken as a barometer of increasing control of the tools of speech.

Another area of important theoretical development in infraphonology will be concentrated in the characterization of the relationship of voluntary and involuntary vocalizations. In collaboration with Barry Lester, I have begun an effort to create an infraphonological characterization of one of the biologically most important involuntary vocalizations, the sounds of infant cry (Oller & Lester, 1989). A major goal of this work is to specify the nature of cry with sufficient clarity that based upon acoustic analysis, cries could be differentiated from all the other sound types infants produce, including voluntary speech-like sounds as well as laughs, coughs, grunts, etc. The task will not be simple, since it is already clear that although there do exist cries that are quite unambiguous (i.e., they are not confusable with other sound types), there also exist units (breath-groups) of cries that would be more properly called "fussing," as well as cries that resemble laughter, grunting, quasiresonant sounds, and even coughs. Furthermore, as the infant matures, crying comes under voluntary control and the infant uses cry instrumentally. Such cry sounds can be superimposed upon other sound categories including canonical babbles.

The gradations of cry from involuntary, unambiguous units through voluntary units that are mixed with other sound types and are thus harder to characterize, must be accounted for within the infraphonological framework. In the past, we have often struggled with the categorization of infant vocalization data because it has not been clear how to treat sounds that include a mixture of speech-like and presumably vegetative features. We have vacillated between ignoring all cry or fussy sounds and attempting to categorize speech-like cries and fusses (e.g., those that include canonical syllables) in the same way we would categorize other speech-like sounds. An infraphonology that incorporates acoustic characterization of cry and other sounds in its definitional framework should provide a principled basis upon which to account for the speechiness of sounds that include acoustic features of involuntary vocalizations.

IMPORTANCE OF EMPIRICAL ELABORATION THROUGH LONGITUDINAL RESEARCH

As our descriptions of infant vocalizations become more detailed and insightful, it becomes increasingly important to examine vocalizations in longitudinal studies that consider both within-subject quotidian variability in vocalizations of infants and between-subject variation. Only in the context of close-interval longitudinal studies on infants from a variety of backgrounds can a clear picture of the significance of vocal patterns be obtained. To illustrate this point consider data in Figure 16-1 based on 30 sessions of vocalization recordings from a deaf infant. The data result from categorization of vocal samples (which were spaced across the period from 4 to 18 months of age, a time period prior to the onset of canonical babbling for this child). The figure indicates the proportion of all nonvegetative sounds that were categorized as "glottal sequences." A glottal sequence is a pattern of at least two nuclei (vowel-like sounds) separated by glottal stops (e.g., the utterance "uh, uh" is a glottal sequence).

A trend has emerged in our recent studies indicating that many deaf infants produce glottal sequences in inordinate proportions compared to the proportions occurring in hearing infants. However, it is difficult to be sure of this, given that there are very large quotidian variations in the proportions of glottal sounds that occur in deaf infants that have been studied. Note that this subject showed variations ranging from 0% to over 60% of the utterances in vocal samples occurring across a 14-month period. Furthermore, highly variable proportions of glottal sequences occurred throughout the 14-month period of sampling.

The proportion of glottal sequences in this deaf infant is much higher than in any of 11 hearing infants sampled across two precanonical sessions each (Oller, Eilers, Bull, & Carney, 1985). The highest proportion of glottal

Fig. 16-1. Proportion of glottal sequences in a deaf infant.

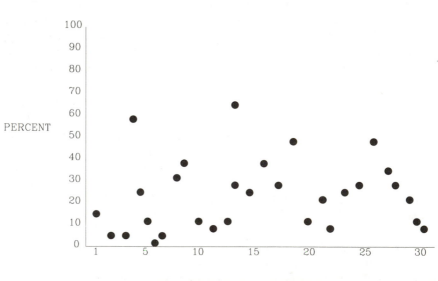

SESSIONS (4–18 MONTHS OF AGE)

sequences occurring in any of these samples was less than 20% and the mean was 4–5%. The mean value across the samples for the deaf child was over 20%. Clearly, then, the deaf child used glottal sequences more than hearing children. The problem is that one is required to collect a substantial body of data in order to prove the point.

If one were to assess the vocalizations of a particular infant on a particular day, trying to compare proportion of occurrence of a particular utterance type against some standard assumed for normal infants, one would be quite likely to be confounded by the occurrence of sample to sample variation. Without longitudinal studies, such variations cannot be anticipated.

Interchild differences in patterns of vocal development are also, of course, problematic for those who wish to provide a perspective on the patterns of vocalization that occur in infancy (cf., Vihman, 1986). A particular problem that has been left aside in previous longitudinal studies concerns the possible role of interchild differences that may be attributable to factors such a socioeconomic status and medical risk due, for example, to premature birth. Without systematic investigation of the roles of such factors in vocal development we are left with a variety of unproven assumptions. Because previous longitudinal work has been focused almost entirely on middle- to upper-middle-class families (the kind of people who commonly participate in longitudinal research projects that require extensive commitments of time and energy), our picture of normal vocal development presumes that small variations in environment (e.g., due to small changes in SES), or in medical risk status would have no effect on vocalization. Future work must assess the validity of this assumption if infant vocal assessments are to be made in a way that includes generality. Only in the context of generally applicable characterizations of the vocal patterns of normal infants can vocalizations of deaf infants be portrayed appropriately.

Interchild variability among hearing-impaired infants is an equally large problem. In particular the role of degree of hearing loss must be assessed. Thus far no infraphonologically rich studies have been conducted on the vocal development of hearing impaired infants who vary systematically in degree of hearing loss. It seems inevitable that differences between profoundly deaf and hearing infants would be greater than differences between moderately impaired and hearing infants.

CONCLUSIONS

Research in infant vocalizations is moving rapidly toward richer characterization of patterns of acquisition. The theoretical developments appear to be as important as empirical ones. Elaborations of infraphonology to include intonational information and sensitive assessments of value-bound signals such as cry and laughter will no doubt greatly enhance descriptive power. Similarly, longitudinal studies within the framework will provide a detailed basis upon which to evaluate the effects of hearing impairment on vocal development.

REFERENCES

Fernald, A. (1988). *Form and function in mother's speech to preverbal infants*. Paper presented at the International and Interdisciplinary Symposium on Origins and Development of Nonverbal Vocal Communication, Max Planck Institute for Psychiatry, Munich.

Irwin, O. C. (1947). Development of speech during infancy. *Journal of Experimental Psychology, 37*, 187–193.

Jakobson, R. (1941). *"Kindersprache, Aphasie, und allgemeine Lautgesetze."* Uppsala, Germany: Almqvist and Wiksell.

Kent, R., Osberger, M. J., Netsell, R., & Hustedde, C. (1987). Phonetic development in identical twins differing in auditory function. *Journal of Speech and Hearing Disorders, 52*, 64–75.

Locke, J. (1984). *Phonological acquisition and change*. New York: Academic.

Lynip, A. (1951). The use of magnetic devices in the collection and analysis of the preverbal utterances of an infant. *Genetic Psychology Monographs, 44*, 221–262.

Oller, D. K. (1980). The emergence of the sounds of speech in infancy. In G. Yeni-Komshian, J. Kavanagh, & C. Ferguson (Eds.), *Child phonology: Vol. 1. Production*. New York: Academic.

Oller, D. K. (1986). Metaphonology and infant vocalizations. In B. Lindbloom & R. Zetterstom (Eds.), *Precursors of early speech*. Basingstroke, Hampshire, England: Macmillan.

Oller, D. K., & Eilers, R. E., (1988). The role of audition in infant babbling. *Child Development, 59*, 441–449.

Oller, D. K., Eilers, R., Bull, D., & Carney, A. (1985). Prespeech vocalizations of a deaf infant: A comparison with normal metaphonological development. *Journal of Speech and Hearing Research, 28*, 47–63.

Oller, D. K., & Lester, B. M. (1989). Structure of cry and noncry sounds of infants: Metaphonological comparisons. NICHD Cry Conference, Mary Woodward Lasker Center, Bethesda, MD.

Oller, D. K., Wieman, L. Doyle, W., & Ross, C. (1975). Infant babbling and speech, *Journal of Child Language, 3*, 1–11.

Papousek, M., & Papousek, H. (1988). *Vocal dialogues between mother and infant*. Paper presented at the International and Interdisciplinary Symposium on Origins and Development of Nonverbal Vocal Communication, Max Planck Institute for Psychiatry, Munich.

Stark, R. E. (1980). Stages of speech development in the first year of life. In G. Yeni-Komshian, J. Kavanagh, & C. Ferguson (Eds.), *Child phonology: Vol. 1, Production*. New York: Academic.

Stoel-Gammon, C., & Otomo, K. (1986). Babbling development of hearing impaired and normally hearing subjects. *Journal of Speech and Hearing Disorders, 51*, 33–41.

Vihman, M. M. (1986). Individual differences in babbling and early speech. In B. Lindbloom & R. Zetterstom, (Eds.) *Precursors of early speech*. Basingstroke, Hampshire, England: Macmillan.

PART D

Language Processes

CHAPTER 17

Models of Language Disorder

ROBIN S. CHAPMAN

The root metaphors that we use in viewing the world often determine what we find, just as less pervasive metaphors—even dead and well-buried ones—may influence the way a problem is understood and the inferences we are likely to draw. Even now the reader may be thinking that this chapter will exhume that old corpse of a problem in the field—are children language disordered, or deviant? So the metaphorical reference hints, and so the chapter will.

Metaphors go far beyond poetic language and folk sayings. Time is money, goes the American proverb—so I spend or save it, waste it, invest it, spare it, use it, lose it, try to budget it through hosts of one-minute managers, borrow a minute of yours (Lakoff & Johnson, 1980) to make this argument. Arguments can be thought of as containers—and critiqued for their amount of content, the presence of holes, what's central, whether they will hold water. Or argument is war: defended, attacked, shot down, demolished, won, or lost. Or argument is a journey—and we note its progress, the amount of ground covered, where we have strayed off the path or gone in circles, whether listeners have followed it. Our models of language disorders, too, conceal metaphors that end up committing us,

Preparation of this chapter was supported in part by Core Support Grant No. 5 P30 HD03352 to the Waisman Center on Mental Retardation and Human Development and NIH Grant R01 HD23353 to the author. I thank my colleagues Rhea Paul, Dolores Vetter, and Susan Weismer for comments.

more or less willingly, to models of the world and the ways of knowing it: the nature of mind and its functioning, the world that is represented and that brings about the representation, the subjective and objective worlds, the role and ways of action.

Some years ago the philosopher Stephen Pepper (1942), in his search for truth, tried to evaluate the various dogmatic positions about the nature of the world that, one by one, he had explored: theology, physics, idealism, Gestalt psychology, psychoanalysis, political democracy and Marxism, logical positivism. In rooting out the metaphors at the heart of these different theories of the way the world is, he identified four root metaphors that, he suggested, led to relatively adequate hypotheses about the world. These hypotheses were mechanism, formism, organicism, and contextualism. (Two inadequate root metaphors for world hypotheses were also derived, animism and mysticism; of these, more later.)

All four adequate hypotheses were reasonable ways of looking at the world, he argued. All four have both the subjective and objective world as their scope. However, the four are autonomous, mutually exclusive, and different in their results. What are pure facts for one theory are highly interpreted evidence for another. It is illegitimate, he proposed, for one of these world theories to be criticized in the categories of the other, or to attempt to demonstrate the truth of one by showing the shortcomings of another. Further, he argued, combining the theories based on different root metaphors is simply confusing conceptually, even if eclecticism arises in practice.

I want to discuss these four world hypotheses here because I believe that we are the inheritors of all four in our attempts to model language disorders. Much of what our students find confusing in the differing definitions of language disorders, and the differing approaches to assessment and intervention, arises, I will argue, from the inherent tension in these differing world hypotheses. Much that is useful comes from entertaining each of the four models in turn as a way of understanding the individual case, rather than accepting one to the exclusion of the other. I am advocating practical eclecticism, as Pepper did.

Ultimately, we may find a view of the world that makes unified sense; until then, the testing of different viewpoints gives us at least a cubistic, fractured sense of the whole. Although it may be cognitively stressful, I believe it is clinically desirable to entertain this multiple vision, if we want to account for the heterogeneous group of children we label "language disordered."

What are these different ways of looking at the world, their root metaphors, and the corresponding models entertained in our own accounts of language disorders (as offered, for example, in Bloom & Lahey's 1978 seminal text)?

MECHANISM: THE ETIOLOGICAL MODEL

Mechanism is a world view associated with the philosophies of Galileo, Descartes, Hobbes, Locke, and Hume among others. The root metaphor of mechanism is a machine. Mechanistic accounts of the physical world have been highly successful; of the mental world, hotly debated. A mechanistic model of language disorders in children would reveal their causes: what has gone wrong in the causal workings of the world and the brain. The etiological model provides a starting basis for defining specific language disorders by ruling out language disorders associated with (presumedly) known causes: retardation (including a variety of more specific syndromes—Down, Fragile-x, Prader-Willi, Williams, Fetal Alcohol), hearing impairment, blindness, emotional disturbance (including autism and thought disorders), seizures and other central nervous system dysfunction, acquired aphasia, and environmental impoverishment. It also rules out language differences associated with differences in culture and dialect. If these factors have been ruled out, then specific language impairment can be diagnosed, with its cause, currently, unknown.

This listing points to major causes of language disorder or difference: cognitive delay or difference, social delay or difference, reduced amount or inappropriateness of linguistic input (through whatever modality) and world experience, impaired short- or long-term memory for that experience, attention disorders, sensory and motor system dysfunctioning. The presumption of the etiological model is that a cause—or causes—can also be found for specific language impairment. The model requires the assessment of the presence or absence of these causally related factors.

The etiological model can make preventive steps clear: keep phenylalanine out of the diet of PKU children; don't drink if pregnant; vaccinate the population for rubella; offer genetic counseling; wear motorcycle helmets; reduce high fevers; wear hearing protectors in noisy environments. It also makes some intervention steps clear: for the hearing impaired, fit a hearing aid and provide auditory and linguistic experience. For those whose speech, but not comprehension, is severely impaired, provide an augmentative means of communication and opportunities to use it. For the retarded, temper expectations for language-learning progress according to what you know of the cognitive deficit. For the autistic, additionally temper expectations for language comprehension and use according to what you know of the social and linguistic deficits.

What the etiological model does not illuminate is how language disorder is to be detected in the first place, save from its association with causal or predisposing factors; or how it is to be characterized in a given population. For guidance about how language disorder—of known or unknown causes—is to be described, we turn to other models.

FORMISM: THE DEVIANCE MODEL

Formism was Pepper's term for models based on categories and relations between them, either in terms of attributes or normative "best exemplars." Platonic idealism, or Aristotle's classificatory scheme of natural objects, would be examples. The root metaphor of these hypotheses is *similarity*—either the categories of equivalence yielded by common sense perception, as in blades of grass, sets of cups and saucers, spoons; or the categories defined by normative prototypes—children developing language normally, for instance.

Ties other than similarity can link categories; one of relevance to our language-disorder model is that of difference or otherness. Opposed to the category of children developing language normally is that of children who are not: language-disordered children. Formists, however, go on to seek the ways that members of a category are similar to one another. The call for increased breadth and specificity of description of language-disordered children in research studies is a call for empirical evidence of that similarity—or evidence that can be used to construct subcategories of similar children.

A number of subcategories have been proposed through the years. One such distinction focuses on *process*—those children with expressive language problems only, versus those with receptive and expressive language problems (Aram & Nation, 1982). These two categories are encountered with approximately equal frequency in mentally retarded children, for example (Miller, Chapman & MacKenzie, 1981).

A second categorical scheme has involved separate linguistic modalities, treating them as modular—pragmatic disorders, syntactic disorders, semantic disorders, phonological disorders or, following Bloom and Lahey's classification (1978), disorders of content, form, use, and their interactions. These have arisen not just because they are the categories imposed by our analytic tools and tests, but also because children have been found who are different in one of the dimensions but not others. A child may score above average in vocabulary comprehension, for example, and significantly below average in syntactic comprehension. Or a shy child may choose not to talk.

A third way of categorizing subgroups of language-disordered children has grouped them according to similarities in types of errors in spoken language (e.g., Fletcher, this volume, chapter 8; Miller, 1987): (1) sentence formulation problems, (2) word finding problems, (3) rate and fluency problems, (4) discourse and pragmatic problems, (5) hyperverbalism, and (6) problems in making reference. These categories have risen out of clinical experience and pose different problems for intervention. Errors in comprehension, too, may arise and yield a typology; these have yet to be studied as subcategories.

Taken together, the categories of language disorder suggested by these various accounts can be assembled as a three-dimensional matrix, process by linguistic module, with the production categories elaborated for error types.

Our research studies and clinical experience tell us that examples of most cells of this matrix exist, though the extent of the association is uncertain. The formist account offers powerful advice for assessment—it carries with it the implication that a complete description of the language disorder requires assessment of each area.

Our research strategies, however, too often continue to be based on a simpler version of a formist model of language deviance—the inclusive category of language disordered. Other labels get applied, of course—specific language impairment, congenital aphasia, language delayed, language-learning disabled—arising, most often, out of differences in geography, textbook, tests used, or age of child or researcher. But often, the researcher's aim is to draw inferences about a single category of child labeled "language-learning disordered" or "specific language impaired," based on the assumption that the different components of the above matrix will all be normal or nonnormal to the degree that the measured entries are—the belief, then, that there is a single category of such children whose dissimilarity from children developing language normally is accompanied by similarity to each other. Or the researcher may be aware of potential heterogeneity but hope to be studying a causal factor sufficiently robust to show group differences anyway. (Or, of course, the researcher, a mechanist at heart, may be assessing the contribution of multiple factors to the heterogeneity of behaviors observed.)

Those who are formists at heart, then, are always struggling with current research practice in their attempts to achieve a full description of the language disorder that captures similarity within groups—a wish to discover the natural taxonomy of language disorder that can be at odds with the purposes of the mechanist.

ORGANICISM: THE DEVELOPMENTAL DELAY MODEL

Organicism as a world view is associated with the philosophies of Schelling and Hegel. The root metaphors of organicism as a world hypothesis are those of the organism, growing; and the process of integration. It is here that developmental models such as Piaget's find their home, and the classical account of language development, as expressed in the work of Brown (1973) and his colleagues. In the developmental model, one stage of language development leads to the next: new functions are first expressed by old forms, and new forms are first used to express old functions (Slobin,

1979). By function is meant both meaning and communicative goal. Developing concepts arise in the interaction of cognitive structure and the world, and the subsequent integration of structures. Changing goals for communication arise in the interaction of the child in his social world. In addition to function constraints, ordering of syntactic and phonological forms is determined by their perceptual saliency, their ease of reproduction, and the consistency and transparency with which they map currently understood meaning and communicative goal. (Frequency of input is sometimes cited as an additional determiner of acquisition order.) The child's language system becomes systematically more integrated in a predictable way. Consistent errors emerge with, and reflect, particular stages of learning.

According to the developmental model, it is not the child's age but his or her language stage that predicts the next achievements and errors. Social and cognitive levels will constrain the functions attempted and input the forms attempted. The main source of individual difference in the developmental model is that of *rate* of language acquisition, though local individual differences will arise from variations in input and the child's cognitive and social levels, and sometimes more pervasive individual differences are proposed (e.g., Nelson's referential versus expressive children, 1973; Peters's analytic versus gestalt learners, 1984; Kagan's behaviorally inhibited children, 1989).

The first question the developmental model raises about children labeled by the etiological and formist models as language disordered is that of whether they are simply developmentally delayed in language. This question has motivated much of the research in child language disorders, leading to control groups matched for mean length of utterance in the study of syntactic, semantic, and pragmatic acquisition and input. Both longitudinal and cross-sectional findings have affirmed that a major component of the language-disordered child's developing system is predicted by what we know of normal developmental sequence. So too are major components of the developing systems of language-disordered children in other etiological groups—the retarded, the autistic, and the hearing impaired, with varying degrees of exception.

In the developmental model, a communication profile might be developed that showed age-equivalent performance on each of a number of language dimensions contributed by the formist. (Those dimensions on which development was atypical of any age would be so marked, in such profiling.) Note that the classification of developmental *level* requires measures sensitive to developmental change on that dimension. There are other assessment systems for the same dimensions that may allow classification of the child's errors, or inventory adult-like structures, but not permit placement on a developmental continuum; for example, the original grammatical analyses of LARSP, or checklists of appropriate or inappropriate pragmatic behaviors where "appropriate" is not defined for the child's age. It is the shift to the developmental model that leads to the search for developmentally sensitive measures, one ongoing today.

When it is asked if the developmental model yields a picture of overall developmental delay in language and nothing else, the conclusion alters. Many exceptions and atypical performances are noted.

First, articulatory performance may diverge from language development, although phonologically disordered children are often language impaired as well (see Shriberg & Kwiatkowski, 1988).

Second, although grammatical structure inventories are similar in normal and language-impaired children, language-impaired children are observed to use the structures less frequently. However, failures of word retrieval appear to arise not from a particular difficulty in word finding, but from a less elaborated semantic network (Kail & Leonard, 1986).

Third, the extensive assessments called for by the formist models of language disorders reveal other asymmetries between the rate of development in one language component and another—for example, the discrepancies between language production and comprehension noted earlier in some, but not all, specifically language-impaired children.

Fourth, the etiological models of language disorder reveal some atypical characteristics, in addition to the generally slowed developmental sequence, peculiar to specific conditions. These included specific difficulties with the acquisition of inflectional morphology among the hearing impaired; unusual failures to request clarification on referential communication tasks by language/learning disabled children; more frequent formulation problems, secondary to the attempt to express more complex propositional content than younger MLU matched controls, in language impaired (MacLachlan & Chapman, 1988); mutism or echolalia and specific deficits in affective and social uses of language in autism; excessive talking with little content, suggesting the separation of expressive syntax and semantics, in hydrocephalic children; and divergence of semantic and syntactic comprehension skills from each other, accompanied by divergence in nonverbal cognitive skills dependent or not on short-term memory (Chapman, Schwartz, & Kay-Raining Bird, 1988).

How to account for these exceptions? This is a puzzle we are still working out, and its answer may considerably alter our approach to language disorders. Part of the answer comes from considering how the normal acquisition process would behave when variation is introduced into one or more of the subsystems that interact to determine acquisition sequence. What happens, for example, when a language-impaired child with the nonverbal cognitive skills of a 10-year-old and the expressive language skills of a 6-year-old attempts to tell a story? The answer appears to be that more elaborate content is attempted by the 10-year-old than the 6-year-old language match, with a corresponding increase in formulation dysfluencies.

Or when these same two children's pragmatic comprehension skills are compared by giving them a picture of four seals—one with a ring, one with a ball, one with a stand, one alone—and asking them to point to the seal? The 6-year-old asks for clarification. The 10-year-old language-impaired—and a 10-year-old normal child—points to the seal by itself, assuming that the experimenter would have provided additional information if it had been needed.

Or consider what information in the acoustic signal would be consistently degraded by a high-frequency hearing loss; specific effects on sibilant bound morphemes might be expected.

Thus a number of apparent exceptions to the normally encountered developmental sequence can be accounted for when we consider how initial asymmetries between cognition, social functioning, input and the current state of the language system might affect its course—indeed, the course of language acquisition in language-disordered children with these divergent cognitive, social, or sensory skills offers an interesting window on the functional subsystems of language, one not always obtainable in studying variation in normal development. Use of the developmental model in this expanded way helps sort out the facts of performance most likely attributable to normal acquisition processes from those most likely to yield insight into what has gone wrong.

The developmental model, then, offers a powerful tool for assessing the language acquisition of a language-disordered child, for predicting what to work on next. Its account of the factors maximizing acquisition rate at different developmental levels also offers a powerful guide to intervention procedures likely to work most effectively. And it creates a useful framework for identifying those aspects of performance *not* consistent with developmental expectations, that other models may better encompass.

CONTEXTUALISM: THE COMMUNICATIVE EVENT MODEL

Pepper's fourth adequate world hypothesis is that of contextualism, commonly called "pragmatism" and associated with the philosophies of Peirce, James, Dewey, and Mead. Its root metaphor is best conveyed by the historic event, an act carried out in and with its setting, which includes, for the historic event, the current act of re-presenting it. The contextualist categories are derived from the total given event and often lack the orderliness of other theories' hierarchically structured categories. Hymes's (1972) account of the communicative event is such a model in our own field.

The communicative event model leads us to analyze, not the child, not his language, not his history, but the current interaction, from the viewpoint of its communicative success or failure.

The speech event is the focus of analysis in this model (e.g., conversation, narrative, lecture), and the conventions that exist regarding its structure and performance. (Expectations about story structure, content, and delivery would be an example.) Eight general components of the communicative event are identified by Hymes: settings, participants, ends, act sequences, key, instrumentalities, norms, and genres. Settings include the time, place, and physical circumstances of the interaction, and the scene, or psychological setting, of the event. Participants include a speaker or sender, the addresser, audience, and addressee. Ends include communicative goals, both conventional and personal ones, and communicative outcomes, including both conventionally expected and unintended ones. Speech act sequences include the message form, content, and communicative intent of the speech acts making up the event. *Key* is Hymes's term for the tone, manner, or spirit with which a speech act is done, referring to social motives derived from clarity or politeness considerations. Instrumentalities include both the channels and forms of the communication. Channels can include spoken, written, telegraphic, or gestural means, used in varying ways (e.g., singing, whispering, whistling, chanting). Form of speech can be designated as particular language and dialect defined by historical development, a particular code defined by mutual intelligibility criteria, and register or variety defined by specializations in use. Norms include norms for social interaction and for interpretation (e.g., expectations described in the Grecian principle of cooperative conversation and the solutions to risk-taking described as politeness phenomena). Genres refer to categories of communication such as poems, myths, stories, proverbs, riddles, prayers, and commercials that may or may not be identical with the speech event.

Contextualist models such as Hymes's shift our perspective on language disorder radically. They lead to an analysis of what has gone well, or ill, in specific interchanges; the assessment of a variety of speech events in which individuals must, or wish to, participate; and intervention recommendations that may increase communicative effectiveness from a variety of participants' viewpoints. For example, students' comprehension failures in a classroom setting during instruction might be redressed by simplifying teacher language, choosing a different textbook, simplifying lesson content, coaching the students to request clarification from each other or the teacher, or creating an instructional routine, with demonstration and label, with which the children are familiar.

Language disorder is not the central construct of a contextualist theory, nor are children and their developmental histories of primary focus.

Communicative expectations, breakdowns, and their remedies in specific contexts are the main points of analysis.

ECLECTICISM IN PRACTICE

Examples of all four kinds of world hypotheses have been described in our models of language disorders: mechanist, formist, organismic, and contextual. Pepper's point in distinguishing the different classes of world hypotheses was that they were mutually exclusive (and hence needed to be kept conceptually distinct) but approximately equally viable candidates for claims to adequacy (despite the dogmatism of some of their adherents). In practice, he added, we end up using all four points of view—and in addition, the animist view created by applying our metaphor of human action to the world, and the mystic view created by our internal explorations of consciousness (see, e.g., Bruner, 1988). We do so because different cognitive domains are structured differently—and because these different structures are based on differing root metaphors (an idea extended by Lakoff, 1987).

In the field of child language disorders, each of these ways of looking at the world brings its own insight into the problem, suggestions for what to look at, ideas for what to do. To entertain them all in a given case is to benefit from the multiple viewpoints they offer. It is also to pursue, in research and clinical practice, the differing questions they raise—of the causes of language disorder (etiological models), of the natural taxonomy of language disorders (deviance models), of the developmental course of language acquisition in language-impaired children (developmental delay models), and of the severity of communicative failure and the systemic means for altering it (communicative event models).

Experience will prove some frameworks more immediately useful than others in specific circumstances. The contextualist framework may be particularly useful for children encountering radically different expectations—those from different cultures, for example, or severely or profoundly retarded individuals expected to function as adults by the community, or autistic children whose means of communicating intents may be discoverable only from context. It will identify the important communicative needs of the child and allow analysis of the similarity of therapy contexts to other contexts of use.

The etiological framework will suggest children at high risk for language impairment, and define by exclusion the group of specifically language-impaired children. Formist frameworks will specify subgroups of such children who may need very different interventions. The organismic view, incorporating developmental delay as it does, is central to the definitions of disorder and the development of intervention goals and expectations.

From this multiple perspective, it can be seen that the question "language disorder: delay or difference?" is really a metatheoretic debate about which world hypothesis, which root metaphor, to invoke. The practical answer being recommended is "consider both," and the theoretical answer, "it depends on your model of the world."

REFERENCES

Aram, D. M., & Nation, J. E. (1982). *Child language disorders.* St. Louis: Mosby.

Bloom, L., & Lahey, M. (1978). *Language development and language disorders.* New York: Macmillan.

Brown, R. (1973). *A first language.* Cambridge: Harvard University Press.

Bruner, J. (1986). *Actual minds, possible worlds.* Cambridge: Harvard University Press.

Chapman, R. W., Schwartz, S., & Kay-Raining Bird, E. (1988). Predicting comprehension skills in children with Down syndrome. Paper presented at American Speech-Language-Hearing Association Annual Convention, Boston, MA.

Hymes, D. (1972). Models of the interaction of language and social life. In J. J. Gumperz & D. Hymes (Eds.), *Directions in sociolinguistics* (pp. 35–71). New York: Holt, Rinehart and Winston.

Kagan, J. (1989). Temperamental contributions to social behavior. *American Psychologist, 44,* 668–674.

Kail, R., & Leonard, L. B. (1986). Word-finding abilities in language-impaired children. *ASHA Monographs,* No. 25. Rockville, MD: American Speech-Language-Hearing Association.

Lakoff, G. (1987). *Women, fire, and dangerous things: What categories reveal about the mind.* Chicago: University of Chicago Press.

Lakoff, G., & Johnson, M. (1980). *Metaphors we live by.* Chicago: University of Chicago Press.

MacLachlan, B., & Chapman, R. S. (1988). Communication breakdowns in normal and language-learning-disabled children's conversation and narration. *Journal of Speech and Hearing Disorders, 53,* 2–7.

Miller, J. F. (1987). A grammatical characterization of language disorders. In *Proceedings of the first International Symposium on Specific Speech and Language Disorders in Children* (pp. 100–113). University of Reading, England. AFASIC: Association for All Speech Impaired Children.

Miller, J. F., Chapman, R. S., & MacKenzie, H. (1981). *Individual differences in the language acquisition of mentally retarded children.* Paper presented at the 2nd International Congress of the Study of Child Language, University of British Columbia, Vancouver, B.C., Canada.

Nelson, K. (1973). Structure and strategy in learning to talk. *Monographs of the Society for Research in Child Development, 38* (Serial No. 149).

Pepper, S. C. (1942). *World hypotheses.* Berkeley: University of California Press.

Peters, A. M. (1984). *The units of language acquisition.* Cambridge: Cambridge University Press.

Shriberg, L. D., & Kwiatkowski, J. (1988). A follow-up study of children with phonologic disorders of unknown origin. *Journal of Speech and Hearing Disorders, 53,* 144–155.

Slobin, D. I. (1979). *Psycholinguistics.* Oakland, NJ: Scott, Foresman.

CHAPTER 18

Questions About Cognition in Children with Specific Language Impairment

JUDITH R. JOHNSTON

The last decade has brought a dramatic change in our view of the child with specific language disorders. In the mid 1960s, when I began my clinical work with such children, the concept of a *specific* disorder connoted a limited degree of impairment and the possibility of focused remediation. The professional Zeitgeist was hence optimistic and short-visioned. Somewhere in the early 70s, however, as I broadened my disciplinary perspective to include all aspects of human development, I began to question the existence of specific language disorders. Larry, Robin, Jimmy, and all of the other children I had taught, were obviously quite real. But if language was both the product and the tool of human cognition, it seemed unlikely that these children could have serious difficulty learning language and be otherwise intellectually normal. I thus initiated a number of studies designed to examine the "nonverbal" cognitive abilities of language-disordered children. Other investigators, for their own reasons, did likewise.

The subsequent research findings have been sobering. As I concluded in my recent review of this literature (Johnston, 1988, p. 705), "Research on the cognitive abilities of language-disordered children presents a convincing picture of substantial impairment. At many ages, across visual, auditory, and tactile stimuli, across many domains of knowledge, in symbolic and nonsymbolic activities, in tasks with little to no explicit verbal demand, language-disordered children perform below age expectations." It now seems clear that whatever the nature of their disability may be, it is neither limited nor local in its scope and consequences. My task in this chapter is to identify some directions for profitable future cognitive research. As a first step I must note that studies designed merely to document low performance in yet another mental task now seem superfluous. We no longer need to ask whether language-impaired children have learning and performance problems that extend beyond the traditional boundaries of language. They do. Instead, I believe that researchers should either dig deeper into known phenomena, or move to a different territory. In the pages to follow, I will point to opportunities for both sorts of strategy.

QUESTIONS ABOUT ESTABLISHED FINDINGS

Anyone who surveys the first decade of investigation into the cognitive status of language-impaired children will discover a set of disparate, and ultimately unsatisfying, hypotheses about the nature of their disability. This literature is problematic, however, not so much because it is wrong-headed as because it is immature. My initial research suggestions are thus for studies that would extend this work.

SYMBOLIC FUNCTION

One line of research has seemed to point to a modality-free symbolic deficit. Studies of pretend play (e.g., Brown, Redmond, Bass, Liebergott & Swope, 1975; Terrell, Schwartz, Prelock, & Messick, 1984; Thal & Bates, 1988) and visual imagery (e.g., Johnston & Ellis Weismer, 1983; Savich, 1984) have demonstrated that language-impaired children have difficulty with symbols of diverse sorts. Explanations for this finding have appealed to the Piagetian notion of a *symbolic function* (i.e. some general facility for the generation and utilization of symbolic representation). I first met this notion 19 years ago and find it no less mysterious now than I did then. In normal development, the near simultaneous emergence of play, gesture, verbal, and imagistic symbols may well signal the arrival of some important new property of human intellect. However, the nature of this property and its relationship to the emergence of symbolic behavior is, to my knowledge, unknown, and I have yet to figure out an approach to identifying it. Reification of the hypothesized function is clearly not the solution.

Despite our fundamental uncertainty about the mental processes underlying symbolic behavior, I believe that further studies in this domain would be useful, particularly those with a focus on play. Early pretend play is a type of intellectual activity that is both analogous to language and distinct from it. It is symbolic and an important tool for early reasoning, but it doesn't seem to be mediated by inner verbalization, and it certainly doesn't require auditory processing. By studying the specific nature of play deficits, we may be able to learn more about the symbolic side of language disorder and do so with reasonable certainty that we are not studying verbal behavior in disguise.

One aspect of the current play literature seems especially promising. It is seen most clearly in a recent study by Thal and Bates (1988). These researchers used imitation tasks to elicit symbolic gestures from nine toddlers, aged 18–32 months. Although the investigators were reluctant to diagnose language disorder, their subjects were not yet using word combinations and fell below the 10th percentile in the size of their productive lexicon—facts that suggest significant language delay. These late talkers were compared with two groups of children who were developing language more normally: age peers and language peers. In a "lexical" gesture task, children were asked to imitate single symbolic gestures with varying degrees of object and language support. In a "structural" gesture task, children were asked to imitate a series of gestures integrated around narrative scripts such as "putting Teddy to bed." The children's responses were videotaped and later scored. Despite an age appropriate ability to produce ordered pairs of gestures in the "structural" task, the late talkers showed limited success in repeating single, gestural "lexemes," performing only at the level of their younger, language-matched peers. Similar restrictions in gestural repertoire were noted by Skarakis (1982) in her longitudinal observations of spontaneous play in language-disordered children.

Thal and Bates argue that their data point to "retrieval problems" in the late talkers, a sort of early gestural anomia. This explanation implies the prior existence of retrievable gesture symbols, that is, schemes that have been decontextualized and mapped to meanings. Rather than suffering from some difficulty with retrieval, language-impaired children may have constructed a smaller number of such schemes. Data from elicitation tasks repeated several times in various supportive contexts might help us choose between these alternative explanations. Retrieval problems would presumably be ameliorated by repetition and physical cuing in a way that repertoire limitations would not. If language-impaired children indeed prove to have fewer available gesture schemes, training studies could then explore the rate and course of their acquisition, along the lines of recent microdevelopmental experiments in word learning (e.g., Leonard et al., 1982). The differences between language and play symbols would be important in interpreting such data. Unlike slow word learning, slow gesture acquisition could not be attributed to auditory perceptual problems, difficulty in mastering an abstract system of recombinant "phonological" elements, the necessary physical dissimilarity of symbol and referent, or fewer opportunities for communication. Instead, difficulty in the acquisition of gesture symbols would invite us to think about the intellectual conditions that promote the emergence of symbolic behavior. Language symbols have clear social purposes, but what are play symbols good for? What leads a child to generate them out of basic perceptual-action schemes? Can we create therapeutic worlds that compel their use? Studies designed to answer these questions would help us understand not only the acquisition of play schemes, but the less obvious, nonsocial motivation for language as well.

COGNITIVE PROCESSING

A number of findings have increasingly led researchers to question the cognitive processing abilities of language-impaired children. To set the stage for my research suggestions I will mention only a few of the most recent studies and refer readers to my earlier review (Johnston, 1988) for more complete coverage.

Work in *perceptual processing* has focused primarily on children's ability to make order judgments about brief, rapidly sequenced events. In one key study, Tallal and her Baltimore colleagues (1981) reported that language-impaired children had difficulty making such decisions about nonlinguistic stimuli, both auditory and visual, requiring abnormally long inter-stimulus intervals to do so. The importance of these findings was highlighted in their subsequent discriminant analysis of 160 variables designed to identify those characteristics that best identified the language-impaired children (Tallal, Stark, & Mellits, 1985). Five of the six best predictors involved the perception of brief events presented either simultaneously or in succession.

Other researchers have documented processing problems that are more clearly of the "top-down" sort. Ceci (1983), for example, asked 10-year-old language-impaired children to name pictured objects as quickly as possible. Prior to each slide, the children were cued to the class of object they were about to see. Reaction times indicated that the language-impaired children failed to make active use of this information to form an *anticipatory set*. They evidenced little or no facilitation of lexical retrieval. Johnston and Smith (1988) used a complex communication task to explore aspects of *processing capacity*. The task involved describing pairs of objects that either were identical or were similar in size or color. Unlike their normal peers, the language-impaired preschoolers seldom referred to these objects as quantified sets (e.g. "the two red ones"). They used all of the requisite words and grammatical patterns. They gave clear evidence of knowing about physical attributes, dimensions and similarity relations. They further demonstrated that they could construct and quantify sets, and could identify an attribute that was uniquely common to two objects. Nevertheless, the language-impaired children seemed to avoid descriptions that would have required them to implement and coordinate all of these knowledge schemes and operations at once. Such complexity apparently lay on the margins of their processing capacity.

Two final studies illustrate recent work in the organization and use of language knowledge. Kail, Hale, Leonard, and Nippold (1984) used recall tasks to explore memory functions in language-impaired children. They were interested in establishing whether "word finding" problems are best attributed to storage or retrieval aspects of memory. Ten-year-olds were asked to listen to word lists and then try to remember them. In some trials they were prompted with category labels to facilitate recall. The language-impaired children recalled fewer words than the normal children, to an equal extent with and without cues. This suggested that their memory deficits were due to *less "well established" lexical representation* rather than to retrieval processes. If their difficulties had occurred primarily during retrieval access, they should have shown relatively greater success when they could use recall cues. Montgomery, Scudder, and Moore (1987) have recently documented one possible consequence of such impoverished language representation. Their subjects were given a target word and were asked to press a button as soon as they heard that word in a subsequent utterance. This procedure allowed the researchers to look at language comprehension "on-line" (i.e., as it unfolds in real time). Throughout the course of an utterance, there is an increasing amount of semantic and syntactic information that can be used to anticipate subsequent lexemes. Listeners who make use of this information should recognize target words more quickly. In comparison to normal 6-year-olds, Montgomery and colleagues' language-impaired 8-year-olds were either *slower to deploy their language knowledge* in the service of speech perception, or needed more information before doing so.

One important theme in these studies concerns the nature of cognitive deficit. We are reminded here that cognition consists of more than knowledge, that is, representations of organized past experience. It consists also of the way the mind uses and manipulates information, from either within or without, to solve problems of the moment. Language learning is, at its simplest, a set of such problems. There are sounds to be categorized, speech streams to be segmented, words to be interpreted and remembered. Despite recent talk of innate syntax, I remain convinced that it is studies of cognitive processing in language-impaired children that will best illuminate their difficulty with language learning.

As implied by the studies cited above, there is a current abundance of candidate explanatory deficits: misperception of brief events, failure to form sets, capacity limitations, slow deployment of resources, and many others not illustrated here. What may be less obvious is that most of these cognitive processes have been investigated in only one or, at best, a handful of studies, and hence represent an opportunity for further work. I will mention here three problem spaces that seem particularly relevant to language learning, admitting that my selection is biased by my own academic history.

Processing Speed

Studies of cognitive processing deficits often yield group differences in reaction time as their major finding. This will be increasingly true as more on-line experiments are carried out. To paraphrase a critic of my own work on visual imagery (Johnston & Ellis Weismer, 1983), is it at all interesting that language-disordered children process information more slowly? To answer this question, we need studies that demonstrate the price of being slow. Current models in cognitive psychology suggest consequences of at least three sorts: when *signals disappear*, a slow processor may be unable to interpret them; when *signals come in sequence*, a slow and limited capacity processor may be fully occupied with the first segment when the second segment arrives; finally, when a mental task requires *parallel processing in diverse domains*, slow processing in one strand may lead to a discoordination of the whole. Language-learning events, of course, have exactly these characteristics.

Results from the experiments on rapid event perception have sometimes been interpreted as indicative of slow processing, but actual measures of rate have yet to be made. This work will probably require electrophysiological data. In other processing domains, the consequences of being slow seem not to have been addressed. Neural network modeling may eventually offer one approach to this question. I wonder, for example, whether an acquisition model that activated its "meaning nodes" more quickly than its "sound nodes" would arrive at the same steady state representation as one in which both systems operated at the same speed.

Nonverbal Processing

Cognitive processing studies with language-impaired children have thus far made predominant use of verbal tasks. This is especially true of the work on memory processes (see Johnston, 1988, pp. 706–707). Results of such studies have contributed to our understanding of the verbal deficits of school-aged children by pointing to a phase of mastery learning that must occur after the initial acquisition of language schemes. However, research with verbal tasks cannot do much to explain difficulties with language acquisition since any observed processing deficit can as easily be the product as the cause of the problem. I am the first to acknowledge that it is hard to design a convincingly "nonverbal" task. I nevertheless would like to see more use of nonverbal paradigms to study cognitive processes in language-disordered children. The Baltimore team succeeded in developing visual analogues for their auditory perceptual processing task; it should be equally possible to develop nonverbal paradigms for the study of phenomena such as anticipatory set and resource allocation.

Processing Capacity and Automaticity

The notion of processing capacity has proven to be a mixed blessing for developmental researchers (Kail & Bisanz, 1982). The construct provides a reasonable explanation for failure to utilize available knowledge, but its origins and course remain the subject of debate. Some theorists see change in processing capacity as the result of growth in the absolute structural properties of the mind; others see change in capacity as the indirect consequence of experience and increased skill with specific schemes (i.e., automaticity). Research that helped us decide between these alternatives would have crucial implications for our understanding of capacity limitations in language-impaired children: automaticity is tractable in a way that structure is not. Short-term intervention paradigms seem promising. If an observed capacity limitation could be overcome through training in component parts of the task, it would suggest that at least a portion of the initial deficit reflected "soft-ware" rather than "hard-ware" characteristics.

Failure to overcome capacity limitations through training would be harder to interpret. Such failure could stem from structural inadequacies, or from an inability to profit from experience, that is, to automatize, in the normal fashion. Training study data could again be useful, however, if they included periodic measurements of "spare" capacity. Riddle and Johnston (1988) made use of a dual-task paradigm to study processing capacity. Preschoolers were asked to classify pictures and at the same time to listen for a buzzer. Reaction time to the buzzer indicated the amount of "spare" capacity available at various phases of picture processing. Subjects in this study had all succeeded with the basic classification task prior to the dual-task experiment. But what if they had not? This same paradigm could be used to track the acquisition and subsequent automatization of a mental scheme. Such a study with language-impaired children might reveal a slower course of automatization or some plateau effect.

NEW TERRITORY

My opening research suggestions have quite purposely built on current findings. Ours is a field in which a very few, overworked investigators are studying a huge and complex problem. Research with atypical children is, moreover, slow and effortful. The result of all of this is that by the time one or two experiments of a given sort have been completed, new theories and issues have emerged. It takes both discipline and imagination to build programmatic research in this environment.

Having said this, I still choose to close this chapter by suggesting a new research direction—well, perhaps not an altogether new one, but certainly one which has lain dormant for some time. The intriguing and important fact about the Larrys, Robins, and Jimmys of the world is that they do not "clinically present" as globally retarded. We have spent much of the last decade documenting the breadth of their cognitive impairment. In the face of these data, I find myself increasingly curious about their cognitive strengths. What positive qualities of mind and learning style distinguish these children from other clinical groups? One limited answer to this question lies in the analysis of items on performance scales of intelligence. By definition, children with specific language disorder perform these tasks as well as their peers. I suspect, however, that their intellectual strengths are not limited to the figurative, visual judgments typical of these instruments. I recently rediscovered a passage in Inhelder's (1976) case studies of dysphasic children that may provide a key to productive research on this topic: "the child treats the classes of objects not as concepts but as 'schemes of action' . . . because of this transfer of conceptual problems to the level of operational activity, some children succeed in compensating for their linguistic deficiencies" (p. 338). By watching language-impaired children think with their hands, we may regain some of the clinical optimism that we have lost.

REFERENCES

Brown, J., Redmond, A., Bass, K., Liebergott, J., & Swope, S. (1975). *Symbolic play in normal and language-impaired children.* Paper presented to the American Speech and Hearing Association, Washington, DC.

Ceci, S. (1983). Automatic and purposive semantic processing characteristics of normal and language/learning disabled children. *Developmental Psychology, 19,* 427–439.

Inhelder, B. (1976). Observations on the operational and figurative aspects of thought in dysphasic children. In D. Morehead & A. Morehead (Eds.), *Normal and deficient child language* (pp. 335–343). Baltimore: University Park Press.

Johnston, J. (1988). Specific language disorders in the child. In N. Lass, J. Northern, L. McReynolds & D. Yoder (Eds.), *Handbook of speech-language pathology and audiology* (pp. 685–715). Philadelphia: B. C. Decker.

Johnston, J., & Ellis Weismer, S. (1983). Mental rotation abilities in language-disordered children. *Journal of Speech and Hearing Research, 26,* 397–403.

Johnston, J., & Smith, L. (1988). *Six ways to skin the cat: Communicative strategies used by language-impaired children.* Paper presented at the Symposium for Research in Child Language Disorders, University of Wisconsin, Madison.

Kail, R., Hale, C., Leonard, L., & Nippold, M. (1984). Lexical storage and retrieval in language-impaired children. *Applied Psycholinguistics, 5,* 37–49.

Kail, R., & Bisanz, J. (1982). Information processing and cognitive development. In L. Lipsitt & C. Spiker (Eds.), *Advances in child development and behavior: Vol. 17* (pp. 45–81). New York: Academic.

Leonard, L., Schwartz, R., Chapman, K., Rowan, L. Prelock, P., Terrell, B., Weiss, A., & Messick, C. (1982). Early lexical acquisition in children with specific language impairment. *Journal of Speech and Hearing Research, 25,* 554–563.

Montgomery, J., Scudder, R., & Moore, C. (1987). *The temporal structure of language impaired children's comprehension of spoken language.* Paper presented to the American Speech-Language-Hearing Association, New Orleans.

Riddle, L., & Johnston, J. (1988). *Resource allocation in preschool aged children.* Paper presented to the American Speech-Language-Hearing Association, Boston.

Savich, P. (1984). Anticipatory imagery in normal and language disabled children. *Journal of Speech and Hearing Research, 27,* 494–501.

Skarakis, E. (1982). *The development of symbolic play and language in language-disordered children.* Unpublished doctoral dissertation, University of California, Santa Barbara.

Tallal, P., Stark, R., Kallman, C., & Mellits, D. (1981). A reexamination of some nonverbal perceptual abilities of language-impaired and normal children as a function of age and sensory modality. *Journal of Speech and Hearing Research, 24,* 351–357.

Tallal, P., Stark, R., & Mellits, D. (1985). Identification of language-impaired children on the basis of rapid perception and production skills. *Brain and Language, 25,* 314–322.

Terrell, B., Schwartz, R., Prelock, P., & Messick, C. (1984). Symbolic play in normal and language-disordered children. *Journal of Speech and Hearing Research, 27,* 424–429.

Thal, D., & Bates, E. (1988). Language and gesture in late talkers. *Journal of Speech and Hearing Research, 31,* 115–123.

CHAPTER 19

Brain Lesions in Children: Implications for Developmental Language Disorders

DOROTHY M. ARAM

WHAT DO WE WANT TO KNOW?

Why would one who sees herself as a specialist in child language disorders become diverted into studying children with brain lesions? Is there a logical and ultimately useful connection between children with developmental language disorders (DLD) and children with brain lesions, or does this represent an interesting, but essentially irrelevant side track? Clearly, there is heuristic pleasure in exploring relatively uncharted territory and humanistic satisfaction in providing at least partial answers to concrete clinical questions related to prognosis for children with focal brain lesions. In the present chapter I suggest that study of brain lesions in children has the potential not only of addressing questions of behavioral and neural plasticity in young children, but also of speaking to the neurological basis of DLD. This potential has yet to be realized; the present chapter outlines my views on what needs to be done.

Preparation of this manuscript was supported by the following grants from the NIH National Institute of Neurological Disorders and Stroke: NS17366 and NS20489.

Although the study of brain-lesioned children is approached from numerous perspectives, questions pursued typically fall into the following general domains. One concerns the nature of sequelae involving specified behavior following brain lesions; second, the relationship between time since lesion onset or age at onset and behavioral effects; third, how variability in observed behavior can be explained in terms of underlying neuroanatomy and neurophysiology; and finally, what the above tells us about the normal development and the causal basis for abnormal behavior, in this context, developmental language disorders.

WHAT IS THE NATURE OF BEHAVIORAL SEQUELAE FOLLOWING LATERALIZED BRAIN LESIONS?

Learning what happens to speech, language, and other aspects of development following lesions in childhood propels the majority of current studies and appears to be an appropriate starting point. Until the past ten years, few investigators provided more than a global assessment of verbal ability in these children, typically through the report of verbal intelligence. To date, very few studies have addressed specific aspects of speech and language, such as syntax or semantics, nor have they differentiated between comprehension and production abilities. Thus far these few studies document subtle syntactic deficits following left- but not right-hemisphere lesions (Aram & Ekelman, 1987; Aram, Ekelman & Whitaker, 1986; Kiessling, Denckla & Carlton, 1983; Rankin, Aram & Horwitz, 1981; Vargha-Khadem, O'Gorman & Watters, 1985; Woods & Carey, 1979) and contradictory data relative to the relationship between lesion laterality and lexical or semantic abilities (Aram, Ekelman & Whitaker, 1987; Kiessling et al., 1983; Vargha-Khadem et al., 1985; Woods & Carey, 1979). Other than passing mention in case studies, there appear to be no studies addressing phonology or pragmatics among children with verified lateralized brain lesions. (Refer to Aram, 1988, for a recent review of studies addressing speech and language among brain-lesioned children.) The few studies reporting syntactic or semantic data have been limited in scope and typically have been bound to a single point in time. Therefore, at a most basic level we need to gain richer descriptions of multiple aspects of speech and language, including phonology, syntax, semantics and pragmatics, and assessment of comprehension versus productive abilities including motor speech and fluency patterns. Such data provides a beginning that remains largely to be filled in.

Beyond detailing speech and language parameters among children with lateralized brain lesions, other than intelligence scores, we know very little about related aspects of cognition and learning. Unlike the adult aphasiology literature, little is known about an array of cognitive skills such as memory, attention, visual-spatial abilities and the like (see Aram & Whitaker, 1988, for a review of these studies). Even studies reporting IQ scores provide widely variable results (see Aram & Ekelman, 1986, for a discussion of these findings). Although earlier clinicians often commented upon deficits in reading and occasionally mathematics (Hecaen, 1976, 1983), how these deficits relate to language or other aspects of cognition remains almost totally unexplored (Aram, Ekelman & Gillespie, in press). Further, such study among brain-lesioned children may provide evidence for "behavioral plasticity," that is, accomplishing a task through alternative strategies.

WHAT IS THE EFFECT OF TIME ON BEHAVIORAL PARAMETERS?

Given the sparsity of even single snapshots of aspects of speech and language among brain-lesioned children at one point in time, it is not surprising that the developmental course of these children has been tackled in only a few single case or small sample studies (Dennis, 1980; Marchman, Miller & Bates, 1989; Thal, Bates, Marchman & Fenson, 1989; Yeni-Komshian, 1977). We do not know, for example, if the syntactic limitations observed among young left-lesioned children (Aram, Ekelman & Whitaker, 1986; Woods & Carey, 1979) persist over time, mitigate, or, as some have suggested for IQ (Levine, Huttenlocher, Banich & Duda, 1987), increase with advancing age.

The variable effect of age of lesion onset has been considered by numerous investigators; however, the question typically has been cast into whether or not lesions prior to versus after 1 year of age (implicitly or explicitly linked to before or after the onset of language) have a differential effect on behavior. Even when several studies have ostensibly addressed the same question, for example, the relationship between age of lesion onset and verbal and performance IQ, findings are contradictory (see Aram & Ekelman, 1986). While to date our work provides little evidence for a differential effect of lesions prior to versus after 1 year of age on ensuing language performance, this important variable has not yet been fully explored. It appears that no study has treated age of lesion onset as a continuous variable, despite Lenneberg's (1967) provocative yet largely unsubstantiated claims of progressively decreasing plasticity from early childhood to puberty.

While developmental neuroanatomy provides little justification for treating age of lesion onset as a linear variable, little justification also exists for setting 1 year as the comparative fulcrum. Considering a potential interaction between age of lesion onset and the specificity versus global nature of the deficit may prove to be useful in resolving such conflicting findings as has been suggested by several investigators including Aram, Ekelman, and Gillespie (in press).

HOW DOES UNDERLYING NEUROANATOMY AND NEUROPHYSIOLOGY RELATE TO VARIABILITY IN SPECIFIED BEHAVIORS?

Probably the chief deterrent in generalizing from children with known brain lesions to children with developmental disorders of unknown origin is the fact that findings to date involving children with lateralized brain lesions are highly variable and often contradictory. This variability and lack of replicability among studies led us previously to conclude (Aram & Whitaker, 1988) that attempting to disambiguate disparate results among studies of children with lateralized brain lesions is an exercise in futility until investigators begin defining and reporting important subject variables, most importantly specifying the involved neuroanatomy.

To date, most studies have aimed to compare the differential effect of left-versus right-hemisphere involvement. However, with very few exceptions, almost all studies have included children with known or presumed bilateral brain involvement. Most studies of children with lateralized brain involvement have included children with *tumors* (where the tumor may be lateralized but the diffuse effects of chemotherapy and whole head radiation are well known, e.g., Fletcher & Copeland, 1988), *head trauma* (where diffuse white matter lesions, contrecoup lesions and brain stem shearing are all a part of the clinical picture, e.g., Levin, Grafman & Eisenberg, 1987); and *seizure disorders* (where the spread of electrical activity may cross the corpus callosum and therefore involve both hemispheres, in addition to the systemic effects of anticonvulsant medications, e.g., Aicardi, 1988). Unfortunately, few studies acknowledge, much less document, the degree of bilateral or more diffuse brain involvement; rather, subjects are treated as if they present left *or* right brain involvement. This failure to appreciate the degree of more diffuse brain involvement, I believe, is the chief factor underlying contradictory findings among studies of children with lateralized brain lesions. To my knowledge, our work constitutes the only series that is restricted to children with single, unilateral vascular lesions and excludes children with ongoing seizures. I am not suggesting that all investigators follow suit. Rather, we all must explicitly specify the degree of brain involvement, which then may provide a means for interpreting the disparate results reported. While I believe we need to direct much more investigation to the effects of clearly specified focal lesions involving one hemisphere alone, I also recognize that this is only one end of the spectrum. What is needed is not that everyone study only children with rigidly defined left or right lesions, but for investigators to define the degree of brain involvement and to treat degree of neuroanatomic involvement as a major variable related to outcome behavior.

Even grouping children by left, right, or diffuse involvement, however, does not account for within-hemisphere variability. A fundamental tenet of neuropsychology is that lesions involving different locations within a hemisphere will be related to different patterns of behavioral deficits, leading some to propose that when brain-behavior questions are addressed, the appropriate methodology involves single subject designs (Caramazza, 1986). Despite the fact that there is no justification for assuming that all left lesions should be related to comparable behavioral effects, with children there has been almost no attempt to differentiate among lesion sites within a hemisphere. While I would hope we will eventually be able to generalize across specified groups of lesioned subjects, at this point we do not know how best to group subjects.

An approach we have recently adopted (Aram, Ekelman & Gillespie, in press; Aram, Meyers & Ekelman, in press) and advocate is to report both group and individual findings. This approach allows us not only to address more global questions (e.g., do children with left lesions have more dysfluencies than controls), but also to identify, report, and attempt to understand significant within-group variability. Throughout our studies, the marked within-group variability is impressive, even among our carefully defined subjects selected to present circumscribed focal lesions. Of late we are focusing upon those with significant deficits and are attempting to identify factors that differentiate these children from the others with left or right lesions who, in many instances, are performing very adequately (Aram, Ekelman & Gillespie, in press). At this point, it appears that involvement of particular subcortical nuclei and fiber tracts are associated with pronounced language-learning deficits (Aram, 1988). Confirmation of these tentative findings, however, will await additional data from other investigators in which the site of lesion within the hemisphere is specified.

With continually improving resolution of imaging techniques, we now have available means of obtaining relatively good specification of lesion location. Magnetic resonance imaging (MRI) provides the capability of identifying small, deep lesions, previously not detected by computerized tomography (CT). In our series we have had to re-classify six children thought to present single, unilateral lesions on the basis of CT scan, into the bilateral group based on additional findings visualized on MRI. Thus at this writing, MRI would be seen as the imaging technique of choice, although undoubtedly in time MRIs also will be supplanted by even more sensitive techniques.

As conventionally employed, however, MRIs are limited to specifying anatomy and give little information about areas of function and dysfunction. More dynamic imaging techniques such as cerebral blood flow and posititron emission tomography (PET) have been limited in their use with children due to the invasive nature of these techniques, the attendant radioactivity, and the task requirements often involving sustained performance for prolonged periods of time. Nonetheless, as these techniques improve, they are being used with children (Chugani, Phelps & Mazziotta, 1987) and we can anticipate in the future the greater availability of techniques for dynamic imaging applicable for use with children.

Electrophysiological measures, notably evoked potentials, are appropriate for use with children and do provide a noninvasive means of studying brain function as revealed by electrical activity. As of yet, however, few investigators (Neville, Mills & Coffey, 1989; Papanicolaou, DiScenna, Gillespie & Aram, in preparation) have attempted to use this technology with brain-lesioned children despite its demonstrated utility in reflecting laterality effects (Papanicolaou et al., in preparation) and processing stages associated with various linguistic tasks (Kutas & Hillyard, 1988). Such procedures can provide evidence of functional reorganization following brain lesions, information that currently is equivocal and derived from the results of a few studies reporting the results of Wada Tests (Mateer & Dodrill, 1983; Rasmussen & Milner, 1977), or inferences based on dichotic listening paradigms (Pohl, 1979; Yeni-Komshian, 1977).

Finally, although a prime question concerns neural reorganization of plasticity following brain insult, I am aware of no studies reporting neuropathological data for children with focal brain lesions for whom language abilities prior to their death was documented. Unlike dyslexia, where a growing neuropathological database now exists (Galaburda, 1988), our understanding of neural reorganization following early brain injury is based almost exclusively on animal models. Those of us following cohorts of children with early unilateral lesions must plan for the eventuality of some of those children coming to autopsy.

IMPLICATIONS FOR NORMAL AND ABNORMAL LANGUAGE DEVELOPMENT IN CHILDREN

Study of the observed behavioral deficits following lesions involving specified areas of brains has long been a principal means of identifying brain-behavior relationships underlying language processing in adults. As well, study of disruptions among processes thought to be components of an overall domain, such as reading, has served as accident-of-nature tests of the dependence or independence of the various component processes and also has served as the primary data for many models of higher cognitive functions in adults (Coltheart, 1987; McCloskey & Caramazza,

1987). So, too, parallel observations among young children serve to inform us about the underlying neurological substrate during the development of language and related functions, as well as the dependence or independence of component processes during development. For example, phonological segmentation is seen by many investigators as a requirement for fluent reading. Studies of brain-lesioned children permit examination of what lesion sites within the brain interfere with this function, and the effect of age. As well, how lesioned children perform on phonetic segmentation and other reading tasks permits assessment of the degree of dependence or independence between these tasks and/or development of alternative behavioral strategies.

Study of the behavior following lesions to specified areas of the brain in young children not only allows us to draw inferences about brain-behavior relationships during development, but also to compare the behavior observed to that of adults with similar lesions and to children with DLD but no known lesions. The comparisons between behavior observed in adults versus that seen in children following comparably located lesions informs us about the degree of behavioral and presumably neural plasticity present at varying ages. The comparison between language deficits observed among brain-lesioned and DLD children permits parallels to be drawn between comparable language symptomatology, and speculations to be advanced regarding similar or dissimilar causal bases for DLD children.

I have maintained that child language disorders do not concern a single entity, but rather that multiple types of developmental language exists. It may be that different causal bases account for each (Aram & Nation, 1975, 1982). Further, it should be kept in mind that although it has long been assumed that at least some forms of DLD have a neurological basis, few such children have been found to present evidence of discrete brain lesions (Horwitz, 1984). The alternate approach, which I have chosen to pursue (i.e., study of the language of children with known brain lesions as a comparison to the language of DLD), has led me to draw the following conclusions thus far.

First, it is rare for a child with a clear unilateral left or right brain lesion to present a severe language disorder, comparable to that observed among the more severely impaired children with DLD, for example, developmental verbal apraxia or auditory verbal agnosia.

Second, a working hypothesis that may be revised is that when a child with a unilateral lesion does present a significant language and/or learning deficit, this appears to involve either critical subcortical structures or interacts with other potential contributing factors such as familial history for language and learning disorders (Aram, Ekelman & Gillespie, in press). When subcortical structures are spared and other potential causal factors do not appear to be present, my experience suggests that we do not begin seeing pronounced language disorders until some degree of bilateral or more diffuse brain involvement is present.

Third, as preschoolers or during the first year after lesion onset, many of the left-lesioned children do present language deficits sufficiently severe to prompt initiation of language therapy, rarely required for right-lesioned children. For these left-lesioned children requiring language therapy, their deficits typically improve sufficiently so that language therapy is relatively short lived and long-standing clinically significant language disorders are not present (not to be confused with statistically significant language deficits in comparison to control subjects). It appears that for these children, given time, sufficient behavioral and presumably neural plasticity occurs, allowing essentially normal language functions. This observation does not contradict the claim of early left hemisphere specialization for language, for which I believe there is abundant evidence (Aram, 1988; Molfese & Segalowitz, 1988); only that sufficient plasticity ultimately permits relatively adequate language development. Thus, comparing language disorders presented on a developmental basis to those observed after acquired lesions in children, it appears that an unidentified unilateral brain lesion or dysfunction could conceivably underlie the relatively mild, more transient language disorders observed among some DLD children, especially during the preschool years. Unilateral lesions, however, are unlikely to account for the more persistent, severe forms of DLD, requiring extended therapy and educational intervention. These hypotheses, however, are speculative and require further substantiation among lesioned children with increasing degrees of bilateral brain involvement and comparison to DLD children, as well as further study of brain structures and functions of DLD children.

A PARTIAL BLUEPRINT FOR FUTURE STUDIES OF BRAIN-LESIONED CHILDREN

How to proceed? By way of conclusion, I suggest that investigators, in their pursuit of answers to some of the speculations suggested above, provide the following in future studies of brain-lesioned children.

SUBJECT CRITERIA AND SPECIFICATION

Unless subject characteristics are explicitly stated and criterion excluding confounding variables are adhered to, additional studies stand little chance of furthering our understanding of developmental brain-language relationships. Subjects need to be restricted to those whose premorbid status is normal and for whom other factors known to be related to higher cognitive disorders are not present. Therefore, children with any developmental disorder prior to lesion onset need to be excluded, as do children from high-risk pregnancies, premature births or with known genetic metabolic, or other systemic abnormalities. Subjects need to be restricted to those whose development presumably would have been normal; when confounding factors of potential causal import are introduced, it is impossible to draw relationships between the lesion presented and the behavior observed. Second, lesions need to be defined with as much specificity as possible; today that means at a minimum use of MRI scans or equally sensitive images. Concomitant factors also need to be documented and reported in detail. For example, when a seizure disorder exists, the type, presence, duration and frequency of seizures needs to be reported, dosage and history of anticonvulsant use needs to be noted, and (electroencephalography) EEG results documenting seizure focus and pattern need to be provided. Third, in group studies comparison subjects need to be included and appropriately selected to be comparable on variables known to effect brain and language development including age, sex, and social class.

MEASURES

Given the fact that very little description of specific aspects of language have been studied in brain-lesioned children, a full range of potentially important aspects of language remain to be fleshed out, as discussed above. Studies that go beyond report of scores on various standardized psychometric instruments have the capability of offering greater insight into subtle residual deficits as well as into the employment of alternative behavioral strategies adopted by lesioned children. Studies that chart the development of aspects of language over time need to be reported, as do continued consideration of the influence on behavioral variability of the factors of age of lesion onset and time elapsed since lesion onset.

If we are to understand reorganization, investigators also need to undertake electrophysiological studies and more dynamic imaging procedures as these become more applicable for use in young children. Finally, even a few well-done neuropathological studies could directly address many existing questions about neural plasticity in young children.

REPORT OF RESULTS

Although report of group findings probably should not be altogether abandoned, greater emphasis on identifying factors related to within group variability would be of value. It is suggested that lesioned children presenting pronounced behavioral deficits be compared to those with adequate performance and that factors that differ by systematically evaluated. Further, it probably makes little sense to continue establishing a priori groups for comparison based on factors such as age of lesion onset (onset prior to or after 1 year of age) or even site of lesion, given the relative absence of objective data upon which to establish these groups. Rather, comparisons by behavioral deficits may ultimately point to a more rational basis for within group comparisons. Finally, because our subject pools are small, we can report and should make available to other investigators individual subject-by-subject data. At this stage, specific data for a single subject with a lesion sustained at a known age to a known part of the brain are of more use in identifying brain-language relationships which ultimately may be applicable to DLD children, than are data amassed from a heterogeneous, globally defined group of brain-lesioned children.

Hopefully continued study of brain-lesioned children will eventually provide some answers relevant to the causal basis of DLD, lead to more effective differentially applied intervention and, maybe, even to prevention.

REFERENCES

Aicardi, J. (1988). Epileptic syndromes in childhood. *Epilepsia, 29,* S1–S5.

Aram, D. M. (1988). Language sequelae of unilateral brain lesions in children. In F. Plum (Ed.), *Language, communication and the brain* (pp. 171–197). ARNMD Series. New York: Raven.

Aram, D. M., & Ekelman, B. L. (1986). Cognitive profiles of children with early onset of unilateral lesions. *Developmental Neuropsychology, 2,* 155–172.

Aram, D. M., & Ekelman, B. L. (1987). Unilateral brain lesions in childhood: Performance on the Revised Token Test. *Brain and Language, 32,* 137–158.

Aram, D. M., Ekelman, B. L., & Gillespie, L. L. (1988). Reading and lateralized brain lesions in children. In K. von Euler, I. Lundberg, and G. Lennerstrand (Eds.), *Brain and Reading.* Hampshire, England: Macmillan.

Aram, D. M., Ekelman, B. L., & Whitaker, H. A. (1986). Spoken syntax in children with acquired unilateral hemisphere lesions. *Brain and Language, 27,* 75–100.

Aram, D. M., & Ekelman, B. L., & Whitaker, H. A. (1987). Lexical retrieval in left and right brain lesioned children. *Brain and Language, 31,* 61–87.

Aram, D. M., Meyers, S. C., & Ekelman, B. L. (in press). Fluency of conversational speech in children with unilateral brain lesions. *Brain and Language.*

Aram, D. M., & Nation, J. E. (1975). Patterns of language behavior in children with developmental language disorders. *Journal of Speech and Hearing Research, 40,* 229–241.

Aram, D. M., & Nation, J. E. (1982). *Child language disorders.* St. Louis: Mosby.

Aram, D. M., & Whitaker, H. A. (1988). Cognitive sequelae of unilateral lesions acquired in early childhood. In D. L. Molfese and S. J. Segalowitz (Eds.), *The developmental implications of brain lateralization* (pp. 417–436). New York: Guilford.

Caramazza, A. (1986). On drawing inferences about the structure of normal cognitive systems from the analysis of patterns of impaired performance: The case for single-patient studies. *Brain and Cognition, 5,* 41–66.

Chugani, H. T., Phelps, M. E., & Mazziotta, J. C. (1987). Positron emission tomography study of human brain functional development. *Annals of Neurology, 22,* 487–497.

Coltheart, M. (1987). Functional architecture of the language processing system. In M. Coltheart, G. Sartori, & R. Job (Eds.), *The cognitive neuropsychology of language* (pp. 1–25). Hillsdale, NJ: Erlbaum.

Dennis, M. (1980). Strokes in childhood: Communicative intent, expression and comprehension after left hemisphere arteriopathy in a right-handed nine year old. In R. W. Rieber (Ed.), *Language development and aphasia in children* (pp. 45–67). New York: Academic.

Fletcher, J. M., & Copeland, D. R. (1988). Neurobehavioral effects of central nervous system prophylactic treatment of cancer in children. *Journal of Clinical and Experimental Neuropsychology, 10,* 495–537.

Galaburda, A. M. (1988). The pathogenesis of childhood dyslexia. In F. Plum (Ed.), *Language, communication and the brain* (pp. 127–138). New York: Raven.

Hecaen, H. (1976). Acquired aphasia in children and the ontogenesis of hemispheric functional specialization. *Brain and Language, 3,* 114–134.

Hecaen, H. (1983). Acquired aphasia in children: Revisited. *Neuropsychologia, 21,* 581–587.

Horwitz, S. J. (1984). Neurological findings in developmental verbal apraxia. *Seminars in Speech and Language, 5,* 111–118.

Kiessling, L. S., Denckla, M. B., & Carlton, M. (1983). Evidence for differential hemispheric function in children with hemiplegic cerebral palsy. *Developmental Medicine and Child Neurology, 25,* 727–734.

Kutas, M., & Hillyard, S. A. (1988). Contextual effects in language comprehension: Studies using event-related brain potentials. In F. Plum (Ed.), *Language, communication and the brain* (pp. 87–100). New York: Raven.

Lenneberg, E. (1967). *Biological foundations of language.* New York: Wiley.

Levin, H. S., Grafman, J., & Eisenberg, H. M. (1987). *Neurobehavioral recovery from head injury.* New York: Oxford University Press.

Levine, S. C., Huttenlocher, P., Banich, M. T., & Duda, E. (1987). Factors affecting cognitive functioning of hemiplegic children. *Developmental Medicine and Child Neurology, 29,* 27–35.

Marchman, V., Miller, R., & Bates, E. (1989). *Pre-speech, babble and early gesture.* Paper presented at the Society for Research in Child Development Meetings, Kansas City, MO.

Mateer, C. A., & Dodrill, C. B. (1983). Neuropsychological and linguistic correlates of atypical language lateralization: Evidence from sodium amytal studies. *Human Neurobiology, 2,* 135–142.

McCloskey, M., & Caramazza, A. (1987). Cognitive mechanisms in normal and impaired number processing. In G. Deloche and X. Scron (Eds.), *Mathematical Disabilities.* Hillsdale, NJ: Erlbaum.

Molfese, D. L., & Segalowitz, S. J. (Eds.). (1988). *Brain lateralization in children.* New York: Guilford.

Neville, H., Mills, D. L., & Coffey, S. A. (1989). *Event-related potential studies of language acquisition.* Paper presented at the Society for Research in Child Development Meetings, Kansas City, MO.

Papanicolaou, A. C., DiScenna, A., Gillespie, L. L., & Aram, D. M. (in press). Probe evoked potential findings following unilateral left hemisphere lesions in children. *Archives of Neurology.*

Pohl, P. (1979). Dichotic listening in a child recovering from acquired aphasia. *Brain and Language, 8,* 372–379.

Rankin, J. M., Aram, D. M., & Horwitz, S. J. (1981). Language ability in right and left hemiplegic children. *Brain and Language, 14,* 292–306.

Rasmussen, T., & Milner, B. (1977). The role of early left-brain injury in determining lateralization of cerebral speech functions. In S. Dimond & D. Blizard (Eds.),

Evolution and lateralization of the brain. Annals of the New York Academy of Sciences,
     299, 335–369.
Thal, D. J., Bates, E., Marchman, V., & Fenson, L. (1989). *First words and early grammar
     in toddlers.* Paper presented at the Society for Research in Child Development
     Meetings, Kansas City, MO.
Vargha-Khadem, F., O'Gorman, A. M., & Watters, G. V. (1985). Aphasia and
     handedness in relation to hemispheric side, age at injury and severity of cerebral
     lesion during childhood. *Brain, 108,* 677–696.
Woods, B. T., & Carey, S. (1979). Language deficits after apparent clinical recovery
     from childhood aphasia. *Annals of Neurology, 6,* 405–409.
Yeni-Komshian, G. H. (1977). *Speech perception in brain injured children.* Paper
     presented at the Conference on the Biological Bases of Delayed Language
     Development, April, New York.

CHAPTER 20

Augmentative Communication: Directions for Future Research

KATE FRANKLIN
DAVID R. BEUKELMAN

Augmentative communication refers to the variety of communication approaches that are used to assist persons who are limited in their ability to communicate messages through natural modes of communication. These approaches may be unaided, as in manual sign and adapted gestures, or aided, with utilization of communication boards or electronic devices. Regardless of the communication mode employed, the goals of augmented communicators are similar to those of natural speakers, that is, to express wants and needs, to share information, to engage in social closeness, and to manage social etiquette (Light, 1988).

Although augmented and natural communicators are common communication goals, the techniques and strategies that they employ may differ considerably. A few of these differences will be highlighted in preparation for the discussion of research perspectives to follow. First, augmented communicators transfer information much more slowly than natural speakers. It is estimated that their communication rate is one-twentieth of natural speakers. This differential appears to impact on the effectiveness of interactional strategies when augmented communicators attempt dyadic or group interactions with natural speakers. Second, because of their severe communication disorder, augmented communicators, who are not literate, must rely on others to select the vocabulary and symbols to be included in their communication systems. Typically those who devise augmentative communication systems are speech-language pathologists, communication aides, teachers, or parents. These natural-speaking adults bring their own perspectives and communication experiences to the communication system development process. Consequently, inappropriate goals may be encouraged as adults and nonspeaking children differ with respect to communication constraints, options, and strategies. Finally, an inability to speak requires that the augmentative communication system be functional in several different contexts. For example, the system must support daily communication needs in an efficient, accurate, nonfatiguing manner. The system must also assist as children learn the language, acquire knowledge, and gain competencies of their culture. Finally, the system must be used to support academic learning. These multiple augmentation system uses involve a wide range of techniques and strategies, some of which are quite different from natural communication processes.

In this chapter, research perspectives will be developed in three areas: vocabulary selection, symbol selection, and interaction among children using augmentative communication systems. Although there are a number of other issues of relevance in the decision-making process, the areas selected for this endeavor represent, perhaps, those considerations of paramount importance when making decisions about appropriate augmentative communication systems for young children who are nonspeaking.

VOCABULARY SELECTION

Augmentative communication systems only serve a truly communicative purpose if the vocabulary content of the system is carefully and strategically selected. For individuals who are nonliterate, vocabulary selection is particularly crucial because "they are unable to create spontaneously their own lexicon and must operate with a vocabulary selected by someone else or preselected, not spontaneously chosen by themselves" (Carlson, 1981, p. 240). These *coverage vocabulary* or *word sets* should "provide the individual with the ability to communicate most effectively and about the widest range of topics, given the limited word set" (Vanderheiden & Kelso, 1987, p. 196). For persons who are literate and able to communicate through letter-by-letter spelling, *acceleration vocabulary* is selected for inclusion into their communication system in order to enhance the speed of message preparation and the timing of message presentation as messages are retrieved or predicted in part or in their entirety.

Several recent trends in augmentative communication have encouraged research in the area of vocabulary selection. Specifically, technical advancements have increased the flexibility of various devices allowing the selection and programming of vocabulary by augmentative communication facilitators in the field rather than at the factory. Technical advances have also permitted the use of different levels of the symbolic representational strategies (e.g., line drawings, Blissymbols [Blissymbolics Communication Institute, 1984], Picsyms [Carlson, 1985], orthographic forms, etc.) on the same device, thereby making these devices accessible to multiple and varied nonspeaking populations. With these increases in technologic flexibility has come the increased responsibility for germane vocabulary selection for the individual augmented communicator. Additionally, the growing appreciation of the unique needs and capabilities of individuals who are severely communicatively disordered has provided another impetus for careful investigation into the area of vocabulary selection.

SELECTING COVERAGE VOCABULARY

The research related to coverage vocabulary can be divided into two general areas: (1) the selection of specific vocabulary words, and (2) the process of selecting vocabulary. Specific word lists have been suggested as initial vocabularies for nonliterate augmented communicators. Some examples of these include: (a) Makaton—a method of organizing the sign-language system of a country into vocabulary based on developmental and functional guidelines (Walker, 1976); (b) Fristoe and Lloyd (1979) developed a list of vocabulary items that occurred in more than 1 of 20 manuals of signs; and (c) Mein and O'Connor (1960) compiled a list of words that occurred at least in 50 percent of natural speech samples of developmentally delayed adolescents and adults. Attempts at selecting initial vocabulary for training in the area of augmentative communication emerged with the work of Fristoe and Lloyd (1979, 1980) in which initial sign-language vocabulary was selected based upon recurring features of signs.

The process of selecting coverage vocabulary has been addressed by several researchers. In 1984, Karlan and Lloyd reviewed two strategies of initial vocabulary selection for individuals with severe disabilities. The first technique adhered to "behavioral-remedial logic" (Guess, Sailor & Baer, 1978), which suggests that initial vocabulary should be developed through an analysis of student preferences, frequency of occurrence, functional utility across situations, and basic human needs. Using a similar rationale, Carlson (1981) stressed the importance of being responsive to the specific needs of augmented communicators within specific environmental parameters. She encouraged the analysis of the activities and persons within various environments to identify those words and messages that would cover the vocabulary needs of a nonliterate augmented communicator.

The second technique suggested by Lloyd and Karlan (1984) is based on the model of normal vocabulary development (Holland, 1975), which suggests that initial vocabulary should represent those content categories demonstrated to be within the language systems of normally developing children (Lahey & Bloom, 1977). In an effort to incorporate both strategies of coverage vocabulary selection, Fried-Oken (in progress) is currently investigating methods of vocabulary selection for preschool children with cerebral palsy who are severely communicatively disordered. She is comparing the initial vocabulary selected for them with the vocabulary of able-bodied speaking children involved in similar environmental contexts. The intent of this research is to establish a data base from which developmental guidelines can be designed to facilitate appropriate initial lexical choices for communication aides that will stimulate the acquisition of expressive language skills in children using augmentative devices while meeting their unique vocabulary needs because of their disabilities and the augmentative approach.

A recent examination of vocabulary selection techniques was undertaken by Morrow, Beukelman, and Mirenda (in press) in which they compared three commonly used techniques. Essentially, a comparison was made of a vocabulary checklist format; a categorical interview format; and a blank page format. Overall, the checklist format yielded more words than did any other vocabulary selection format and was judged by the informants to be the most satisfactory tool used. Unique words, that is, words offered by only one informant, were most often provided by the blank page format. Of the three informant groups, parents provided a greater number of unique vocabulary words than teachers or speech-language pathologists. Implications of this research indicated that multiple methods of vocabulary selection should be included as they appear to provide the best overall vocabulary to meet the individual's communication needs.

Numerous research directions related to the selection of coverage vocabulary remain to be pursued. These directions encompass the following:

1. There is a need to document the vocabulary use patterns in various environments and contexts of augmented communicators of various ages who use coverage vocabularies. There is little information in the literature about the actual word-use patterns of these individuals to meet their specific communication and learning needs.
2. There is a need to validate the effectiveness with which the various vocabulary selection strategies predict the actual vocabulary needed by persons requiring coverage vocabulary. Although the vocabulary selection process has been investigated in a few studies, the validity of prediction has not been studied.
3. Research about impact of vocabulary selection and use strategies on the vocabulary learning patterns of persons requiring coverage vocabularies has not been addressed. More broadly, there is minimal

information about how augmented communicators learn vocabulary or about those factors that influence the efficiency of their learning.

SELECTING ACCELERATION VOCABULARIES

Acceleration vocabularies are utilized to enhance the speed and efficiency of communication by literate augmentated communicators through message retrieval and message prediction. Recently there has been an emphasis on the use of standardized vocabulary lists in the development of initial selection of acceleration vocabularies for individuals using augmentative communication devices. Beukelman, Yorkston, Poblete, and Naranjo (1984) collected communication samples from language-intact adults using Cannon Communicators. From an analysis of the frequency of word occurrence, they suggested that core vocabulary lists could be developed to provide a framework upon which to build unique messages in addition to vocabulary items that are not used frequently enough to be included in the core. A recent research endeavor by Yorkston, Dowden, Honsinger, Marriner, and Smith (1988) indicated that there was a lack of congruence between readily available standard word lists and the vocabulary needs of the augmentated communicator. They eluded to the idea that composite lists of augmented communicator vocabularies may function to form a large source vocabulary list from which appropriate core and fringe vocabulary may be chosen. Additionally, Yorkston, Smith and Beukelman (in press) conducted research comparing and contrasting the relative benefits of individualized word lists versus standardized vocabulary sources. Results of this study indicated that "short lists" derived from natural communication samples of augmented communicators can represent a large proportion of necessary vocabulary for these individuals. They concluded by stressing that standardized vocabularies for augmented communicators in various age ranges should not be an abandoned research effort. Rather, they suggest that these lists can provide sources of potential words to be included within augmentative communication applications. Beukelman, Jones, and Rowan (in press), Fried-Oken (in progress), McGinnis (in progress), McGinnis and Beukelman (1989), and Trevor and Nelson (in progress) continue to study the spoken and written language of preschoolers, elementary school students, high school students and college students on selected social, academic, and vocational tasks in an attempt to develop a variety of standardized vocabulary lists of persons in various age ranges and communicative situations.

In an attempt to move beyond the level of single-word vocabulary, Yorkston, Beukelman, Smith, and Tice (in press) conducted research in order to determine the feasibility of identifying and utilizing word sequences in facilitating vocabulary selection and reducing the required number of keystrokes necessary for message retrieval. In their analysis of linguistically intact augmented communicators utilizing a vocabulary frequency analyzer, they found that word sequences of three to five words in length did not occur frequently in extended communication samples of individual subjects nor was there much overlap between subjects. However, frequently occurring one- and two-word sequences may facilitate keystroke savings.

Several research directions in the area of communication acceleration would support augmentative communication interventions and technique development.

1. There is a need to document language-use patterns in the various contexts in which augmented communicators may wish to participate and compete. Two types of vocabulary studies appear to be necessary to clarify the vocabulary requirements of literate augmented communicators who are participating and competing in integrated settings. First, word-usage patterns of natural speakers who are successful students, employees, and so on, are necessary to provide the augmented communicator with access to the language forms commonly associated with a specific context or task. Second, the word-usage patterns of augmented communicators who are successful participants in a particular task or context will provide information about the unique vocabulary requirements of augmented communicators.
2. Currently, several message storage/retrieval and prediction strategies are utilized to enhance the speed and timing of augmented communication. Additional research to develop strategies that maximize communication efficiency and minimize the cognitive and learning requirements of the strategies is required.
3. The learning requirements of various message coding/retrieval and prediction strategies is of concern in the augmentative communication field. Studies that document the relative cost-benefit relationships among learning costs and communication efficiency benefits are a pressing research need.

SYMBOL SELECTION

Perhaps one of the greatest challenges in developing augmentative communication systems for young children and for those with intellectual disabilities is determining the symbol level that can be used to represent their vocabulary to enhance communication expression and comprehension. Symbols can be operationally defined as those arbitrary entities that stand for and can take the place of a real object, event, person, action, or relationship (Savage-Rumbaugh, 1986). In the acquisition of language, it is essential that an individual realize that symbols refer to environmental referents, that is, they must be internally represented (Sevcik & Romski, 1986).

Two primary considerations have prevailed in the literature, to date, relating to symbolic functioning. The first consideration reflects how to determine most accurately the symbols that best parallel a person's internal representations. The second relates to the development of strategies to teach students successfully how to use symbols communicatively and what process of assessment most adequately tests symbol level.

The issue of "matching" symbol level to a student's internal representation has been a pervasive research topic within the literature. Vanderheiden and Lloyd (1986) discussed the various kinds of symbols that can be used in communication. Generally, all symbols can be divided into two categories: dynamic and static. Static symbols best lend themselves to augmentative communication systems as they are relatively permanent in nature and are considered to be the easiest to use although there are data that contradict this assumption (Harris-Vanderheiden, Brown, MacKenzie, Reinen & Scheibel, 1975; Romski, Sevcik & Pate, 1988; Romski, White, Millen & Rumbaugh, 1984). Additionally, there is a body of research surrounding the notion of a symbol's transparency, translucency, and opaqueness (Mizuko, 1987) or what Vanderheiden and Lloyd (1986) refer to as the iconic or abstract nature of symbols. Transparent symbols are those that are most iconic, that is, their meaning can be readily guessed by naive viewers. Symbols that are not so obvious but still enable the viewer to perceive a relationship between the symbol and its meaning are considered to be translucent. Finally, symbols that are abstract in nature, that is, have no obvious relationship to meaning, are opaque.

Several studies have been undertaken that address the issue of symbol "learnability" involving both normally developing children and those with varying degrees of intellectual disability. Results of research with normally developing children indicate that there is a predictable developmental progression in the order in which students recognize and learn various types of symbols. Mizuko (1987) found that nonhandicapped preschool children found Picsyms and PCS symbols (Mayer-Johnson Co., 1986) to be more transparent and more learnable than Blissymbols. Musselwhite and Ruscello (1984) found Picsyms and Rebus symbols (Clark, Davies & Woodcock, 1974) are more easily identified by children than Blissymbols. Additionally, Clark (1981) and Ecklund and Reichle (1987) found that children were able to learn symbol-word associations more easily with iconic symbol sets. Both of these studies found that Rebus were easier than Blissymbols, followed by NonSLIP (Carrier & Peak, 1975) and finally written words. The conclusion that can be drawn from this research is that normally developing preschool children (ages 3–5 years), who already understand speech, recognize iconic representations more easily than abstract symbols.

Research involving learners with varying levels of intellectual disability indicates that symbols judged to be high in iconicity were more easily learned by individuals with intellectual disabilities than symbols with low iconicity (Clark, 1984; Goossens, 1983; Hurlburt, Iwata & Green, 1982). Symbols that represent high to medium levels of iconicity would include actual objects, photographs, colored line drawings, and black and white line drawings (e.g., Rebus, PCS, and Picsyms). Similar results were obtained by Reichle and Yoder (1985) in a study in which they taught the use of iconic symbols to individuals with severe intellectual disabilities.

Mirenda (1985) addressed the need for iconicity when developing augmentative communication systems for learners with intellectual disabilities although she very cogently points out that "the type of pictorial system selected must be determined on an individual basis for each student, after consideration of a number of interrelated factors. These include, but are not limited to: (1) the student's developmental status and symbolic ability, (2) the student's prior knowledge and experience base, and (3) the student's visual processing abilities" (p. 59).

In research investigating the "learnability" of abstract symbols, Harris-Vanderheiden, Brown, MacKenzie, Reinen, and Scheibel (1975) determined that Blissymbols could be taught to individuals with severe intellectual disabilities. They found that the students were able to respond to the symbols but were not using them expressively. Romski, White, Millen, and Rumbaugh (1984) and Romski, Sevcik, and Pate (1988) also support the use of abstract symbols with individuals who have intellectual disabilities. Romski, Sevcik, and Pate have successfully taught three out of four subjects to use lexigrams (geometric shapes used to form symbols) to request food and, subsequently, objects. In short, there appears to be substantiation for the use of both iconic and abstract symbol use among individuals with intellectual disabilities. One might conjecture that individual differences may be a potential reason for the ability of students to use one method over another. However, another potential explanation might reflect some noted inconsistencies in strategies used for the assessment and teaching of symbol use.

Inconsistencies in the research findings appear to fall into two general categories. First, the symbol assessment measures utilized among normally developing children and in those with intellectual disabilities vary across studies. More specifically, a number of visual matching and verbal labeling assessment protocols have been used (Clark, 1981; Ecklund & Reichle, 1987; Mirenda & Locke, 1989; Mizuko, 1987; Musselwhite & Ruscello, 1984; Musselwhite & St. Louis, 1982, 1988). Second, the symbol system training methods employed to instruct persons with intellectual disabilities reflect the use of a number of divergent learning strategies. The literature reports a variety of symbol training strategies ranging from basic verbal labeling tasks to multiple match-to-match strategies (Carrier & Peak, 1975; Keogh & Reichle, 1985; Reichle & Yoder, 1985; Sevcik & Romski, 1986; Romski, Sevcik, & Pate, 1988).

As outlined above, there is a good deal of variation in the assessment and training protocols used in the identification and teaching of appropriate communication symbols. Although this is not necessarily inappropriate, comparisons across the research findings are difficult as a result. Specifically, it is uncertain whether the findings of existing research are the result of differences in the iconicity and/or "learnability" of symbols or whether variations in the assessment and training protocols differentially effect the outcome of the research.

Another issue of emerging importance involves the receptive language levels of individuals being assessed and trained symbolically. Sevcik and Romski (1986) identified two groups in their research involving identity and nonidentity matching. One group was classified as having functional language skills defined as having a minimum vocabulary of 10 spoken words, manual signs, or visual-graphic symbols used spontaneously in both comprehension and production. Results of their research found that those with functional language skills performed better on both the identity and nonidentity matching conditions than those determined to not have functional language skills. Additional support for perhaps beginning to systematically investigate the influence of receptive language levels on the acquisition and assessment of various symbols emerged from the research looking at a training strategy to teach abstract symbol use (Romski, Sevcik & Pate, 1988). Results of this research indicated that the student who had speech comprehension prior to the onset of the study demonstrated accelerated acquisition and generalization of lexigrams.

Clearly, there is considerable need for future research in the area of symbol selection. The following research directions reflect evidence from available literature that demonstrates the need for investigation into a variety of issues in symbol selection.

1. There is a need to identify the assessment strategies that will best predict a symbol level paralleling the internal representation of the individual. To date, there are a variety of visual-matching and auditory-matching tasks used to establish symbol level functioning. However, there is a lack of research quantifying the validity of these various methods as appropriate predictors of symbol level functioning.

2. Currently, there is little information related to the linguistic functioning of the individual who is nonspeaking when making symbol selection decisions. The level at which the individual is functioning in terms of receptive and expressive language skills may impact on the

symbol system determined to be most appropriate to the augmented communicator. This information may also influence the sequence in which these individuals learn to use the symbol systems chosen.
3. To date, there is a plethora of research supporting a predictable developmental progression in the order in which students recognize and learn various symbols. There is, however, a need to investigate the effectiveness of various teaching strategies and evaluate how they impact on the relative learnability of various types of symbols.

COMMUNICATIVE INTERACTION

Historically, the study of the communication interaction patterns of augmented communicators has been associated with a good deal of controversy. Researchers continue to struggle as they develop strategies to appropriately operationalize terms within this arena. For the purposes of this chapter, research in the area of communicative interaction will be divided into three perspectives, including (a) a production perspective—developed to investigate aspects of the adequacy of "operating" the linguistic and augmentative communication systems, (b) a social perspective—which addresses issues of social context variables as well as attitudes and perceptions toward the augmented communicator, and (c) a personal perspective—one that focuses on the feelings and perceptions of the augmented communicator. A discussion of each of these perspectives follows.

In an initial attempt to define communicative interaction within the augmentative communication field, Kraat (1985) utilized information from a variety of disciplines including psychology, sociology, and linguistics, in order to adequately represent the various considerations related to interaction. Beyond being an exchange of semantic meaning or the transmission of information, Kraat indicated that "the speaker utters a particular sentence and attempts to get the 'listener' to understand what is meant" (p. 7). From a *production perspective* Kraat indicated that it is important to examine the intentions of the speaker from a "speech acts" framework. Within this framework one must look beneath the surface structure to establish the speaker's intentions (i.e., to discover how the utterance affects the listener). Light (1988) attempted to delineate the production competencies of augmentated communicators in a "communicative competencies" framework defined as "the state of being functionally adequate in daily communication, or having sufficient knowledge, judgement or skill to communicate" (p. 4). Within the production perspective, Light identified linguistic competence (adequate mastery of the linguistic code), operational competence (proficient use of the augmentative communication system), and strategic competence (appropriate compensatory strategies that facilitate effective communication) as being of primary concern. One might further operationalize this overall concept of communicative competence by considering the aspects of linguistic, operational, and strategic competence within the "listener" or communication partner. All of these competencies are required of partners in order for the conversational interaction to be functional and adequate.

To date, the majority of research in conversational interaction involving augmentated communicators has attempted to describe the characteristics of interactions among individuals who are nonspeaking and normal-speaking communication partners. This research has been largely conducted at a microanalytic level in which the focus has been on specific aspects or strategies within a given interactional situation. Primarily, research has considered communication interactions from a perspective in which the partner and the augmented communicator engaged in a dyadic interaction. The majority of the literature has reported asymmetrical communication interactions in which the augmented communicators clearly did not interact in the same manner as their normal-speaking partners. Results of a number of studies have indicated that augmented communicators are primarily responders rather than initiators, have limited number of turns, have limited length of turn, do not initiate, have reduced contribution to the topic, exhibit limited speech act range, rely on more immediate means of communicating (gestures, vocalizations, eye gaze, spoken or handwritten communication), experience communication breakdowns, and are limited in communication repair strategies (Beukelman, Yorkston, Gorhoff, Mitsuda & Kenyon, 1981; Beukelman & Yorkston, 1980; Buzolich & Weimann, 1988; Calculator & Dollaghan, 1982; Calculator & Luchko, 1983; Colquhoun, 1982; Culp, 1982; Farrier, Yorkston, Marriner & Beukelman, 1985; Harris, 1978; Light, Collier & Parnes, 1985a, 1985b, 1985c; Lossing, 1981; and Wexler, Blau, Leslie & Dore, 1982). Research looking specifically at the communication partner within a dyadic situation generally revealed that they were dominant in the conversation, had control of the turn size and topic, structured the interaction to result in one- to two-word responses from the augmentated communicator, rarely modeled communication strategies, and were infrequent in responding to the initiations of the augmentated communicator (Kraat, 1985; Light, 1988).

Earlier in this chapter, the authors eluded to the notion that the majority of research in the area of communicative interaction has been microanalytic in nature. From this information we know that there are subject variables, partner variables, contextual variables, augmentative communication system variables, and experiential and/or training variables that all influence the interactional process. One cannot diminish the value of this research, but the time has arrived in which exploration of communicative interaction must be addressed from a macroanalytic level as well. That is, the interactional process must be investigated as a whole; within the realm of the *social perspective*. In this perspective, researchers should not only look at the quality of various competencies within an interaction, but focus is necessary on the social contexts in which the interaction takes place. Additionally, Kraat (1985) revealed that there should be considerations of the augmentated communicator from a psychosocial perspective. This perspective would constitute utilizing language as a vehicle to reflect aspects of an individual's personality. This was further supported by Light (1988) who indicated that one of the necessary considerations in the area of communicative interaction lies in the acquisition and development of skills in the social rules of communication. Further, societal issues such as labeling effects, aspects of bias toward the augmentated communicator may, at a macro level, be limiting their opportunities as communicators. This in turn may adversely affect the nature of the conversational interaction. Kraat (1985) perceptively suggested that "we need to develop an understanding of what those attitudes are, and how they are translated into interactional behaviors and experiences. Of primary importance seems to be how to alter inappropriate perceptions of augmented speakers and systems" (p. 144).

Within the realm of communication system implementation and training, Warrick (1988) suggested that responsible intervention should address not only the linguistic but also the social issues of conversational interaction. She stated, "In order to address the sociocommunicative issues more effectively, intervention should consider the following: (a) the promotion of meaningful tasks; (b) appropriate environmental feedback; (c) affective relations which encourage self-esteem; (d) the promotion of common perceptions; and (e) encouragement of socially acceptable communication modes" (p. 49).

The *personal perspective* is a necessary component in a discussion of conversational interaction as it qualifies the perceptions and attitudes of the augmentated communicator within the context of an interaction. Using the methods of qualitative research, Smith-Lewis and Ford (1987) illustrated the importance of making certain that the augmentated communicator was instrumental in all aspects of decision making. This article clearly illustrated the variability in levels of perceived communicative competence and how it impacts on the conversational interaction process.

The communicative interaction perspectives outlined above reflect a need within the augmentative communication field to consider the influence of elements relating to production strengths and constraints, as well as elements relating to society and those elements specific to the augmentated communicator. Through the use of microanalytic and macroanalytic research methodologies, perhaps more information can be obtained relative to the interactional processes between augmentated communicators and natural speakers.

Essentially, current research is inadequate to make any conclusions regarding aspects of communicative interaction in the field of augmentative communication. The future research considerations regarding communication interaction and augmented communication are extensive. The following outlines some suggestions for preliminary investigation into the area of communicative interaction.

1. There is a pressing need to study the performance of successful as compared to unsuccessful augmented communicators to determine the interaction strategies that successful persons use. The constraints and options imposed by augmentative communication approaches seem to require at least some unique interactional strategies. Although authors have hypothesized some of these strategies, there is little empirical evidence to support these suggestions. Light (1988) has suggested that macroanalysis and microanalysis be combined to identify those strategies used by augmented communicators to achieve successful interaction patterns.
2. There remains a need to compare the performance of successful augmented communicators to that of natural speakers in an effort to determine the similarities and differences in interactional strategies in these two groups. To date, the research has largely compared the overall interactional outcomes of augmented and natural speakers; however, little attention has been paid to the interaction strategies that each use.
3. Extensive study is needed of the impact of specific augmentative communication issues, such as message presentation speed, message output mode, and message timing on interaction patterns.
4. Opportunities for interaction appear to be influenced by listener and potential listener perception of speaker competence. Research is needed that identifies the impact of augmentative communication issues such as high technology versus low technology, quality of speech synthesis, symbol strategies, message completeness, and age appropriateness of messages on perceptions of augmented communicator competence.
5. Finally, consideration of the personal perceptions and attitudes of the augmented communicator must be incorporated into all aspects of the interaction process in order to fully realize the impact of augmentative communication on an overall communicative interaction.

FINAL COMMENT

The augmentative communication field is dynamic—providing persons with severe communication disorders the access to effective communication options. In 1989, a relatively large number of individuals communicate entirely or in part using an augmentative mode as they attempt to participate in their homes, schools, recreational activities, and employment settings. The number of augmented communicators is growing rapidly. The language issues associated with the augmentative communication effort are extensive—far exceeding the capability of the researchers already associated with this field to pursue. The need for trained research personnel to address language issues that relate to the augmentative communication field is urgent, as much of this research can have immediate clinical or technical impact.

REFERENCES

Beukelman, D. R., Jones, R. S., & Rowan, M. (in press). Frequency of word usage by non-disabled peers in integrated preschool classrooms. *Augmentative and Alternative Communication.*

Beukelman, D. R., & Yorkston, K. M. (1980). Nonvocal communication: Performance evaluation. *Archives of Physical Medicine and Rehabilitation, 61,* 272–275.

Beukelman, D. R., Yorkston, K. M., Gorhoff, S. C., Mitsuda, P. M., & Kenyon, V. T. (1981). Cannon communicator use: A retrospective study. *Journal of Speech and Hearing Disorders, 46,* 374–388.

Beukelman, D. R., Yorkston, K. M., Poblete, M., & Naranjo, C. (1984). Frequency of word occurrence in communication samples produced by adult communication aid users. *Journal of Speech and Hearing Disorders, 49,* 360–367.

Blissymbolics Communication Institute. (1984). *A supplement to Blissymbolics for use.* Toronto: Blissymbolics Communication Institute.

Buzolich, M., & Weimann, J. (1988). Turn taking in atypical conversations: The case of the speaker/augmented-communicator dyad. *Journal of Speech and Hearing Research, 31,* 3–18.

Calculator, S., & Dollaghan, C. (1982). The use of communication boards in a residential setting: An evaluation. *Journal of Speech and Hearing Disorders, 47,* 281–287.

Calculator, S., & Luchko, C. (1983). Evaluation of the effectiveness of a communication board training program. *Journal of Speech and Hearing Disorders, 48,* 185–191.

Carlson, F. (1981). A format for selecting vocabulary for the nonspeaking child. *Language, Speech, and Hearing Services in the Schools, 12,* 240–245.

Carlson, F. (1985). *Picsyms categorical dictionary.* Lawrence, KS: Baggeboda Press.

Carrier, J. K., & Peak, T. (1975). *Non-SLIP (Non-speech language initiation program).* Lawrence, KS: H & H Enterprises.

Clark, C. (1984). A close look at the standard Rebus system and Blissymbols. *Journal of the Association for the Severely Handicapped, 9,* 37–48.

Clark, C. R. (1981). Learning works using traditional orthography and the symbols of Rebus, Bliss, and Carrier. *Journal of Speech and Hearing Disorders, 46,* 191–196.

Clark, C. R., Davies, C. O., & Woodcock, R. W. (1974). *Standard Rebus glossary.* Circle Pines, MN: American Guidance Service.

Colquhoun, A. (1982). *Augmentative communication systems: The interaction process.* Paper presented at the American Speech, Language and Hearing Association Annual Convention, Toronto, Canada.

Culp, D. (1982). *Communication interactions—nonspeaking children using augmentative systems.* Unpublished manuscript, Callier Center for Communication Disorders, Dallas, TX.

Ecklund, S., & Reichle, J. (1987). A comparison of normal children's ability to recall symbols from two logographic systems. *Language, Speech, and Hearing Services in the Schools, 18,* 34–40.

Farrier, L., Yorkston, K., Marriner, N., & Beukelman, D. (1985). Conversational control in nonimpaired speakers using an augmentative communication system. *Augmentative and Alternative Communication, 1,* 65–73.

Fried-Oken, M. (in progress). Vocabulary needs of the nonspeaking child as determined by caregivers.

Fristoe, M., & Lloyd, L. L. (1979a). Nonspeech communication. In N. R. Ellis (Ed.), *Handbook of mental deficiency: Psychological theory and research* (pp. 401–430). Hilldale, NJ: Erlbaum.

Fristoe, M., & Lloyd, L. L. (1979). Signs used in manual communication training with persons having severe communication impairment. *AAESPH Review, 4,* 364–373.

Fristoe, M., & Lloyd, L. L. (1980). Planning an initial expressive sign lexicon for persons with severe communication impairments. *Journal of Speech and Hearing Disorders, 45,* 170–180.

Goossens, C. (1983). *The relative iconicity and learnability of verb referents depicted in Blissymbols, manual signs, and Rebus symbols: An investigation with moderately retarded individuals.* Unpublished doctoral dissertation, Purdue University, West Lafayette, IN.

Guess, D., Sailor, W., & Baer, D. (1978). Children with limited language. In R. L. Schiefelbusch (Ed.), *Language intervention strategies.* Baltimore: University Park Press.

Harris, D. (1978). *Descriptive analysis of communicative interaction processes involving nonvocal severely physically handicapped children.* Doctoral dissertation, University of Wisconsin–Madison.

Harris-Vanderheiden, D., Brown, W. P., MacKenzie, P., Reinen, S., & Scheibel, C. (1975). Symbol communication for the mentally handicapped. *Mental Retardation, 13,* 34–37.

Holland, A. (1975). Language therapy for children: Some thoughts on context and content. *Journal of Speech and Hearing Disorders, 40,* 514–523.

Hurlburt, B. I., Iwata, B. A., & Green, J. D. (1982). Nonvocal language acquisition in adolescents with severe physical disabilities: Blissymbols versus iconic stimulus formats. *Journal of Applied Behavior Analysis, 15,* 241–258.

Keogh, W. J., & Reichle, J. (1985). Communication intervention for the "difficult to teach" severely handicapped. In S. F. Warren & A. K. Rogers-Warren (Eds.), *Teaching functional language* (pp. 157–194). Austin, TX: PRO-ED.

Kraat, A. W. (1985). *Communication interaction between aided and natural speakers: An IPCAS study report.* Toronto: Canadian Rehabilitation Council for the Disabled.

Lahey, M., & Bloom, L. (1977). Planning a first lexicon: Which words to teach first. *Journal of Speech and Hearing Disorders, 42,* 340–349.

Light, J. (1988). Interaction involving individuals using augmentative and alternative communication systems: State of the art and future directions. *Augmentative and Alternative Communications, 2,* 66–82.

Light, J., Collier, B., & Parnes, P. (1985a). Communicative interaction between young nonspeaking physically disabled children and their primary caregivers: Part I: Discourse patterns. *Augmentative and Alternative Communication, 1,* 74–83.

Light, J., Collier, B., & Parnes, P. (1985b). Communicative interaction between young nonspeaking physically disabled children and their primary caregivers:

Part II: Communicative functions. *Augmentative and Alternative Communication,* *1*, 98–107.

Light, J., Collier, B., & Parnes, P. (1985c). Communicative interaction between young nonspeaking physically disabled children and their primary caregivers: Part III: Modes of communication. *Augmentative and Alternative Communication,* *1*, 125–133.

Lloyd, L. L., & Karlan, G. (1984). Nonspeech communication symbols and systems: Where have we been and where are we going? *Journal of Mental Deficiency Research, 28,* 3–20.

Lossing, C. (1981). *A technique for quantification of non-verbal communication performance by listeners.* Unpublished master's thesis, University of Washington, Seattle.

Mayer-Johnson Co. (1986). *The Picture Communication Symbols, Book I.* Solana Beach, CA: Author.

McGinnis, J. S. (1989). *A comparison of spoken and written vocabulary by third grade students in regular classrooms.* Doctoral Dissertation, University of Nebraska–Lincoln.

McGinnis, J. S., & Beukelman, D. R. (1989). Vocabulary requirements for writing activities for the academically mainstreamed student with disabilities. *Augmentative and Alternative Communication, 3,* 183–191.

Mein, R., & O'Connor, N. (1960). A study of the oral vocabularies of severely subnormal patients. *Journal of Mental Deficiency Research, 4,* 130–143.

Mirenda, P. (1985). Designing pictorial communication systems for physically able-bodied students with severe handicaps. *Augmentative and Alternative Communication, 1,* 58–64.

Mirenda, P., & Locke, P. (1989). A comparison of symbol transparency in nonspeaking persons with intellectual disabilities. *Journal of Speech and Hearing Disorders, 54,* 131–140.

Mizuko, M. (1987). Transparency and ease of learning of symbols represented by Blissymbols, PCS, and Picsyms. *Augmentative and Alternative Communication, 3,* 129–136.

Morrow, D., Beukelman, D. R., & Mirenda, P. (in press). Vocabulary selection for augmentative communication systems: A comparison of three techniques. *Augmentative and Alternative Communication.*

Musselwhite, C. R., & Ruscello, D. M. (1984). Transparency of three symbol communication systems. *Journal of Speech and Hearing Research, 27,* 436–443.

Musselwhite, C., & St. Louis, K. (1982, 1988). *Communication programming for the severely handicapped: Vocal and nonvocal strategies.* Austin, TX: PRO-ED.

Reichle, J., & Yoder, D. (1985). Communication board use in severely handicapped learners. *Language, Speech, and Hearing Services in the Schools, 16,* 146–157.

Romski, M. A., Sevcik, R. A., & Pate, J. L. (1988). The establishment of symbolic communication in persons with severe retardation. *Journal of Speech and Hearing Disorders, 53,* 97–107.

Romski, M. A., White, R. A., Millen, C. M., & Rumbaugh, D. M. (1984). Effects of computer-keyboard teaching of the symbolic communication of severely retarded persons: Five case studies. *The Psychological Record, 34,* 39–51.

Savage-Rumbaugh, E. S. (1986). *Ape language: From conditioned response to symbol.* New York: Columbia University Press.

Sevcik, R. A., & Romski, M. A. (1986). Representational matching skills of persons with severe retardation. *Augmentative and Alternative Communication, 2,* 160–164.

Smith-Lewis, M., & Ford, A. (1987). A user's perspective on augmentative communication. *Augmentative and Alternative Communication, 3,* 12–17.

Trevor, K., & Nelson, N. (in progress). Vocabulary use by children in first, third, and fifth grade classrooms. Kalamazoo: Western Michigan University.

Vanderheiden, G., & Kelso, D. (1987). Comparative analysis of fixed vocabulary communication acceleration techniques. *Augmentative and Alternative Communication, 4,* 196–206.

Vanderheiden, G. C., & Lloyd, L. L. (1986). Communication systems and their components. In S. W. Blackstone (Ed.), *Augmentative communication: An introduction* (pp. 49–161). Rockville, MD: American Speech-Language-Hearing Association.

Walker, M. M. (1976). *The revised Makaton vocabulary.* London: Royal Association in Aid of the Deaf and Dumb.

Warrick, A. (1988). Sociocommunicative considerations within augmentative communication. *Augmentative and Alternative Communication, 4,* 46–52.

Wexler, K., Blau, A., Leslie, S., & Dore, J. (1982). *Conversational interaction of nonspeaking cerebral palsied individuals and their speaking partners, with and without augmentative communication aids.* Unpublished manuscript, Helen Hayes Hospital, West Haverstraw, NY.

Yorkston, K. M., Beukelman, D. R., Smith, K., & Tice, R. (in press). Extended communication samples of augmented communicators II: Analysis of multiword sequences. *Journal of Speech and Hearing Disorders.*

Yorkston, K. M., Dowden, P., Honsinger, M., Marriner, N., & Smith, K. (1988). A comparison of standard and user vocabulary lists. *Augmentative and Alternative Communication, 4,* 189–210.

Yorkston, K. M., Smith, K., & Beukelman, D. R. (in press). Extended communication samples of augmented communicators I: A comparison of individualized versus standard single word vocabularies.

CHAPTER 21

Lexical Acquisition and Processing in Specific Language Impairment

RICHARD G. SCHWARTZ

As with so many comparisons of children with specific language impairment (SLI) and their normal-language (NL) peers, we have found many instances of similarities in lexical acquisition and use. However, some closer examinations of word learning, production, and comprehension reveal differences that may provide insights into the nature of the language-learning difficulties faced by these children. They also may reveal some less obvious, but critical, features of language acquisition. In this chapter I will briefly describe some key differences between children with SLI and their younger NL peers. I will then argue that these finer grained investigation of lexical acquisition and on-line lexical processing by these children is a fruitful avenue of pursuit in revealing more about the nature of language acquisition and the constraints on language acquisition facing SLI children.

In at least two senses, the lexicon is a crossroads at which we may observe the interaction of several aspects of language and language acquisition. The first involves the developmental interactions among phonology, semantics, phonology, and syntax. The second concerns the lexicon as it is represented mentally and the role it plays in the active processing of language for immediate use and for learning. With respect to the latter perspective, the interaction in which I am most interested is among input, perception, and output.

PHONOLOGICAL FACTORS IN LEXICAL ACQUISITION

Over the last 10 years I have been engaged in a program of research with Laurence Leonard and a number of our former doctoral students employing an experimental approach to the learning of novel words by both normal and language-impaired children. In various studies we have included children ranging in linguistic level from production vocabularies of under 5 words to vocabularies of up to about 75 words. All of these children were limited to predominantly single-word productions. The characteristics of the experimental words employed and their referents varied depending on the particular questions of interest. Generally, the children were presented with the experimental words and their referents over a period of about three weeks, under controlled conditions in play-like sessions. We have then examined their acquisition of these words in various ways, depending on the specific goal of the experiment.

I want to focus on one particular set of studies in which we found that, both for NL and SLI children, words with consonants and syllable structures that were produced accurately (IN words) were more readily added to the child's productions than were words with consonants or structures that either never appeared in productions or targets (OUT words) or appeared in adult targets, but never in the child's productions (ATTEMPTED words). There were no differences among the word types in terms of the children's comprehension. This of course is not the interesting finding as it adds to the large number of similarities found to exist in comparisons of SLI children and younger, NL peers. The provocative findings emerged when the productions of these words were examined.

In general, IN words were produced more accurately than either OUT or ATTEMPTED words. The children differed, however, in the distribution of what we considered to be unusual productions—patterns that fell outside common substitution errors. The NL children exhibited more errors of this type on OUT words than on ATTEMPTED words (there were some errors of this type on IN words, but they were few in number). In contrast, the errors made by the SLI children were equally likely to be unusual across the three word types, with relatively large numbers in productions of IN and ATTEMPTED words. Recall that these words had sounds that the children had attempted and produced correctly and incorrectly, respectively. They already had an available production pattern to apply to novel words including those sounds. The NL children took advantage of these available patterns. The SLI children tended to employ unusual production errors that had not appeared in their spontaneous speech.

In a separate experiment, NL and SLI children were presented with novel words that were potentially homophonous with a word in the child's existing lexicon (e.g., if the child omitted final consonants, the experimental word *baf* would be a potential homophone for *back*). There was a tendency for the children to produce the potential homophones in ways that made them distinct. Again, the NL children seemed to rely on existing production patterns, whereas the SLI children's productions did not reflect existing regularities in their production lexicon.

Though these lexical learning experiments were intended to examine some observed phenomena in young children's speech, they have yielded unexpected returns. They revealed something about a child's lexical structure and its relationship to the new words in the language-learning environment. Furthermore, they provided an indirect glimpse of input-output relationships in the language acquisition. The SLI children did not take advantage of regularities in their existing lexicon in the mappings between input and output to the extent that we saw in the NL children. By itself, that seems to me to be an important finding. Certainly it may be a hint of some of the difficulties faced by these children in learning new lexical items and, perhaps, in other aspects of language.

If we consider what is involved in acquiring and producing a new word when a child does take advantage of regularities in the existing lexicon, we can see where the process might go awry. First, we assume that the adult's production of the new word is comparable to earlier produced words with the identical sounds. The child must then perceive this new word in a fashion consistent with the way in which similar words were previously perceived and then stored. Of course, neither the perception nor the storage need be accurate. A perceptual representation (i.e., some type of recognition/comparison template) must be extracted and compared with the perception-based representations of existing lexical entries. In cases where a match (using the child's criteria) in characteristics between a new representation and an existing representation(s) is found, the motor pattern(s) associated (accurate productions of targets or previously produced substitutions/errors) can be adapted for production of the new word. Even without a match, the child could associate an available motor pattern with the new word.

In discussing these findings elsewhere (Leonard, Schwartz, Swanson & Frome Loeb, 1987; Schwartz, Leonard, Frome Loeb & Swanson, 1987) we have identified three possible loci of deviation from this scenario in which a child capitalizes on the regularities of an existing lexicon. Recall that this is seen occasionally in NL children but frequently in SLI children. Relatively peripheral perceptual or motor factors may be responsible for variations from existing production patterns. For some reason children may not perceive related adult words as similar or may not be consistent in motor production. An important factor that may affect this consistency of production and perception is the "age" of a lexical item. Because of developmental changes, the representations of older words may differ from related, but more recently acquired words. If this is a contributing factor, it would put SLI children at a distinct disadvantage for developing a regularity-based system because of the temporal spread of their acquisition.

Analysis of the perceptual information, establishment of an underlying representation, and comparison of that representation to those of previously acquired words may be other points of departure from existing regularities. There may be inconsistencies in analysis, access to existing representations for comparison, or comparison variations (either in the process or in the criteria for recognition of congruities).

We also considered that the failure to capitalize on existing regularities may not reflect some deficiency or inconsistency in the process of acquiring and producing novel words. Instead, these findings may indicate something about the developmental organization of a lexicon. Rather than a lexicon that is phonetically and phonologically homogenous, there may be some advantage in maintaining contrast among the entries in a lexicon (e.g., Charles-Luce & Luce, 1985; Tversky & Hutchinson, 1986). Adult lexicons may be organized phonologically, semantically, and syntactically (at least in terms of grammatical role) into related neighborhoods. As a child initially constructs a mental lexicon, maintenance of contrast may be beneficial either in production or in perception (even at a lower, segmental level in the building of a phonetic inventory).

This is comparable to the distinction between the Quantal Theory of Speech (Stevens, 1989) and the Theory of Adaptive Dispersion (Lindblom, MacNeilage, & Studdert-Kennedy, in press). Stevens posits that languages tend toward regions representing physical correlates of phonological distinctive features in a universal phonetic space that have high acoustic and auditory stability and homogeneity. Lindblom and his colleagues argue that the selection criterion for a language is "sufficient perceptual contrast." The same principles may apply to the development of a phonology and a lexicon in the sense of an ontogeny recapitulating phylogeny. However, in development, the "universal space" is much narrower—the input and the child's perception and analysis of that input.

My sense is that, for both languages and for individuals, there is some natural tension between these criteria. Multiple factors including linguistic constraints (semantic, syntactic), communicative requirements, and biological constraints (neurologic, sensory, and motoric) drive the resolution of this tension toward an endpoint. However, a disturbance in these naturally occurring constraints, such as an underlying cause of SLI or the impairment itself, may disrupt the developmental structuring of the lexicon.

This paradigm has provided us with important glimpses of the influence of existing lexical structure on the acquisition of new words. It remains for us to further explore these issues. However, our lexical learning paradigm, particularly in its dependent measures, has thus far provided a periscopic view. Several steps are needed to permit a more direct view.

INPUT-OUTPUT RELATIONSHIPS

A key issue in describing the acquisition of new words, as well as other morphological, syntactic, phonological, or semantic units, is the relationship between the input to the child and the child's output. This is true regardless of the magnitude of the role ascribed to input. There are multiple steps between these two endpoints, all of which should be subject to empirical study rather than assumption. For example, there is a set of inherent presuppositions when we describe phonological and transcribed phonetic characteristics of children's productions of words in relation to adult citation forms. We assume something about the nature of the adult input, the child's perception, the child's storage of the perception-based information, the relationship of this information to information about other words in the lexicon, its association with a set of motor instructions, and the execution of those motor instructions. Similar examples may be constructed for the referent categories and concepts underlying words, for affixes, and for the syntactic categories in which words occur.

The point is that we must specify, not assume, the characteristics of the input, its perception and storage, the characteristics of the output, and the mappings among the intermediate stages between these endpoints to better understand the nature of both typical and atypical language acquisition. The questions thus become empirical and methodological. Essentially, they are a series of Watergate questions: What information is available to the child? What does the child know (perceive and store) and when does she know it? What does the child do (i.e., produce)?

The first and the third questions may be somewhat easier to answer than the second. But even then, we need to grind somewhat smaller than we have in the past. For example, both NL and SLI children may be exposed to input that is generally comparable. However, the relationship of that input to the child's linguistic system may not be the same for both populations. As mentioned earlier, SLI children accumulate a lexicon over a longer period of time so the input set may actually be larger. Adults may abandon some input characteristics (e.g., certain phonetic features such as exaggerated vowel duration differences, or certain syntactic/discourse features) because of reduced responsiveness from children, chronological age/language discrepancies, or because of a temporal limitation on the tendency to make child-directed speech adjustments. Regardless of an explanation for any differences, we still know relatively few details about the nature of input to children, particularly as they may relate to perceptual, to storage, and to output characteristics.

Young children's perception of meaningful speech is also something about which we know relatively little, in contrast to what we know about their perception of nonmeaningful stimuli. It is important to understand the developmental transition from prelinguistic perception in infancy to true linguistic perception in childhood. There is also good reason to believe these conditions will not yield isomorphic results. Furthermore, there are questions that can be addressed with meaningful stimuli that cannot be considered otherwise. For example, we can determine, for a given lexical item, what segments, subphonemic phonetic characteristics, or suprasegmental characteristics are critical for the child's recognition of a given word. In order to accomplish this, particularly for younger children of an age/language level at which this type of question is of greatest interest, new paradigms were needed. Specifically, we turned to perception paradigms that would tie an auditory stimulus to a referent. By adapting cross-modal perception paradigms in which children are presented with a visual stimulus and an auditory stimulus and examining gaze behavior (in cases of older children, pointing or screen touch) for habituation, for novelty, for preference between two visual stimuli, we are now beginning to examine some of these questions. The experimental word-learning paradigm mentioned at the beginning of this chapter provides an opportunity for greater control over the stimuli in such experiments. It will also be critical to design experiments in which the dimensions of perception examined are tied to suspected dimensions of difficulty for NL and SLI children relative to input and to output. These types of experiments are necessary to determine whether any of the auditory perceptual limitations of SLI children are in fact related to lexical learning.

Children's output and production learning also need to be further examined in relation to input, to perception, and to storage. When we do more than simply paint a picture of output with broad strokes, we may find that SLI and NL children diverge in the relationship between the existing structure of their lexicon and their lexical learning and production. The correspondence between input and output may also differ from that seen in NL children. We already know this to be generally true in terms of the volume of input in relation to the language level of SLI and NL children.

A final and key piece in this puzzle is the relationships, both dynamic and static, among input, perception and storage, and output. From a dynamic perspective, the recent convergence of two bodies of literature, speech perception and spoken word recognition, represents the potential for important advances in understanding these relationships. For example, several different proposals generally agree in postulating that, individuals perceive and process speech at a sub-lexical level primarily for the purpose of phoneme identification, they then recognize words, and, once that is accomplished, they must deal with larger units to permit semantic analysis and syntactic parsing. There is a good deal more that could be said about this literature, but I want to raise only a few key points (see Curtiss & Tallal, chapter 9, for additional discussion).

First, it is hard to guess how SLI children would perform on various tasks requiring this kind of processing. SLI children may be at a distinct disadvantage because of the limitations imposed by their impairment on processing that might occur in a top down direction. Alternately, they may have some advantage in that they have known at least some lexical items over a longer period of time. Without speech perception tasks that involve meaningful stimuli such as spoken word recognition experiments, we won't be able to evaluate these possibilities.

Some auditory perceptual deficits have already been identified in SLI children. However, these deficits do not seem to influence speech production (i.e., limitations in perceiving temporally brief stimuli do not seem to entail production difficulties). Speech processing may reflect these deficits more directly. For example, SLI children may have difficulty perceiving or identifying sub-lexical features involving temporally brief cues, larger units (e.g., bound morphemes, functors) that are unstressed (and thus short in duration), cues to phrase structure boundaries or to syntactic categorization of words. One step up the processing line children may often be faced with situations in which they have to perceive, store, and compare utterances (words or larger units) to existing representations or to the other member of a pair of utterances (e.g., the child says, "Want cookie." The mother says, "You want what?"). An impairment affecting any part of this processing is likely to have a cascading effect and thus may circumscribe the accessibility of input information for learning syntactic, semantic, morphological, and phonological features. Research that focuses on these processes and on the synchronic mappings between input and output is a critical area of need in understanding the constraints on lexical acquisition and, more broadly, language acquisition by SLI children.

MODELING

One direction that holds great promise for the not-too-distant future is the capability to model developing mappings between input and output. Architectures referred to as parallel distributed processing (PDP), or connectionist networks (CN) seem more relevant than traditional artificial intelligence (AI) architectures because of some basic differences. Briefly,

CNs are composed of layers of relatively similar, highly connected units, that operate in a parallel rather than a serial fashion. They have activation levels that are determined by the sum of weights of the excitatory connections to the unit minus the weights of any inhibitory connections. Representations are generally distributed over a number of units instead of having a single location. Perhaps the greatest appeal is that CNs are, using various procedures, adaptive—AI architectures are not. One can create an architecture and a learning algorithm and provide some input and the network "learns." Finally, CNs do not have explicit rules provided to them. Instead their "rule behavior" results from a pattern extraction from input and probabilistic or frequency-based output behavior. They thus can discover structure in the input much as a number of cognitive, constructivist models of language acquisition suggest.

Initial attempts to create such simulations focusing on the acquisition of English past tense marking and on text-to-speech conversion have been crude and will require refinement to yield heuristically valuable simulations. Much of the current controversy centers around the breadth of the claims and counterclaims concerning this architecture as an adequate representation for human cognition. Though I do not believe that, in their present form, such architectures alone can adequately represent all aspects of language acquisition, subsets of this domain may be adequately simulated. This requires two steps beyond our present abilities. First, satisfactory architectures must be developed that deal with issues such as hierarchically related units, temporally sequential information, and semantics. Architectures are rapidly becoming more sophisticated in addressing these issues. Second, we need detailed longitudinal and experimental data from young children. The former is becoming more readily available through the CHILDES data base. The latter type of information needs to be collected following some of the directions discussed in this chapter. With all this in hand, such models will need to be validated by comparing the mappings between input and output they yield against data from children. It may then be possible to simulate variations representing individual differences and various types of impairments. As we have found in our own work with these networks, some of the potential sources for output variations become more obvious. In other disciplines, mathematically based models have played an important role in advancing the understanding of structure and change. Connectionist networks may be an important first step in this direction for both typical and atypical language acquisition.

CONCLUSION

Though I have focused almost exclusively on phonological factors in lexical acquisition, I would argue that my points apply more generally to semantic and syntactic aspects of lexical learning in SLI children. Furthermore, some of the constraints we encounter in these more detailed studies of input-perception-output relationships may reveal some of the general constraints in language learning that characterize specific language impairment.

REFERENCES

Charles-Luce, J., & Luce, P. (1985). *Some structural properties of words in young children*. Paper presented to the Child Phonology Meeting, Purdue University, West Lafayette, IN.

Leonard, L., Schwartz, R., Swanson, L., & Frome Loeb, D. (1987). Some conditions that promote unusual phonological behaviour in children. *Clinical Linguistics and Phonetics, 1,* 23–34.

Lindblom, B., MacNeilage, P., & Studdert-Kennedy, M. (in press). *Evolution of spoken language*. Orlando, FL: Academic.

Schwartz, R., Leonard, L., Frome Loeb, D., & Swanson, L. (1987). Attempted sounds are sometimes not: An expanded view of phonological selection and avoidance. *Journal of Child Language, 14,* 411–418.

Stevens, K. (1989). On the quantal nature of speech. *Journal of Phonetics, 17,* 3–45.

Tversky, A., & Hutchinson, J. (1986). Nearest neighbor analysis of psychological spaces. *Psychological Review, 93,* 3–22.

CHAPTER 22

English Literacy Development in Deaf Children: Directions for Research and Intervention

PETER A. DE VILLIERS

The study of language acquisition and intervention with deaf children remains a contentious area because of major schisms in the field over the appropriate mode(s) of communication to be used in the educational or intervention setting. More heat than clarity has been generated in the debate over whether oral English alone, simultaneous spoken and manually encoded English (and which signed English system), or full American Sign Language should provide the primary face-to-face communication system used with the deaf child. Relevant data to these issues are scarce and open to many different interpretations, since most studies attempting to address the relative success of lack thereof of different communication systems have taken only global measures of educational achievement, such as standardized reading comprehension scores. These are determined by

The research in this chapter was supported by a grant from the National Institute on Disability and Rehabilitation Research and by the Language Acquisition Project at Clarke School for the Deaf. Much of it was carried out in collaboration with Sarah Pomerantz.

multiple variables, many of which have nothing to do with the modes of communication being compared and which are practically impossible to equate across the different populations of students being studied. As a result, the different factions in the debate end up simply disagreeing about the data and arguing largely on ideological and cultural considerations or on the basis of practicalities (or impracticalities) of implementing a particular approach. Unfortunately, I think this condition of turmoil in the language intervention field is unlikely to change over the next 5 to 10 years, since there is no agreement as to what would be relevant empirical data or how to collect it, and indeed it does not seem to be an issue readily resolved by empirical data.

On the other hand, all of the major factions in the debate, while disagreeing passionately about the best face-to-face communication system for the deaf child, agree that effective English *literacy* skills are of central importance for the integration of deaf individuals into the wider hearing society in postsecondary education, vocational training, and job placement (see Commission on the Education of the Deaf, 1988). In this area of English reading and writing skills in deaf students, several major research questions based on recent progress in our understanding of the acquisition of fluent reading and writing skills in normally hearing children have begun to impact the field and will provide the focus for much of the research on English language acquisition in deaf children over the next decade.

In this chapter I will address these research issues and directions and contrast them with the data on English language acquisition collected from deaf children through the 1970s and early 1980s.

ENGLISH LITERACY IN
DEAF STUDENTS: A BRIEF REVIEW

READING

Extensive research over the past 20 to 30 years has documented the limitations of the average deaf student's reading comprehension over the course of his or her schooling. Although a review of demographic data by Allen (1986) indicates a statistically significant improvement in reading achievement scores for the population of deaf students between 1974 and 1983, the increase is small: reading comprehension levels for the average profoundly deaf child continue to increase about 2 grade equivalents in 5 to 6 years of schooling (age 10 to 16), and tend to asymptote between ages 15 and 18 at third to fourth grade level, some 5 years behind their normal-hearing peers. Numerous demographic and research studies have described this slow growth and low plateau in reading comprehension (see

King & Quigley, 1985; and Quigley & Paul, 1984; for detailed reviews), although some have questioned the validity and usefulness of the standard norm-referenced tests of reading achievement (e.g., Ewoldt, 1982).

WRITING

Comparable demographic data assessing achievement in writing are not available, but several research studies have characterized deficiencies in the written language of deaf students. In the typical study, written productions (letters, or stories elicited by picture stimuli) were analyzed for frequency and type of lexical or grammatical error, variety and number of words and syntactic constructions, and the length and complexity of sentences appearing in the text (e.g., Heider & Heider, 1940; Myklebust, 1964). More sophisticated studies have employed linguistic models of the structure of English, such as transformational grammar, as the basis for analysis of written language (e.g., Kretschmer & Kretschmer, 1978; Quigley, Wilbur, Power, Montanelli & Steinkamp, 1976; Taylor, 1969). In this way, the average deaf student's written English has been described as significantly less developed than that of hearing peers. More syntactic and lexical errors are made, and the structure of the compositions is characterized as stereotypic, repetitive, employing more simple sentence patterns, and lacking many of the more complex syntactic forms found in hearing children's writing above a third- or fourth-grade level (such as nominals, relative clauses, or complement constructions). (See Quigley & Paul, 1984, for a detailed review). Some of the characteristic patterns of written language (e.g., repetitive use of particular phrases and simple construction types) and areas of particular difficulty (anaphoric pronouns, definite and indefinite reference, and ellipsis) have been attributed to particular formal instructional methods frequently employed and to an overemphasis on the structure of the single sentence in English language classes for deaf students (van Uden, 1977; Wilbur, 1977).

Nevertheless, several studies of both reading achievement and writing have shown that some children with profound hearing loss do acquire satisfactory English literacy skills more closely comparable with their hearing peers. High English achievement levels have been reported in groups of deaf children in highly structured, intensive oral programs (Geers & Moog, 1987; Moog & Geers, 1985; Ogden, 1979); in integrated classrooms (Pflaster, 1980); and in some Total Communication programs (Brasel & Quigley, 1977; Delaney, Stuckless & Walter, 1984; Moores, 1987). These good readers tend to come from families of above average socioeconomic status, and have parents who are particularly involved in the educational process and have high educational expectations for their children. A subgroup of them have parents who are themselves deaf (see Moores, 1987, for a review).

ANALYSIS OF LANGUAGE
SKILLS UNDERLYING LITERACY

The poor literacy levels of many deaf children can be viewed in the context of current theories of the reading and writing process in normal-hearing children and adults. Many theorists analyze the global skills of reading and writing into specific psycholinguistic components or subskills. Although there is some disagreement about the relative weighting that each of the component skills should receive in an account of fluent reading, the dominant models of the reading process stress an interaction between "bottom-up" processes (word recognition and text decoding) and "top-down" processes (inferential processes involving the use of syntactic, semantic, and experiential knowledge to generate hypotheses or predictions about what the text means) (e.g., Beck & Carpenter, 1986; Just & Carpenter, 1980; Rumelhart, 1977; Samuels & Eisenberg, 1981).

An influential developmental model (Chall, 1983) suggests that bottom-up or top-down processes may predominate at different stages in the acquisition of reading skills. Thus the prereading or early reading child may be able to interpret or "tell" the story of a passage of the text using top-down processes almost exclusively, if the events are particularly well known to the child or highly predictable and redundant. At a later point in development, with the beginning of formal phonics or word recognition instruction, the child's reading will be dominated by bottom-up decoding processes. Reading in this stage tends to be slow and word by word.

Finally, as the decoding processes become more automatic, both word recognition and inferential processes interact in determining fluent reading. The extent to which each process is then employed by the skilled reader will depend on the familiarity and complexity of the text in its semantic, syntactic, and organizational properties.

Looking at the component skills underlying fluent reading, we can identify several domains in which problems for deaf students have been reported that could contribute to limitations in reading comprehension.

VOCABULARY

One standard measure of reading ability is vocabulary comprehension, usually testing through the child's ability to pick out the definition corresponding to the meaning of a word from several other alternatives in a multiple choice format. Studies of deaf children using these formats typically conclude that their vocabulary growth is significantly slower and ultimately quantitatively reduced when compared to their hearing peers (Quigley & Paul, 1984; Walter, 1978). Deaf students understand and use fewer English words across all the different form classes: nouns, verbs, adjectives, adverbs, and connectives.

The discrepancy between the deaf and hearing students becomes even more marked when infrequent or abstract words are tested (Walter, 1978); or when the children are required to indicate the various meanings of a word with multiple meanings (Paul, 1984). Several lines of research have implicated these vocabulary limitations in the poorer reading comprehension of the deaf student (e.g., LaSasso & Davey, 1987). A recent National Institute of Neurological and Communicative Disorders and Stroke (NINCDS)–sponsored study of the relationship between reading and writing and various measures of language achievement in 16- to 18-year-olds found the highest correlations were between reading comprehension scores on the Stanford Achievement Test-HI and vocabulary scores on the California Achievement Test (Geers & Moog, 1987; Moores, 1987).

Failure to grasp that words may have more than one meaning will interfere with comprehension of text in which secondary or less common meanings of multimeaning words are used. Poorer understanding of the semantic interrelationships between words, such as antonym or synonym relationships, or subordinate and superordinate relationships (Collie, sheepdog, dog, mammal, animate being, and so on) will restrict the child's ability to anticipate or predict ahead the meanings to expect as they read a passage. These semantic relationships between words are crucial for understanding and producing the lexical cohesion that binds a passage together into a coherent text (Halliday & Hasan, 1976).

SYNTAX

Another central factor in fluent reading and writing is the child's productive mastery of the various grammatical processes of English. The study of syntax within a psycholinguistic framework has thrown considerable light on the areas of English grammar that provide particular difficulty for deaf students. For example, Quigley and his collaborators carried out extensive research on the reading comprehension, judgment, and production in written sentences of a wide range of syntactic processes central to a transformational generative grammar of English (Quigley et al, 1976; Quigley & King, 1980). Most of the older students in these studies (18 years old) performed at a significantly lower level than 8- to 10-year-old hearing children, yet the difficulty ordering of the syntactic processes and the nature of the errors made was similar in the two populations of students. Quigley et al. concluded that while the syntactic development of the deaf students was quantitatively slower and often ultimately arrested at a lower point in development, it was qualitatively similar to that of the hearing subjects in the study. Looking at the syntactic processes in detail, the deaf students were found to have particular problems with verb inflectional processes and auxiliaries; with embedded structures, such as relative clauses; and with any sentences in which the basic subject-verb-object

(SVO) order of English was violated (such as in the passive voice and some relative clause constructions).

Similar findings on embedded or initialized subordinate clauses and sentence structures that deviate from an SVO sequence have been reported by Engen and Engen (1983) in a text of "through-the-air" language comprehension (simultaneously signed and spoken English sentences). Most important, several analyses have shown that while many of these complex syntactic forms are infrequent in spoken English, they are far more common in written text (see Chafe, 1985; Perera, 1984). Quigley et al. reported that they emerge in increasing numbers in reading materials frequently used with deaf students above a third-grade level.

Finally, the NINCDS study (Moores, 1987) found that performance on Test of Syntactic Abilities Quigley et al. was among the best predictors of both reading comprehension on the SAT-HI and judged sophistication and effectiveness of written English essays. Thus comprehension and judgments of written syntactic structures in isolation is highly correlated with reading and writing skills in text.

CONNECTED DISCOURSE AND TEXT

Mastery of the grammar of single sentences is necessary but is not sufficient for fluent reading and writing of connected discourse and narrative. There has therefore been extensive recent work on hearing children's ability to deal with extended written text. Much of this research has studied children's production, comprehension, and retelling of stories (e.g., Geva & Olson, 1983; Peterson & McCabe, 1983). The structure of these narratives can be approached from a variety of perspectives (Johnston, 1982): either looking at the story grammars or thematic rules that organize them into suprasentential discourse units (Stein & Glenn, 1979); or examining the linguistic cohesion devices like anaphoric pronouns, definite and indefinite reference, or conjunctive adverbs and connectives that refer across sentence boundaries and so build cohesive ties between the element in the text (Bamberg, 1987; Halliday & Hasan, 1976; Karmiloff-Smith, 1981).

Finally, the notion of "scripts," or "schemata," has been applied to the analysis of the reader's conceptual knowledge and experience that is brought to bear in understanding the content of the narrative and allows the skilled reader to draw inferences about events that are not stated in the text itself (Anderson, 1985; Nelson & Gruendel, 1979; Tannen, 1979). These inferences away from what is stated to what is presupposed or implied by the events mentioned in the text are central to reading comprehension at the higher grade levels.

There is far less research in this domain with deaf children. However, a few studies implicate deficiencies at the level of discourse skill in the reading and writing difficulties of deaf students. For example, Wilbur (1977) reanalyzed passages of text from the Quigley et al. (1976) study using a pragmatic analysis of new versus old information. She found that discourse devices that signal coreference across propositions (pronouns, articles, and ellipsis), were better controlled at a within-sentence level than they were between sentences. Wilbur argued that the students understood these forms in single-sentence contexts, but did not know how or when to use them in discourse. She attributed the problem to the overemphasis in most of the language instruction experienced by deaf students on the structure of the single sentence removed from its pragmatic function in discourse.

More recently, Yoshinaga-Itano and Snyder (1985) analyzed written stories from deaf and hearing students aged 10–15 years. They demonstrated that the ability to provide appropriate discourse cohesions and to elaborate the propositional structure of the story clustered together as a single semantic factor underlying variations in the deaf students' written narrative skill. This semantic factor was more closely related to reading comprehension levels for the students that were measures of syntactic development (words per theme-unit and words per main clause). Yoshinaga-Itano and Downey (1986) have argued that the deaf child's limited organization of his or her semantic knowledge as well as less elaborate scripts of everyday experiences may underlie poorer narrative comprehension and production.

Finally, in a study of persuasive text written by deaf 17-year-olds categorized by their teachers as good or poor writers, Gormley and Sarachan-Deily (1987) found no significant differences between the two groups on what they termed the mechanics of writing—spelling, punctuation, and inflectional morphology. However, good writers produced text that was more cohesive, clarifying intersentence links for the reader and providing more appropriate content for the persuasive message with an introduction and more elaborated suggestions, reasons, and conclusions. Poor writers were more likely to use a rigid, highly structured organization, but provided few cohesive links between propositions. Both groups used incorrect sentence structures (e.g., omitting required sentence constituents or using incorrect word order) and inappropriate pronominalization, but better writers were less likely to make these major syntactic errors than were the poorer writers.

NEW DIRECTIONS FOR RESEARCH

The above review of the descriptive literature on deaf students' English language abilities implicates a number of specific domains of English as crucial for fluent reading and writing skills. However, several important questions must be answered before we will be in a position to understand the nature of deaf students' difficulties in these domains and make strong recommendations about the kind of language-intervention methods that are most effective at maximizing the deaf child's English language skill.

Whereas there is ample documentation of deaf children's quantitative delay and lower levels of performance on particular measures of English achievement (e.g., size of receptive and productive vocabulary or comprehension of syntactic features of English in isolated sentences), there is very little in-depth psycholinguistic data on the pattern and process of their English language acquisition.

Part of the problem has been the kind of testing methods and materials that have been used in studies of English language acquisition in deaf children. As shown above, much of the data from deaf children come from performance on English language achievement tests that provide scores to compare with normal developmental norms or other deaf students, but do not lend themselves to psycholinguistic analysis (although there is now much richer data on the acquisition of several aspects of ASL; see Newport & Meier, 1985 & Wilbur, 1987, for reviews).

For example, in the area of vocabulary, research has focused on the lexical knowledge of the deaf child but we know little, if anything, about the *process* by which that knowledge is acquired. Studies of deaf students' grammatical development have primarily investigated knowledge of the syntactic rules by which single sentence constructions are formed, that is, *syntactic competence*. But a considerable amount of recent research in language acquisition with normal-hearing children has distinguished between the acquisition of sentence structures in isolation and the employment of syntactic devices in plurifunctional ways for discourse purposes, that is, *communicative competence* (e.g., Karmiloff-Smith, 1981, 1986).

In collaboration with research teams at the Rhode Island School for the Deaf and the Boston University Center for the Study of Communication and Deafness, and funded by the National Institute on Disability and Rehabilitation Research (NIDRR), I have begun a major research project on the development of English literacy skills in deaf students from different backgrounds and in a wide variety of educational programs employing different modes of communication. The major focus of the Literacy Acquisition Project is to determine the patterns and processes of reading and writing development in deaf students aged 7 to 15 years and to relate their English literacy skills to their primary language skills in English or ASL and to the ways in which English language is taught in different programs.

In the remainder of this chapter I will address some of the questions around which our research is designed and describe some of the results from initial studies on the process of English vocabulary acquisition in deaf students and the development of narrative skills in their writing, especially the mastery of discourse cohesion devices that are essential for fluent comprehension and production of text in English.

VOCABULARY ACQUISITION

The magnitude of the problem of vocabulary development for the deaf child can best be understood by reference to the incredibly rapid process of vocabulary acquisition in normal-hearing children. Summarizing a number of studies over the years attempting to estimate the size of a child's written English vocabulary at different points in development, Nagy and Herman (1987) conclude that the average twelfth grader has a vocabulary of the order of 40,000 word families (counting closely related words like "persecute," "persecution," and "persecutor" as a single-word family). Estimating that the average third grader's reading vocabulary is between 5 and 10,000 words, this means that the average normal-hearing child learns the meanings of around 3,000 words per year, or 8 to 10 words a day (more if only school days are counted).

How does the child do this? Not by explicit instruction of word meanings. Even the most ambitious of vocabulary programs does not provide direct instruction on more than a few hundred words per year. In fact, given the magnitude of the task and the time available for instruction, even extensive teaching of individual words cannot cover enough words to bring a student with an inadequate vocabulary up to average (Miller & Gildea, 1987; Nagy & Herman, 1987). Each year the average normal-hearing reader encounters upwards of 10,000 unknown words in text (Anderson & Freebody, 1983).

Most vocabulary is learned from context. Several elegant studies have established that this process of acquiring new meanings for words from the context (linguistic and nonlinguistic) in which they occur operates at an early age in spoken English. Carey and Bartlett (1978) showed how a 2- or 3-year-old could establish a "fast-mapping" of the meaning of a new word from the first time they heard it, especially if it was produced in explicit contrast with a familiar word to which it was related. For example, told to bring and adult "the chromium tray, not the blue tray," a 3-year-old would later be able to show that they knew at least that the new word "chromium" referred to the dimension of color, and even in some cases the general type of color that it was. Heibeck and Markham (1987) reported similar findings for form and texture words, and showed that the explicit contrast with a known word need not be provided for the child to make an appropriate fast-mapping of the meaning of the word (see also Dickinson, 1984).

Studies of this process of acquiring new vocabulary from written contexts have employed two major paradigms. In one, the students read words (shown on pretests to be unknown) embedded in sentences or short paragraphs. The students' attention is explicitly drawn to the unknown words and they are asked to derive a meaning for the word, either in a multiple-choice task or by giving a definition (e.g., Carnine, Kameenui & Coyle, 1984; McKeown, 1985; Werner & Kaplan, 1952).

In the second, more naturalistic, approach, students read extended passages of text containing words that they are unlikely to know; later, the change in their knowledge of the words' meaning is assessed relative to other students who did not read the passages or relative to their own knowledge of the words before reading the passages (Jenkins, Stein & Wysocki, 1984; Nagy, Anderson & Herman, 1987).

These studies have shown that incidental learning of word meanings from written text probably accounts for more than 1,500 words per year for the average normal-hearing child. Several factors determine how much is learned about a word:

1. One is the degree of contextual support for the word or the informativeness of the context about the word's meaning. The more explicitly the meaning is determined by the context, the number and type of contextual cues (such as explicit equivalences or contrasts stated, or both grammatical and semantic clues provided), their proximity to the unknown word, and the centrality of that word to the gist or theme of the passage are all implicated in how well children can use the context to determine at least a partial meaning for the new word (Carnine et al., 1984; Jenkins et al., 1984; Sternberg & Powell, 1983).

2. Another is the degree of prior understanding of the concept(s) underlying the word's meaning. If the student is learning a new word that refers to a familiar concept (such as "ire" for "anger"), incidental learning from context is much more likely than in cases where the student must acquire both a new concept and the word that refers to it (such as "fascism") (Nagy et al., 1987). In other words, the extent to which the child can slot the new word into an established lexical network of word relationships contributes to the likelihood that new words are incidentally learned from merely being encountered in context in text. When both the word and concept are unknown or obscure, explicit instruction or many exposures to the word in a variety of contexts may be needed.

3. Third, the conceptual complexity of the passage in which the unknown word appears and the explicitness of the relationships between propositions in the text also determines the ease with which a meaning can be derived for the word. That is, the more the student can fit the word into an integrated schema or theme that ties together the elements of the passage, the better he or she can establish its likely meaning (Nagy et al., 1987).

4. Finally, there is a close relationship between reading skill and ability to derive meaning from context. Better readers are more skilled at integrat-

ing meaning across several propositions into a schema from which the meaning of an unknown word might be established and are also more able to use sequential contexts to limit or switch possible meanings for a word (McKeown, 1985).

Given the importance of this process for vocabulary acquisition, a major direction of our research on the development of literacy in deaf students concerns their derivation of word meanings from context.

In one study of this process (carried out with Sarah Pomerantz), 36 hearing-impaired students took part, 31 of them with profound degrees of hearing loss (>90 dB). Twenty-one of them attended an oral school for the deaf (average age = 12:6 [9:2–14:8]; hearing loss = 100.8 dB [80–120]; and reading comprehension grade level on the SAT-HI = 2.8 [1.6–3.9]). The remaining 15 students attended a school for the deaf using Signed English in a Total Communication program (average age = 13.2 [10:11–15:4]; hearing loss = 94.8 dB [71–110]; and reading level = 3.1 [2.2–4.8]).

The students were given a pretest of their knowledge of 30 words—10 nouns, 10 verbs, and 10 adjectives. The words were taken from *A Cluster Approach to Vocabulary Instruction* (Marzano & Marzano, 1988) and varied from second to sixth grade in the level at which they became relatively frequent in reading materials commonly assigned in schools (such as basal readers and subject-area texts). In the pretest the students were asked to give a meaning for each word ("What do these words mean? Write as much as you know about each word.") In addition, they were asked to guess at the general connotation of the word ("Do you think the word means something good or bad?").

The six nouns, six verbs, and six adjectives that fewest of the students knew were then embedded in short two- or three-sentence passages to test the students' ability to derive a meaning for the words from context. For each word three contexts were created that varied in how informative they were about the meaning of the unknown word. The *lean* contexts provided very little information about meaning other than the word's grammatical category. An example of this condition for the word "eerie" is: "The boy painted a picture of an *eerie* house in his art class. He took it home to show his mother and father." The *rich* context condition supplied a great deal of semantic information about the word: "The old house on the hill was an *eerie* place. It was dark and had broken windows and it looked like ghosts lived in it." And the *explicit* condition provided a clear contrast and/or equivalence statement, such as, "In the daytime the woods look safe and friendly, but at night they can be an eerie place. The trees look strange and scary in the dark."

In the meaning derivation task, one test word appeared at the top of each page in bold print and capital letters. Below the word was a passage containing the word (underlined and in bold type), and providing either a lean, rich, or explicit context. On each test form, a lean context was given for two nouns, two verbs, and two adjectives, a rich context was given for another two nouns, two verbs, and two adjectives, and an explicit context was provided for the remaining nouns, verbs, and adjectives. The context type given for each word varied on the different test forms, so a word with a lean context on Form 1 would have a rich or explicit context on Form 2 and yet a different context on Form 3. Directly below the passage containing the unknown word the student was again instructed to give a meaning for the word ("What do you think _____ means?") and to guess at its positive or negative connotations ("Do you think it means something good or bad?").

Pretest and in-context meaning derivation tasks were given about a week apart in class groups of four to seven students and administered by the students' teachers. Instructions were both read and signed and/or spoken for the students. For the in-context task the students were ranked according to reading score and grouped by threes. One of each trio then received Form 1, a second received Form 2, and the third received Form 3 of the task. In this way children of approximately equal reading level were given each of the three forms, so if one child received a particular word in a lean context, a child of comparable reading level received that word in a rich context, and a third matched child read it in an explicit context.

Responses on the give-a-meaning task were scored on a 2-point system: 0 points for no answer or a totally wrong answer, 1 point for a partially right answer (such as "nice" or "good" for *honest*), and 2 points for a completely correct answer (for example, "tells the truth" for *honest*). For analysis of the results, the students were divided into two groups, those with reading levels below third grade (n = 21), and those above third grade (n = 15). No significant differences between the oral and TC students or significant interactions involving school mode of communication were observed.

Figure 22-1 shows the relationship between reading level and the ability of the students to provide a meaning for the unknown words read in context. There was a significant interaction between reading level and success at using context to derive meaning (F[1,32] = 15.8, p = .0004). While there was no significant difference between the two reading groups in their knowledge of the meanings of the words in the pretest (p = .36), there was a significant difference in the number of words for which they could derive a meaning from the context (p < .001). Both reading groups showed statistically significant gains in their knowledge of the words' meanings from reading them in context, but the better readers were much more skilled at the task.

The differential effects of the amount of information provided by the types of context is shown in Figure 22-2. There was a significant interaction between the effects of context and the type of context in which the word

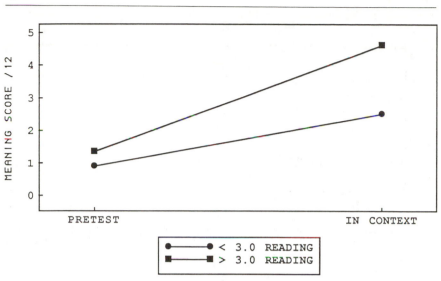

Fig. 22-1. The relationship between reading comprehension grade level and the ability of deaf students to derive a meaning for unknown words read in context.

appeared (F[2, 64] = 11.9, p < .0001). While lean contexts provided sufficient information for the students to derive some appropriate partial meanings for the words (Newman-Keuls comparison with pretest scores: p < .01), the rich context and explicit context scores were significantly better than the lean context scores (p < .01). There was no difference between the rich and explicit contexts, so once sufficient semantic information was provided in a passage context, setting up an explicit contrast or equivalence statement in the context did not improve the students' ability to assign the unknown words a meaning. Figure 22-2 shows that although the better readers were much more skilled at using context to derive word meanings, the differential effects of the context conditions were the same for the two reading groups.

In the positive versus negative connotation task, the effects of the different context types were somewhat more complex and differed between the two reading groups (see Figure 22-3). For the better readers the effects of the different contexts mirrored those for giving a meaning: rich and explicit contexts were better than lean contexts but no different from each other (see lower panel). However, for the students reading below a third-grade level, only the rich context could be used with any degree of effectiveness to determine whether the word had a good or bad meaning. In the give-a-meaning task, the students had the option of not providing any answer, but

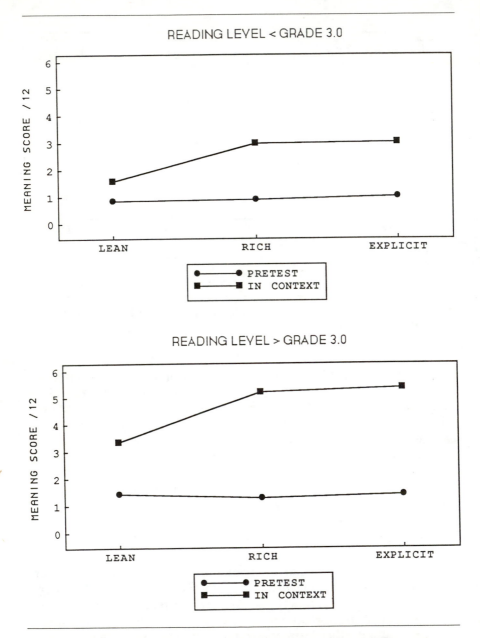

Fig. 22-2. Effects of different types of context on deaf students' ability to give a meaning for unknown words read in passages of text. Passages varied in the number and type of semantic cues given for the meaning of the words. This relationship is shown for both better readers (reading grade > 3.0) and poorer readers (reading grade < 3.0).

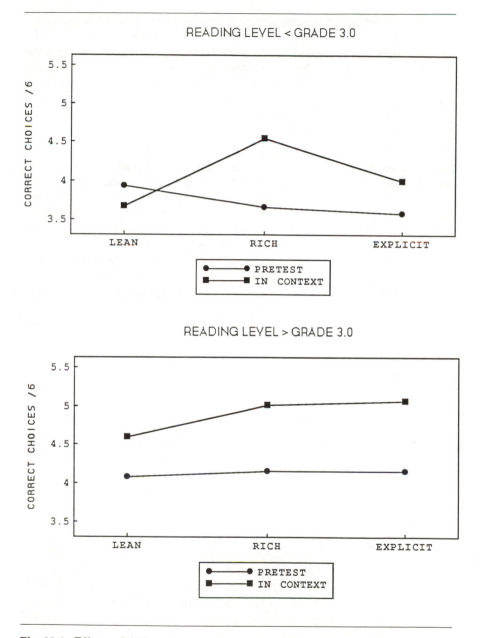

Fig. 22-3. Effects of different types of context on deaf students' ability to determine the positive or negative meaning connotations of unknown words embedded in passages of text. This relationship is shown for both better (reading grade > 3.0) and poorer readers (reading grade < 3.0).

in the good versus bad connotation task we required the students to guess at an answer for each of the words. Only the rich contexts enabled the poorer readers to do this better than in the pretest. The decline in performance with the explicit contexts is interesting since it suggests that in many cases the poorer readers were unable to process the explicit meaning contrasts provided in the sentences, either through a failure to understand the syntactic devices employed in such sentences (e.g. "not X but Y"), or through a failure in integrating the passage meaning into a single schema of related propositions. Instead they apparently located a word or two of familiar meaning near to the unknown words and used them to assign the good or bad connotation. In cases of explicit contrast such as the lean context for the word "drab," "The woman's dresses were very different. One had bright colors, but the other one was a *drab* grey color," a student who did not process the contrast could easily assign a positive connotation for "drab" on the basis of the expression "bright colors."

Thus deaf students can use highly informative contexts to derive at least partial meanings for unknown words, but this skill is closely related to the student's reading comprehension level. Many deaf children are in a vicious circle: their impoverished vocabularies limit their reading comprehension, and poor reading strategies and skills limit their ability to acquire adequate vocabulary knowledge from context.

Sternberg and Powell (1983) suggest that three processes apply to learning new words from context:

1. Selective encoding—separating relevant from irrelevant information to the meaning of the word.
2. Selective combination—combining relevant cues into a working definition.
3. Selective comparison—relating new information about the word given in the text to old information about that or related topics already stored in memory.

Drum and Konopak (1987) argue that the usefulness of a cue depends on the prior knowledge of the student about the topic domain. "Although the within text cues can refine and enrich previous meanings for words, if the reader has no understanding of the topic, then learning will be confined to a possible recognition memory for the words. Word knowledge accrues with domain knowledge. Context without contextual understanding will not suffice" (p. 85).

Deaf students with poor skills in deriving meanings for new words from context could have problems in any or all of these areas: identifying relevant cues, combining cues to delimit the meaning, integrating passage meaning into a general gist or schema, and background knowledge about word relationships or about the topic matter of the passage (see Yoshinaga-Itano & Downey, 1986, on semantic schema limitations of deaf students). Our research over the next few years will attempt to clarify the sources of the poorer readers' problems in this crucial process of vocabulary acquisition and to explore the possible value of explicit instruction in how to use written context to assign at least partial meanings to unknown words (Sternberg, 1987).

Most teachers of the deaf believe that vocabulary learning is important for English language development, but they tend to think of it as teaching words or dictionary skills. So there is a proliferation of word lists in language curricula for the deaf that the students are to be taught, usually by being given definitions or synonyms to memorize. However, Miller and Gildea (1987) have shown how ambiguous and inefficient dictionary-based vocabulary learning is for normal-hearing children, and several studies have demonstrated that words are best taught and learned in meaningful passage contexts by both normal-hearing (Gipe, 1979; Miller & Gildea, 1987) and deaf students (Pomerantz & de Villiers, in preparation). Finally, as Sternberg (1987) forcefully points out, teaching students specific vocabulary items can at best only be a "small drop in a very large bucket," but teaching students how to learn vocabulary from context will allow them to expand their vocabularies independent of direct instruction. Therefore, research into methods of facilitating this process in deaf students will be of major significance for the development of new instructional methods to enhance the students' English literacy skills.

COHESION IN WRITTEN NARRATIVE

A second major direction in our research concerns the development of effective written discourse in deaf students, in particular, the mastery of syntactic devices that are central to the production of cohesive and coherent narratives and various types of expository text.

Several features are involved in creating cohesive stories. Stories are typically organized around characters and their interaction, requiring the introduction, specification, and maintenance of reference to them throughout the narrative. Events or episodes in the story are most frequently temporally organized (and sometimes causally or spatially related). Thus the writer needs to establish a time line and relate events to each other along this time line. A variety of linguistic devices is used for these purposes: definite and indefinite articles and personal pronouns for reference cohesion; adjectives, prepositional phrases, and relative clauses for reference specification; and tense and aspect markers and adverbial phrases and clauses for temporal cohesion (Bamberg, 1987).

To study referential and temporal cohesion in deaf students' written narratives we designed several picture sequence stories based loosely on those described by Karmiloff-Smith (1981) for her study of the oral narratives of normal-hearing 4- to 9-year-olds. One is shown in Figure 22-4.

The sequences all included at least two characters of the same sex so that the child could not simply contrast male and female pronouns to distinguish between the possible referents; some reference-specifying expressions were needed to unambiguously identify the character that the writer had in mind. The focal character involved in the events depicted in each picture in the sequence was sometimes maintained from event to event and sometimes switched from one character to another so that the appropriate discourse context was provided for the use of pronominal or nominal expressions to indicate referent maintenance or change. Finally, transitions between pictured events were designed to motivate temporal, adversative, and causal linking expressions—major conjunctive discourse cohesion devices discussed by Halliday and Hasan (1976).

Sixty-six normal-hearing first- and second-graders, and fifteen orally taught deaf students were given three picture sequence stories and asked to write the story that each of them showed. The sequences were given to the students in class by their teachers as part of their writing assignments and they wrote one story in each of three writing sessions spaced a week or two apart. The normal-hearing students came from two first- and two second-grade classes at the Smith College Campus School and varied in age from 6:8 to 9:7. The deaf students were in the lower and middle school at the Clarke School for the Deaf and varied in age from 9:5 to 14:4. Their hearing loss varied from 85 to 120 dB with a mean of 96.3, and all were prelingually deaf and of normal performance IQ.

For analysis of the data the students were divided into reading levels as well as by grade. The reading levels for the normal-hearing students were determined by the class teachers' allocation of the students to reading groups over the course of the year. Grade levels for the reading groups were estimated by the teachers based on the reading materials in use with each group. No students in the school were given standardized achievement tests until the middle of third grade, so these were not available.

Reading levels for the deaf students were established by their scores on the SAT-HI. The matching between the deaf and normal-hearing children on reading comprehension levels is at best then only approximate, but the groupings do serve to order the students within each group by general reading ability. Table 22-1 shows the distribution of students across reading levels. Examples of the stories written by normal-hearing children and deaf students of similar ages but at different reading levels are given in Table 22-2.

We are continuing to analyze the written samples from all of the picture sequences, but the findings on temporal and reference cohesion on the

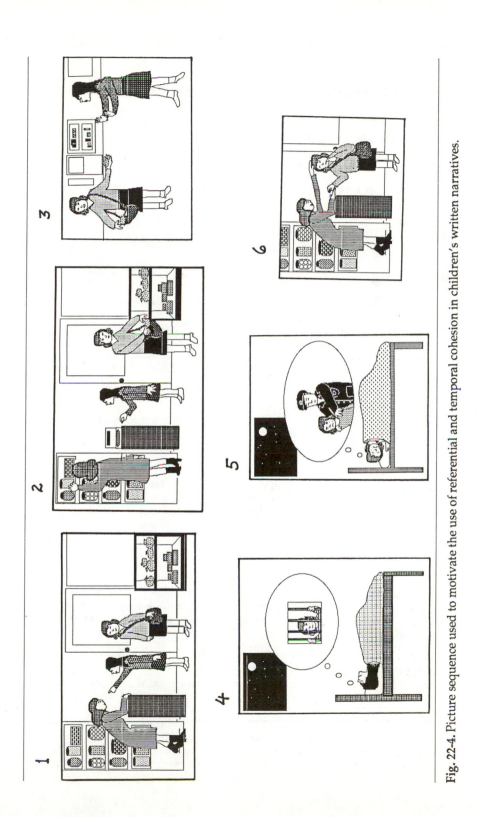

Fig. 22-4. Picture sequence used to motivate the use of referential and temporal cohesion in children's written narratives.

Table 22-1. Average age and number of students at each reading level in narrative discourse study

	Reading Level (Grade Equivalence)				
	1	2	3	4	5+
NUMBER AND AGES ( ) OF STUDENTS					
1st Grade	12	11	11		
	(7:3)	(7:2)	(7:3)		
2nd Grade		8	8	8	8
		(8:8)	(8:1)	(8:2)	(8:1)
Deaf		3	→ 7 (Grade Levels 3.0–5.3)		
		(12:5)	(9:10)		

Table 22-2. Written narrative samples from normal-hearing and deaf students on the candy stealing picture sequence

NORMAL-HEARING STUDENTS

7:10 years. Reading level: 2nd grade.
Ann seas some candy. Sea takes some. sea ofers some to her friend susan. Her friend Susan says no. That night anns friend dreams that ann is in jail. Susans friend drems that same thing.

8:0 years. Reading level: 4th grade.
Two girls went to a store. While the women was not whatching one of the girls stole something. When they got home the girl told the other girl what she did. That night she dremped that she was arsted. So the next day she went to the store and gave it back.

DEAF STUDENTS

10:7 years. Reading level: 2nd grade.
Christie said may I have chocolate chip cookie please. The woman said yes you may have. The woman went to get the chocolate chip cookie for the girl. The woman did not see Nocole stole the cookie. The woman gave some cookie and the girl said no thank you I don't want it. The girl is dreamed about her. Christie gave the money to the woman.

10:0 years. Reading level: 4th grade.
Nancy and her sister Susan went to the store. Nancy bought some jelly beans. Susan saw some popcorns. She stole one bag of popcorn. When they got home Susan gave Nancy one bag of popcorn. Nancy did not want it. When Susan went to bed she dreamed that she was in jail and a policeman let her go. When she woke up she went to the store to gave the woman some money for the popcorns.

candy stealing incident pictured in Figure 22-4 illustrates the way in which those processes develop in the different groups of students.

Temporal Cohesion

To examine the way in which the students used adverbial expressions to provide temporal settings and connections between major events in the story we looked at four pictured events: the stealing of the candy in the store, when the girl who stole the candy offers some to her friend, that night when the two girls have nightmares, and the following morning when the girl who stole returns to the store to make amends. The data from this analysis are given in Table 22-3. As can be seen from the table, there was a close relationship between the children's reading level and the likelihood that they would provide a temporal setting or linking phrase for each of the pictured events. Thus for the stealing of the candy, more and more students provided a "when" or "while" clause in sentence-initial position to indicate the event setting in which the stealing took place, most of them indicating that "*While the woman was looking away,* the girl stole some candy." or "*While*

Table 22-3. Temporal cohesive expressions provided by students at different reading levels

Pictured Event	Reading Level (Grade)				
	1	2	3	4	5+
STEALING (% OF STUDENTS USING INITIAL "WHEN" OR "WHILE" CLAUSE)					
Normal-hearing	0	5.3[a]	53.6	37.5	75
Deaf		0	→ 14.3[b]		
OFFERING (% OF STUDENTS USING INITIAL "WHEN" OR "AFTER" CLAUSE)					
Normal-hearing	8.3	15.8	31.6	62.5	62.5
Deaf		0	→ 42.9		
DREAMING (% GIVING A TIME SETTING, E.G., "THAT NIGHT")					
Normal-hearing	50	68.4	68.4	87.5	100
Deaf		25	→ 71.4		
PAYING BACK (% GIVING A TIME SETTING, E.G., "THE NEXT MORNING")					
Normal-hearing	33.3	42.1	78.9	75	100
Deaf		12.5	→ 57.1		

[a]Another three students (15.8%) used a "when" or "while" clause in sentence-final position.
[b]Reading grade levels for these seven deaf students varied from 3.0 to 5.3.

her friend was buying some candy, the other girl stole some candy." For the scene in which the stolen candy is offered to the friend, most better readers provided a setting with a temporal adverbial clause like "When they got outside" or "After they left the store." Finally, for the dreaming and paying back events, simpler adverbial phrases such as "That night" or "In the morning" could be used and more students at each reading level provided them in their stories.

The relationship between reading comprehension level and the providing of temporal cohesion links was very similar for the deaf and the normal-hearing students. Deaf students with reading levels above third grade provided the appropriate links with about the frequency expected for their reading level from the normal-hearing student samples. Deaf students with reading levels below grade three only provided a few of the simplest phrasal cohesions.

There were two interesting differences between the deaf and normal-hearing students on their description of the stealing scene, however. First, all except one of the adverbial clauses provided by the normal-hearing students to set the scene for the most important incident for the story, the stealing, were initialized "while" clauses. None of the deaf students provided a "while" clause, for either this scene or the offering scene.

Second, the normal-hearing students who did not use an adverbial clause to describe the fact that the stealing took place while the shopkeeper had turned away to fetch the candy off the shelf (so that she did not see it take place) did not mention that fact at all. Since we know that normal-hearing 7- and 8-year-olds do have mastery of the syntax of "when" and "while" clauses, at least in their spoken English, the relationship between reading level and the use of initialized adverbial clauses for temporal cohesion in this group may reflect differences in their understanding of narrative form more than mastery of the use of syntax.

In contrast, 11 of the 15 deaf students stated in one way or another that the woman did not see the girl steal the candy. Perhaps these students had an appropriate understanding of the importance of that fact in telling the story, to set the stage for the stealing, but they did not have mastery of the appropriate syntactic device for backgrounding that information and providing a cohesive link between the two events.

Reference Cohesion

To explore the development of reference cohesion in the students' stories, the text was divided into theme-units (T-units) following Hunt (1965). Hunt defined the T-unit as a unit of discourse capable of functioning as a sentence. Each T-unit thus consisted of one main clause and any subordinate clauses attached to it. For the first graders whose punctuation was erratic or nonexistent, the division into T-units was decided by two independent scorers who judged which elements of text could function as separate sentences. Agreement between the two scorers was over 95%.

We then examined the noun phrase that was the subject or focus of the T-unit main clause and determined its referential relationship to the referents mentioned in the previous T-unit. Focal NPs could either introduce or *switch* to a new referent not mentioned in the previous T-unit, *maintain* the same focal referent as the previous T-unit, or *continue* a referent that was mentioned in the previous unit but was not the focus of that unit (for example, it may have been the object of the previous main clause). This three-way classification follows that used by Sachs (1988) to study pronominal cohesion in the oral stories of normally hearing preschoolers.

Table 22-4 shows the percentage of personal pronouns used to refer to the focal character of each T-unit in the candy-stealing stories in the three different referential conditions. There is a clear contrast between nominal expressions being overwhelmingly provided when there was a switch to a new referent, and pronouns predominating when the focal referent maintained the same character as the previous T-unit. This contrast is even more marked for the deaf students than for the normal-hearing students, with the latter being somewhat more likely to use nominal expressions for referent maintenance even when it would have been unambiguous for the child to use a personal pronoun. The deaf students in this study therefore seemed to have a clear discourse rule to use a pronoun when they were writing about the same referent as had been the subject of the last sentence main clause but to provide a nominal expression if a new referent was being introduced that had not been mentioned in the last sentence.

However, these data are somewhat misleading without determining whether the pronominal expressions provided unambiguous identification of the referents for the reader who could not see the picture sequence. When this analysis is carried out, the mastery of pronominal use obeying the discourse requirement for unambiguous reference is related to grade level and reading level, and the deaf students have a far poorer understanding of these discourse rules than the normal-hearing students of comparable reading levels (see Table 22-5).

Table 22-4. Use of nominal and pronominal expressions in different referential contexts (percent pronominal expressions)

	Normal-hearing		Deaf
	2nd Grade	1st Grade	
Switch to new referent	1.7	10.3	5.2
Maintain same focal referent	61.9	65.3	83.5
Continue nonfocal reference from previous T-unit	21.3	27.3	29.0

Table 22-5. Percentage of students using at least one referentially ambiguous pronominal expression

	Normal hearing	
	2nd grade	15.6
	1st grade	47.1
	Deaf	73.7

	Reading Level (Grade)				
	1	2	3	4	5+
Normal hearing	41.7	36.8	36.8	12.5	0
Deaf		87.5	→ 57.1		

All of the ambiguous pronouns for the deaf students were in referent-continue cases where the referent for the pronoun had been mentioned in the previous T-unit. This suggests that many of the deaf students had a simple rule for the use of pronouns: if the referent had been mentioned in the previous sentence, a pronominal expression should be used, but if there was a switch to a new referent a nominal expression was necessary. However, this rule is not sufficiently conditioned by the communication need of the reader for unambiguous reference and leads to referential confusion.

It is our experience that pronominalization is frequently taught to deaf students as just such an explicit rule: substitute a personal pronoun for a noun when the noun has just been mentioned. It is only from a great deal of experience with real communicative discourse that the *contextual* rules for referential expressions can be acquired.

This study is somewhat limited in scope since it considers only narrative writing based on short sequences of pictures that are in front of the students when they write, but the materials provided a strongly motivating context for these types of cohesive devices, and the stories give us a detailed view of the development of discourse cohesion in children's writing. The results presented here suggest that there is a close relationship between reading ability and the writing of cohesive text, that is, in the use of linguistic devices such as adverbial clauses and pronominalization for their appropriate discourse functions.

The data presented here are also limited to orally taught deaf students, not representative of the full range of deaf students. However, as part of our Literacy Acquisition Project in the coming year we are collecting written samples in this task from a wide range of deaf students in different day and residential programs for the deaf employing a variety of communication modes. Samples of longer stories written by the same students in a story-retelling task will provide additional information about their mastery of discourse cohesion and aspects of narrative structure, while samples of expository text will be collected to examine the student's writing of informative text of different types.

FURTHER DIRECTIONS FOR RESEARCH

These two studies represent changes in the approach to English language acquisition in deaf students away from measures of achievement toward studies of the *process* of acquisition, and away from sentence level processes toward the analysis of *discourse skills*. We believe that this change will provide us with a far better understanding of English literacy development and more useful implications for intervention strategies with deaf students. Knowing that deaf students have vocabulary limitations of particular types has far less direct implications for instructional practice than does understanding the constraints that operate on the process of vocabulary learning in deaf children. Similarly, knowledge of particular syntactic structures is necessary for literacy skills, but the deaf child has also to master the form-function mappings of those devices in various forms of discourse if he or she is to develop effective reading and writing.

Several important issues remain that we intend addressing in the next few years of our research program. The literature that I reviewed earlier in the chapter implicates particular subcomponents of English language competence as major factors in the literacy problems of deaf students, yet these have typically been studied in isolation. We know little of the relationships between these factors and the overall weighting of each as contributors to the child's competence with English text. Our project will provide a wide range of information on vocabulary, sentence syntax, and discourse-level language processes from the same children, so we will be able to relate skills in these language domains to each other.

Most studies have failed to distinguish between primary language skills ("through the air" communication) and reading and writing English. Although language ability in these two domains is closely related in normal-hearing children, especially in early stages of literacy (Wells, 1985), there is a great deal of recent work documenting important differences between the characteristics of English in face-to-face communication and in written text (see Chafe, 1985; Perera, 1984; Rubin, 1987; & Tannen, 1985). Normal-hearing children begin with better spoken than written English skills. They soon begin to use similar language in the two domains, but by the age of 9 or 10, there is a marked difference between their spoken and written English along a variety of vocabulary, syntactic and textual measures (Perera, 1984).

The implications of this for the development of literacy in deaf students is not clear. The only large-scale study of the relationship between primary language (English, ASL, & Signed English) and reading and writing achievement in deaf students (the NINCDS study: Geers & Moog, 1987; Moores, 1987) studied 16- to 18-year-old deaf students at high average levels of achievement (around an average reading comprehension level on the SAT-HI of eighth grade for the orally taught group, and 6.5 grade for the two signing groups). That study also used rather global measures of achievement in writing (the ETS rating of the sophistication and effectiveness of a written essay) and conversational fluency (an overall rating of competence in an interview situation like that developed by the Foreign Service for second-language learners). Many of the more detailed measures of primary language competence that they used do not lend themselves to psycholinguistic analysis. Another goal of our project is therefore to investigate the relationship between primary language competence in a number of domains of receptive and expressive language, and reading and writing ability in those domains for deaf students at different stages of language development.

The distinction between primary and secondary language development is not an easy one to make for deaf children. For normal-hearing children this represents the distinction between *spoken* (primary) and *written* language (secondary). Spoken language is primary for these children in two senses: (1) it is acquired first and the development of literacy is based upon it; (2) it is the medium through which the printed word is represented or encoded. In the case of the deaf language learner this distinction is more complicated. For many oral-only deaf children the case is similar to the hearing child, with spoken language primary and literacy secondary; nevertheless it is possible that some orally taught children are dealing with two systems, oral system of linguistic knowledge including articulatory, visual (lip-reading), and (for some) acoustic components, and a separable, visually based written English system.

For native ASL signers the situation is similar in the sense that ASL is the primary linguistic system in both priority and representational senses; but the secondary literacy skills will represent a second-language system for these children, for which they may or may not also have an incomplete oral, phonologically based representation. The case of deaf children exposed to simultaneous communication in spoken English and some manually coded form of English is still more complicated since the initial language system that they acquire will contain features of both the spoken and the manual forms of English.

Our project will explore the relationship between the level of linguistic competence in various domains of ASL or manual English systems (such as SEE2) and English language competence in the written mode. The signing assessment will employ not only sentence-level comprehension and production tasks (e.g., Newport & Meier, 1985; Supalla, 1989), but will also collect extended discourse samples in Sign comparable to the written

English samples described in this chapter. In the light of heightened interest in bilingual approaches to the education of deaf students using ASL (Johnson, Liddell & Erting, 1989; Strong, 1988), it is essential to determine the relationship between the development of signing skills in deaf children with either normal-hearing or deaf parents and the acquisition of English literacy skills.

CONCLUSION

Future research on English literacy development in deaf students must be informed by current theoretical and empirical work on the nature of the reading and writing process and its development in normal-hearing children. In this chapter I have argued that we need a more process- and discourse-oriented approach to language development if we are to illuminate the characteristics of deaf students' acquisition of reading and writing skills in a way that has clear implications for intervention.

Finally, future studies must answer the difficult questions posed by the relationship between deaf children's face-to-face language skills and their English literacy development. It is only from this type of research that implications of different modes of communication for the language acquisition of deaf students can be addressed.

REFERENCES

Allen, T. E. (1986). Patterns of academic achievement among hearing-impaired students. In A. N. Schildroth & M. A. Karchmer (Eds.), *Deaf children in America.* Austin, TX: PRO-ED.

Anderson, R. C. (1985). Role of the reader's schema in comprehension, learning and memory. In H. Singer & R. Ruddell (Eds.), *Theoretical models and processes in reading.* New York: International Reading Association.

Anderson, R. C., & Freebody, P. (1983). Reading comprehension and the assessment and acquisition of word knowledge. In B. Hutson (Ed.), *Advances in reading/language research: A research annual.* Greenwich, CT: JAI Press.

Bamberg, M. G. (1987). *The acquisition of narratives: Learning to use language.* New York: Mouton de Gruyter.

Beck, I., & Carpenter, P. (1986). Cognitive approaches to understanding reading. *American Psychologist, 41,* 1098–1105.

Brasel, K., & Quigley, S. P. (1977). The influence of certain language and communication environments in early childhood on the development of language in deaf individuals. *Journal of Speech and Hearing Research, 20,* 95–107.

Carey, S., & Bartlett, E. (1978). Acquiring a single new word. *Papers and Reports on Child Language Development, 15,* 17–29.

Carnine, D., Kameenui, E. J., & Coyle, G. (1984). Utilization of contextual information in determining the meaning of unfamiliar words. *Reading Research Quarterly, 19,* 188–203.

Chafe, W. (1985). Linguistic differences produced by differences between speaking and writing. In D. Olson, N. Torrance, & A. Hildyard (Eds.), *Literacy, language and learning*. New York: Cambridge University Press.

Chall, J. S. (1983). *Stages of reading development*. New York: McGraw-Hill.

Commission on the Education of the Deaf. (1988). *Toward equality*. A report to the President and the Congress of the United States. Washington, DC: GPO.

Delaney, M., Stuckless, E. R., & Walter, G. (1984). Total communication effects: A longitudinal study of a school for the deaf in transition. *American Annals of the Deaf, 129*, 481–486.

Dickinson, D. K. (1984). First impressions: Children's knowledge of words gained from a single exposure. *Applied Psycholinguistics, 5*, 369–373.

Drum, P. A., & Konopak, B. C. (1987). Learning word meanings from written context. In M. McKeown & M. Curtis (Eds.), *The nature of vocabulary acquisition*. Hillsdale, NJ: Erlbaum.

Engen, E., & Engen, T. (1983). *The Rhode Island test of language structure*. Austin, TX: PRO-ED.

Ewoldt, C. (1982). Diagnostic approaches and procedures and the reading process. In R. E. Kretschmer (Ed.), *Reading and the hearing-impaired individual. Volta Review, 84*, 83–94.

Geers, A. E., & Moog, J. S. (1987). *Factors predictive of the development of reading and writing skills in the congenitally deaf: Report on the oral sample*. NIH-NINCDS-83-19. Bethesda, MD: National Institutes of Health.

Geva, E., & Olson, D. (1983). Children's story-retelling. *First Language, 4*, 85–110.

Gipe, J. (1979). Investigating techniques for teaching word meanings. *Reading Research Quarterly, 20*, 624–644.

Gormley, K., & Sarachan-Deily, A. (1987). Evaluating hearing-impaired students' writing: A practical approach. *Volta Review, 89*, 157–170.

Halliday, M., & Hasan, R. (1976). *Cohesion in English*. London: Longmans.

Heibeck, T. H., & Markman, E. M. (1987). Word mapping in children: An examination of fast mapping. *Child Development, 58*, 1021–1034.

Heider, F., & Heider, G. (1940). A comparison of sentence structure of deaf and hearing children. *Psychological Monographs, 52*, 42–103.

Hunt, K. W. (1965). Grammatical structures written at three grade levels. *National Council of Teachers of English Research Reports* (No. 3).

Jenkins, J. R., Stein, M. L., & Wysocki, K. (1984). Learning vocabulary through reading. *American Educational Research Journal, 21*, 767–787.

Johnson, R. E., Liddell, S. K., & Erting, C. J. (1989). Unlocking the curriculum: Principles for achieving access in deaf education. *Gallaudet Research Institute Working Paper* 89–3, Washington, DC: Gallaudet University.

Johnston, J. R. (1982). Narratives: A new look at communication problems in older language-disordered children. *Language, Speech and Hearing Services in Schools, 13*, 144–155.

Just, M., & Carpenter, P. (1980). A theory of reading: From eye fixations to comprehension. *Psychological Review, 4*, 324–354.

Karmiloff-Smith, A. (1981). The grammatical marking of thematic structure in the development of language production. In W. Deutsch (Ed.), *The child's construction of language*. New York: Academic.

Karmiloff-Smith, A. (1986). Some fundamental aspects of language development after age 5. In P. Fletcher & M. Garman (Eds.), *Language acquisition* (2nd ed.). New York: Cambridge University Press.

King, C., & Quigley, S. P. (1985). *Reading and deafness*. Austin, TX: PRO-ED.

Kretschmer, R. R., & Kretschmer, L. (1978). *Language development and intervention with the hearing impaired*. Baltimore: University Park Press.

LaSasso, C., & Davey, B. (1987). The relationship between lexical knowledge and reading comprehension for prelingually, profoundly hearing-impaired students. *Volta Review, 89*, 211–220.

Marzano, R. J., & Marzano, J. S. (1988). *A cluster approach to elementary vocabulary instruction.* New York: International Reading Association.

McKeown, M. (1985). The acquisition of word meaning from context by children of high and low ability. *Reading Research Quarterly, 20*, 482–496.

Miller, G., & Gildea, P. M. (1987). How children learn words. *Scientific American, 257*, 94–99.

Moog, J., & Geers, A. E. (1985). EPIC: A program to accelerate academic progress in profoundly deaf children. *Volta Review, 87*, 259–277.

Moores, D. (1987). *Factors predictive of literacy in deaf adolescents.* NIH-NINCDS-83-19. Bethesda, MD: National Institutes of Health.

Myklebust, H. (1964). *The psychology of deafness* (2nd ed.). New York: Grune and Stratton.

Nagy, W. E., Anderson, R. C., & Herman, P. A. (1987). Learning words from context during normal reading. *American Educational Research Journal, 24*, 237–270.

Nagy, W. E., & Herman, P. A. (1987). Breadth and depth of vocabulary knowledge: implications for acquisition and instruction. In M. McKeown & M. Curtis (Eds.), *The nature of vocabulary acquisition*, Hillsdale, NJ: Erlbaum.

Nelson, K., & Gruendel, J. (1979). At morning it's lunchtime: A scriptal analysis of children's stories. *Discourse Processes, 2*, 73–94.

Newport, E., & Meier, R. (1985). The acquisition of American Sign Language. In D. Slobin (Ed.), *Cross-linguistic studies of language acquisition: Vol. 1, The data.* Hillsdale, NJ: Erlbaum.

Ogden, P. (1979). Experiences and attitudes of oral deaf adults regarding oralism. Unpublished doctoral dissertation, University of Illinois, Bloomington.

Paul, P. (1984). The comprehension of multi-meaning words from selected frequency levels by deaf and hearing subjects. Unpublished doctoral dissertation, University of Illinois, Bloomington.

Perera, K. (1984). *Children's writing and reading.* Oxford, England: Basil Blackwell.

Peterson, C., & McCabe, A. (1983). *Developmental psycholinguistics: Three ways of looking at a child's narrative.* New York: Plenum.

Pflaster, G. (1980). A factor analysis of variables related to academic performance of hearing-impaired children in regular classes. *Volta Review, 82*, 71–84.

Pomerantz, S. B., & de Villiers, P. A. (in preparation). Teaching vocabulary in narrative context.

Quigley, S. P., & King, C. (1980). Syntactic performance of hearing-impaired and normal-hearing individuals. *Applied Psycholinguistics, 1*, 329–356.

Quigley, S. P., & Paul, P. (1984). *Language and deafness.* Austin, TX: PRO-ED.

Quigley, S. P., Wilbur, R., Power, D., Montanelli, D., & Steinkamp, M. (1976). *Syntactic structures in the language of deaf children.* Urbana: University of Illinois, Institute for Child Behavior and Development.

Rubin, D. L. (1987). Divergence and convergence between oral and written communication. *Topics in Language Disorders, 7*, 1–18.

Rumelhart, D. (1977). Toward an interactive model of reading. In S. Dornic (Ed.), *Attention and Performance VI.* New York: Academic.

Sachs, J. (1988). *Pronominal cohesion in children's oral narratives.* Talk to staff at the Rhode Island School for the Deaf, Providence, RI.

Samuels, S. J., & Eisenberg, P. (1981). A framework for understanding the reading process. In F. J. Piaozzolo and M. C. Witterock (Eds.), *Neuropsychological and cognitive processes in reading.* New York: Academic.

Stein, N., & Glenn, C. (1979). An analysis of story comprehension in elementary school children. In R. Freedle (Ed.), *New directions in discourse processing.* Norwood, NJ: ABLEX.

Sternberg, R. J. (1987). Most vocabulary is learned from context. In M. McKeown & M. Curtis (Eds.), *The nature of vocabulary acquisition.* Hillsdale, NJ: Erlbaum.

Sternberg, R. J., & Powell, J. S. (1983). Comprehending verbal comprehension. *American Psychologist, 38,* 878–893.

Strong, M. (1988). A bilingual approach to the education of young deaf children: ASL and English. In M. Strong (Ed.), *Language learning and deafness.* New York: Cambridge University Press.

Supalla, E. (1989). *An assessment battery for ASL.* Paper presented to the Boston University Conference on Language Acquisition, Boston, MA.

Tannen, D. (1979). What's in a frame? Surface evidence for underlying expectations. In R. Freedle (Ed.), *New directions in discourse processing.* Norwood, NJ: ABLEX.

Tannen, D., (1985). Relative focus on involvement in oral and written discourse. In D. Olson, N. Torrance, & A. Hildyard (Eds.), *Literacy, language and learning.* New York: Cambridge University Press.

Taylor, L. (1969). A language analysis of the writing of deaf children. Unpublished doctoral dissertation, Florida State University, Tallahassee.

van Uden, A. (1977). *A world of language for deaf children: Part 1, Basic principles.* Amsterdam: Sevets & Zeitlinger.

Walter, G. (1978). Lexical abilities of hearing and hearing-impaired children. *American Annals of the Deaf, 123,* 976–982.

Wells, G. (1985). Oral and literate competencies in the early school years. In D. Olson, N. Torrance, & A. Hildyard (Eds.), *Literacy, language and learning.* New York: Cambridge University Press.

Werner, H., & Kaplan, E. (1952). The acquisition of word meaning: a developmental study. *Monographs of the Society for Research in Child Development* (No. 15), 3–120.

Wilbur, R. (1977). An explanation of deaf children's difficulty with certain syntactic structures in English. *Volta Review, 79,* 85–92.

Wilbur, R. (1987). *American Sign Language: linguistic and applied dimensions.* Austin, TX: PRO-ED.

Yoshinaga-Itano, C., & Downey, D. M. (1986). A hearing-impaired child's acquisition of schemata: something's missing. *Topics in Language Disorders, 7,* 45–57.

Yoshinaga-Itano, C., & Snyder, L. (1985). Form and meaning in the written language of hearing-impaired children. In R. R. Kretschmer (Ed.), *Learning to write and writing to learn. Volta Review, 87,* 75–90.

CHAPTER 23

The Cross-Linguistic Study of Language-Impaired Children

LAURENCE B. LEONARD

In this chapter I try to show that cross-linguistic research can provide important insight into the nature of language impairment in children. I will argue that the types of hypotheses that one can explore with this line of research are not easily approached in studies of only one language group. Further, I hope to show that this work can even reveal flaws in current conceptualizations of the disorder.

The paper begins with examples of how cross-linguistic study might contribute to our understanding of language impairment in English. In the sections to follow, I discuss the contributions of English to the study of language impairment in other languages, as well as some of the limitations of cross-linguistic research.

Preparation of this paper was supported in part by Research Grant NS25883 from the National Institutes of Health. I wish to thank the following individuals for their helpful comments on an earlier draft: Kathleen Kangas, Sue Young Kim, Diane Frome Loeb, Karla McGregor, James Montgomery, Parimala Raghavendra, Richard G. Schwartz, Lori Swanson, and Jennifer Windsor.

UNDERSTANDING
LANGUAGE IMPAIRMENT IN ENGLISH

Let us consider the rather heterogeneous group of children who are given the label "specifically language impaired" (SLI). A common profile among English-speaking (E) SLI children is a moderate deficit across a range of language areas with a more serious difficulty in the use of grammatical morphemes. Even when these children are matched with younger, normally developing children on the basis of mean utterance length, ESLI children are more likely to omit grammatical inflections (e.g., -s, -ed) and function words (e.g., *the, is*) (see Johnston, 1988 for a recent review).

There are a number of plausible hypotheses for these children's especially poor morphology. Unfortunately, a study of English alone does not provide much basis for evaluating them. I shall consider some of these hypotheses below, and suggest ways in which data for other languages can shed additional light on the matter.

PERCEPTUAL SALIENCE

The grammatical morphemes of English are nonsyllabic consonant affixes and unstressed syllables. Because these morphemes are shorter in duration than adjacent morphemes in the sentence, they are less salient perceptually. According to a number of investigators, this property of English grammatical morphemes contributes to the telegraphic look of children's early sentences (e.g., Gleitman, Gleitman, Landau, & Wanner, 1988). Given that grammatical morphemes pose extraordinary problems for ESLI children, it is possible that these children are especially limited in their ability to perceive, and thus hypothesize, morphemes that have this acoustic property.

One test for this hypothesis would be to examine the speech of SLI children who are acquiring a language that contains a number of perceptually salient grammatical morphemes. One such language is Hebrew. A number of grammatical morphemes in Hebrew take the form of stressed syllables at the end of the word (e.g., plurals) or within a word (e.g., vocalic infixes marking place, number, and gender of the verb), and show correspondingly longer relative durations. If SLI children acquiring Hebrew do not show the same weakness in morphology (relative to other features of language) that we see in ESLI children, the "perceptual salience" hypothesis would pass an important first test.

SEMANTIC SALIENCE

Language-learning theories of all persuasions seem to have some means of accounting for the fact that English-speaking children's early sentences are composed of open-class words that form semantically definable relationships. In some theories, the semantic roles themselves are assumed to be the operative feature; in others, it is assumed that the child merely uses reliable semantic role-form class associations as an initial means of identifying grammatical categories. However framed, each proposal describes the early stage of development as one of acquiring the basic predicate-argument structure of the sentence. Because English grammatical morphemes fall outside this basic structure, they are acquired later.

Given that the relative difficulty of grammatical morphemes is even greater for ESLI children than for younger normally developing English-speaking children, one might hypothesize that these children are occupied with predicate-argument structure to a fault. Perhaps their attention to this basic structure is so rigid that they ignore, or disregard as frills, the grammatical morphemes of the language.

An hypothesis of this type can be tested without much difficulty. Some languages employ grammatical morphemes to express basic arguments of the verb. That is, although the form is structurally dependent and incapable of standing alone in an utterance, it represents an obligatory argument in the sentence. For example, in Italian one uses a clitic (in the form of an unstressed syllable) for an obligatory direct object or indirect object whose referent has already been established. Support for the "semantic salience" hypothesis would be seen if Italian-speaking SLI children have no special problems expressing direct and indirect objects when they involve clitics. On the other hand, finding that Italian-speaking SLI children have grave difficulties with clitics would suggest that it is more than the peripheral nature of grammatical morphemes that pose problems for these children. Such a finding, in fact, would be in keeping with the "perceptual salience" account.

Of course, it could be the case that both the "perceptual salience" and the "semantic salience" hypotheses are correct to a degree. If two forms are equivalent in semantic salience, the one that is more salient perceptually might be acquired earlier; if, instead, the two forms are comparable perceptually, the one that serves as an obligatory argument or predicate might be acquired first. But such findings would not tell us which of these two factors has the more powerful influence. Through judicious selection of languages, one could probably make this determination. In certain languages with complex morphology, major semantic elements of the sentence are considerably less salient perceptually than the inflections attached to them. In Quiché, verb roots are often low in perceptual salience, with stress falling on the syllabic verb suffixes (see Pye, 1983). If SLI children acquiring such a language showed greater use of unstressed verb roots (relative to stressed suffixes) than normally developing children, this would constitute strong support for the "semantic salience" hypothesis, at the expense of its rival.

IDENTIFICATION OF GRAMMATICAL ROLE

A third hypothesis is that ESLI children are capable of understanding the types of abstract notions entailed in grammatical morphemes, but have problems sorting out which notion is expressed by which morpheme. There are two characteristics of English morphology that make this job rather difficult. A number of morphemes in English are homophonous. Most notably, -s can be a plural suffix, a third person singular verb inflection, a contracted auxiliary or copula, or a possessive marker. The other characteristic (more true of many other languages than of English) is that certain morphemes simultaneously code two grammatical notions. The verb inflection -s marks not only third person but also singular. It will not be sufficient for the child to hypothesize one of these grammatical notions without the other.

There are languages whose structure avoids both of these problems. Turkish is a commonly cited example (see Aksu-Koc & Slobin, 1985). There are relatively few homophonous morphemes in Turkish. Further, it is an agglutinating language; strings of morphemes, each marking a single grammatical notion, are attached to the stems of nouns and verbs. For example, to express past, a past tense affix is appended to the verb. If the subject is plural, a plural affix is then added to the end of the past affix, and so on. Because these characteristics of Turkish should greatly facilitate identification of the grammatical role played by each morpheme, SLI children acquiring Turkish should not be especially weak in morphology, at least, if this hypothesis were correct.

AVOID EXCEPTIONS

Many languages are said to be morphologically uniform, but they can express this uniformity in two different ways. Some languages, such as Spanish, are uniform because verb stems must have inflections. Others, such as Chinese, are uniform because verb stems never have inflections. English is not uniform, for it has a "mixed" morphology; verb inflections occur, but bare stems are permitted. It is reasonable to consider the possibility that ESLI children are initially swayed by the frequent appearance of bare stems in English, and consequently they treat their language as uniform in the sense of Chinese (viz., that all stems must be bare) (see Hyams, 1987).

Such an "avoid exceptions" hypothesis must be tested by examining SLI children acquiring a language such as Russian. This language has a rich morphology, but it, too, is "mixed" because in certain instances bare stems occur. Because bare stems are the exceptions to the rule, support for the hypothesis would take the form of Russian-speaking SLI children adding suffixes to grammatically appropriate bare stems. For example, rather than using the bare stem for singular accusative masculine nonhuman and neuter nouns, these children might add the feminine accusative suffix to the stem (see Slobin, 1973).

CUE OVER-RELIANCE

Relative to other languages of the world, English is rather extreme in its word order rigidity. Presumably because word order is such a powerful cue in English (see Bates & MacWhinney, 1987), both normally developing and SLI children acquiring English show rather strict adherence to the highly dominant subject-verb-object order of the language from the very outset of grammatical development. At some point English-speaking children must focus their attention on those few grammatical morphemes that do appear in the language. Given that ESLI children are especially slow in acquiring these morphemes, it is possible that these children have great difficulty shifting their focus to another cue type (inflectional morphology) once one type (word order) has been established.

It seems that such an hypothesis could be tested by examining SLI children acquiring a language such as Hungarian. This language has a rich morphology and, although it has a "basic" word order (subject-object-verb), it is very flexible in this regard, with word order varying according to pragmatic factors. In languages of this type, morphology is acquired very early by children, for it is the dominant grammatical cue (MacWhinney, 1985). Given the hypothesis that SLI children become overreliant on the dominant cue type in the language, we could expect SLI children acquiring Hungarian to disregard word order to the point where word orders are sometimes produced that can be explained by neither canonical word order nor pragmatic appropriateness.

LENGTH OR SEQUENCE CONSTRAINTS

A final hypothesis is that SLI children have a severe limitation on the length or sequence of morpheme strings that they can process. If this were the case, it would follow that grammatical morphemes would be the most expendable, at least in English where they do not constitute part of the predicate-argument structure of the sentence. Central to this proposal is the assumption that the notions reflected by grammatical morphemes are not difficult in and of themselves; the problem is that their inclusion would result in a sentence that exceeds the length that the child can handle.

One means of testing the plausibility of this hypothesis would be to examine the speech of SLI children acquiring a tone language in which morphological marking is accomplished by pitch variations. For example, in Bini, a (monosyllabic) verb expressed as a habitual action would be produced with a low tone, whereas the same verb expressed as an action in the past would be produced with a high tone (see Ladefoged, 1975). Because tone is a suprasegmental feature that is superimposed on the syllables of a sentence, it should not have the same cost to a child with a length or sequencing limitation that an additional affix would have. Thus, we would expect to find that SLI children acquiring a language of this type would express many grammatical features that ESLI children fail to use.

The "length-sequence constraint" hypothesis might also be evaluated against some of the hypothesis already discussed. As noted earlier, Turkish makes use of inflections whose grammatical roles are quite clear. Given the "identification of grammatical role" hypothesis, then, SLI children acquiring this language should not have special difficulty with morphology. On the other hand, the agglutinating property of Turkish requires that strings of morphemes, in a particular sequence, be added to stems. Thus, in contrast to the "identification of grammatical role" hypothesis, the "length-sequence constraint" hypothesis would predict significant morphological limitations in Turkish-speaking SLI children.

CONTRIBUTIONS OF ENGLISH

Thus far, the focus has been on how the study of other languages might permit us to evaluate hypotheses about specific language impairment in English. But, of course, the influence is bi-directional. Data from ESLI children can help guide investigations in other languages toward hypotheses that hold real promise, and away from those unduly influenced by the peculiarities of the language under study.

An example from German can serve as an appropriate illustration of the contribution of English data. In adult German, transitive finite verbs appear in second position in canonical declarative sentences, reflecting a basic order of subject-verb-object. Yet, the early sentences of German-speaking SLI children show a disproportionate number of transitive verbs in final position (Grimm & Weinert, 1987). This finding has prompted some researchers to propose that German-speaking SLI children have great difficulty with word order. However, an alternative account is that these children's verb-final usage is attributable to the appearance of other kinds of sentence constructions in the ambient language. Most notably, transitive as well as intransitive infinitives that follow modals or auxiliaries appear in sentence-final position in German. Because English also employs subject-verb-object as its canonical word order, yet does not place transitive verbs in final position in other constructions, the speech of ESLI children represents an excellent test case. In fact, ESLI children do not show much evidence of word order errors, and transitive verbs are rarely, if ever, placed inappropriately in final position.

SOME LIMITATIONS

It is clear that proposals such as those made here face significant obstacles of a practical nature. I would argue that the most obvious one—the logistics of traveling to Guatemala to study Quiché or Nigeria to study Bini—is not the most important. I see nothing on the horizon to lead me to believe that the continued study of a single language will be a faster route to uncovering the nature of language impairment in children.

A more serious concern is that the culture of the people who speak the language of interest does not recognize the notion of language impairment, or defines impairment in such a different way that cross-linguistic comparison is meaningless. A related concern is whether there are professionals within the culture who assume responsibility for identifying children with deficient language skills. Even when there are highly competent professionals engaged in clinical practice, the profession might be so new to the country that standardized language tests do not exist. In such cases, the collection of normative data will need to be the first step in the research process.

CONCLUDING REMARKS

In summary, I tried to make the case that a deeper understanding of language impairment in children can come about from cross-linguistic research. Although the examples provided dealt only with one group of language-impaired children—those with specific language impairment— the questions pursued in these examples are applicable to other language-disordered groups as well.

It is possible that some of these same research questions can be approached without recourse to cross-linguistic comparisons. For example, studies of miniature language learning might be used to determine if ESLI children can acquire morphemes more readily if they are perceptually salient, or nonhomophonous. Of course, because miniature language learning usually represents a type of second language learning, it is not without its interpretive limitations.

Perhaps the strongest justification for pursuing cross-linguistic research comes from considering the limitations in not doing so. By focusing only on one language, the confounds within the language compel us to examine factors outside of language (e.g., lower-level auditory processing, anticipatory imagery) for possible insights into the basis of the problem. It is possible that the source of difficulty rests in such factors. However, the study of factors external to language necessarily requires assumptions about how these factors are meaningfully related to specific features of language. Subsequent investigation may fail to support the direct relationship assumed. For this reason, the research approach discussed in this paper represents an essential complement; the factors examined are within language itself, and confounds are separated by comparing different languages.

REFERENCES

Aksu-Koc, A., & Slobin, D. (1985). The acquisition of Turkish. In D. Slobin (Ed.), *The crosslinguistic study of language acquisition: Vol. 1; The data* (pp. 839–878). Hillsdale, NJ: Erlbaum.

Bates, E., & MacWhinney, B. (1987). Competition, variation, and language learning. In B. MacWhinney (Ed.), *Mechanisms of language acquisition* (pp. 157–193). Hillsdale, NJ: Erlbaum.

Gleitman, L., Gleitman, H., Landau, B., & Wanner, E. (1988). Where learning begins: Initial representations for language learning. In F. Newmeyer (Ed.), *The Cambridge linguistic survey* (pp. 150–193). New York: Cambridge University Press.

Grimm, H., & Weinert, S. (1987). *Deviant processing in dysphasic children: A longitudinal study*. Paper presented at the Fourth International Congress for the Study of Child Language, Lund, Sweden.

Hyams, N. (1987). *The setting of the null subject parameter: A reanalysis*. Paper presented at the Boston University Conference on Language Development, Boston.

Johnston, J. (1988). Specific language disorders in the child. In N. Lass, L. McReynolds, J. Northern, & D. Yoder (Eds.), *Handbook of speech-language pathology and audiology* (pp. 685–715). Toronto: B. C. Decker.

Ladefoged, P. (1975). *A course in phonetics*. New York: Harcourt, Brace, Jovanovich.

MacWhinney, B. (1985). Hungarian language acquisition as an exemplification of a general model of grammatical development. In D. Slobin (Ed.), *The crosslinguistic study of language acquisition: Vol. 2; Theoretical issues* (pp. 1069–1155). Hillsdale, NJ: Erlbaum.

Pye, C. (1983). Mayan telegraphese: Intonational determinants of inflectional development in Quiché Mayan. *Language, 59*, 583–604.

Slobin, D. (1973). Cognitive prerequisites for the development of grammar. In C. Ferguson & D. Slobin (Eds.), *Studies of child language development* (pp. 175–208). New York: Holt, Rinehart and Winston.

CHAPTER 24

Metalinguistic Abilities and Language Disorder

PAULA MENYUK

It has been hypothesized that children with specific language impairment suffer a delay in their language development but that the sequence of their development mirrors that of normally developing children (Leonard, 1972). Longitudinal studies of these children's language development indicate that, despite a slowed pace and some plateaus in development, the path they follow is similar to that of normally developing children. From these data one can hypothesize that their knowledge of language changes in the same way, although not at the same time as normally speaking children. Overall, a similar picture has been presented for the language development of developmentally delayed children (Miller, 1987). These children also follow a path similar to that of normally developing children but exhibit, in their case, severe delays in development.

Some have argued that the latter group of children may suffer delays in language development because they also suffer delays in cognitive development (Bricker & Bricker, 1974). However, there is still a great deal of controversy about the exact relation between cognitive and linguistic development (Menyuk, 1988), and different relations have been found between cognition and language in developmentally delayed children (Curtiss, 1981). Presumably, with SLI children cognitive delay cannot be posited as the reason for delays and plateaus in language development because, by definition, these children are cognitively normal. The reasons for these delays and plateaus have yet to be determined for both groups of children.

Several causes other than across-the-board cognitive delay have been pointed to as causes for linguistic delay. It has been argued that language-disordered children have a reduced rate of processing fast-fading stimuli (Tallal & Stark, 1980). Because of this, they have difficulty in categorizing speech sound units and sequences and, therefore, in progressing normally in language development. It has also been suggested that these children have memorial difficulties. They cannot keep in mind the categorizations they have made of the speech units and, therefore, need many more instances of these units in order to establish linguistic categories and relations (Menyuk, 1978). The hypothesis to be explored here is that these children are delayed because they do not achieve an awareness of linguistic categories in the process of acquiring them. They have difficulties in metaprocessing. This is a highly speculative hypothesis for which there is only indirect evidence at present.

In this chapter I will first discuss some recent findings concerning the metalinguistic processing of SLI children and children with matched-language knowledge abilities from two other populations. I will then discuss data from the normal language development literature to support the hypothesis that difficulties in metaprocessing lead to these children's language development delays. Finally, I will discuss what I believe are the important questions still to be asked about the relations between difficulties in metalinguizing and language development delay.

LANGUAGE PERFORMANCE AND PROCESSING

There are relatively few studies that have explicitly examined the language awareness of language-disordered children. The language knowledge of SLI children is often measured by a battery of tests that examine varying aspects of language, or by collecting and analyzing language samples by various experimental procedures. In a recent study (Liebergott, Menyuk, Chesnick & Korngold, 1988) we asked several questions about the metalinguistic abilities of a group of language-disordered children. One of the questions we asked was concerned with the pattern of development of these children's meta-abilities over a 3-year period in early childhood.

A group of SLI children was given a battery of standard tests. An additional population in the study were children who had evidenced delay in language development at an early age but who had largely, but not completely, outgrown their difficulties ("iffy children"). Also included in the study were a group of very-low-birth-weight (VLB) premature children. All 135 children were initially tested when they ranged in age from

4.6 to 5.6 years. The test scores of these three groups of children on these standard tests are presented in Table 24-1. As can be seen from this table, the SLI children consistently had the lowest scores, the iffy children had the next highest scores, and the premature children had the highest scores.

Almost immediately after the standard testing all the children were given a battery of language metaprocessing tasks. All of these tasks required conscious awareness of categories and relations at various levels of language: morphophonology, semantax, lexicon, and discourse. The three subject populations differed from each other on this experimental battery, and they differed in the same way as they had on the standard tests. The SLI children performed worst, the iffy children better than the SLI children, and the VLB children best. Table 24-2 lists the tasks that were included in the battery.

A cluster analysis of the scores on the battery measures was carried out to determine which children in the other two groups were performing as poorly as the SLI children on the metalinguistic tasks in the battery. It was found that 44 of the iffy and 9 of the VLB children clustered with the SLI children on the battery measures. Thus, the cluster analysis based on the metalinguistic measures indicated that some children in the other two groups were, in fact, performing as poorly as the SLI children on linguistic metaprocessing tasks.

Table 24-1. Mean age equivalent scores on the standard measures

Language Tests	SLI Group	Iffy Group	Premature Group
RECEPTIVE			
Token	45.7	59.8	69.2
TACL (%ile)	35.8	51.7	67.8
PPVT	51.1	61.2	69.3
EXPRESSIVE			
DSS	39.0	51.9	59.1
Reporters	.2	1.0	2.2
ITPA	52.9	69.4	78.1
Gardner	53.7	71.0	79.8
SUPPLEMENTARY			
TOLD Discrim.	55.3	66.2	66.6
Templin Darley	41.7	57.9	69.3
Verbal Fluency	52.9	61.9	61.6

Table 24-2. List of metalinguistic tasks and aspects of language assessed

Task	Aspects of Language
Syllable segmentation	Phonological
Phonological segmentation	Phonological
Sentence judgment and correction	Semantactic
Comprehension of complex sentences	Semantactic
Related items recall	Lexical
Nonrelated items recall, Uninterrupted	Lexical
Nonrelated items recall, Interrupted	Lexical
Rapid automatized naming	Lexical
Oral cloze procedure	Semantactic
Story recall	Discourse

Metalinguistic abilities, as measured on the battery, were accessed at three points in time over a 2½-year period. Developmental changes in metalinguistic abilities with varying aspects of language were measured, and the abilities of the SLI children (now composed of SLI, iffy, and VLB children) were compared with those of the other children in the study. There were significant differences between this lowest performing group and the other children on almost all tasks at all three points in time. All the children, other than the SLI children, steadily improved in their metalinguistic abilities. With this group of children one general pattern of development could be observed, and this pattern was associated with almost all aspects of language. The tasks were collapsed as metaprocessing tasks, which require awareness of phonological, semantactic, lexical, and discourse units. In the lowest performing group of children, semantax and phonological processing abilities increased remarkably slowly over the time of the study. This was particularly true of lexical processing abilities. All the abilities not only increased slowly but, also, plateaued at the midpoint of the study. This was not true of story recall. The number of propositions recalled at time 2 almost doubled, and, although not as dramatically, increased at time 3. Nevertheless, this group performed significantly more poorly than the other children even on this task. These developmental patterns are shown in Figure 24-1.

The children were given a battery of exit measures. One of these was a standard test of oral language development. These children still performed significantly more poorly on a standard measure of language development than did the other children in the study. The data obtained indicate that SLI children at age 4.6 to 5.6 years are delayed in language development, as indicated in performance on a standard battery of tests. Their performance

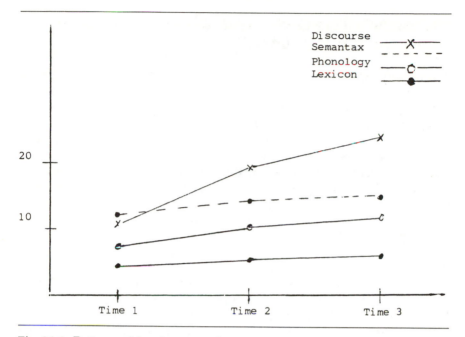

Fig. 24-1. Patterns of development of meta-processing various aspects of language.

on the exit measure indicated that they do develop further linguistic knowledge but that they do not catch up to their normal-speaking peers over a 3-year period. These data also indicate that SLI children have marked difficulty in bringing to awareness their knowledge of categories and relations in language. They exhibit some slow growth in awareness and, also, plateaus in some aspects of awareness. One might assume that further growth in metalinguistic abilities will be observed, and with more complex aspects of language when the children in this study are older, but this is just a speculation. However, other researchers have found these metaprocessing difficulties in younger language-disordered children, and with less complex aspects of language (Kahmi, Lee & Nelson, 1985).

Despite the findings of this and some other studies that language-disordered children have metaprocessing difficulties, the cause-effect relation between difficulty in metaprocessing of language and language delay is unclear. Thus far, all that the data indicate is that these children have delays in language development and particular difficulties in metalinguizing. Below, a logical argument will be presented to support the notion that these children are delayed in language because of metalinguizing difficulties.

METALINGUIZING DIFFICULTIES AND LANGUAGE DELAY

Several researchers have discussed the development of metalinguistic abilities (Bialystok, 1986; Karmiloff-Smith, 1986; Menyuk, 1983). There are both similarities and differences in the descriptions of these various researchers of the developmental changes that occur in metalinguizing. All researchers describe these abilities as being able to become consciously aware of the different units and levels of language. Overall it has been suggested that three stages occur in this development. The first is intuitive use of linguistic knowledge, then there is awareness and executive use of such knowledge in various tasks that require such awareness. One of these tasks is, of course, reading. The third and final stage is automatic use of knowledge.

Differences arise among researchers concerning the timing of such developments. Some believe that awareness begins only during the middle childhood period when children can talk about what they know. Others hypothesize that metalinguizing is a continuous process that constantly changes as the child linguistically matures, and that the ability to talk about knowledge is, perhaps, only the end stage of awareness. It is this latter view that might explain the relation between metalinguizing and development in language. A hypothetical model of developmental changes in processing linguistic data, knowledge acquisition, awareness, and automaticity appears in Table 24-3.

The above view suggests that the child achieves awareness of linguistic categories and relations as knowledge of language is being acquired. This awareness may occur as the child compares what is known about language with what he or she hears. As what is known is compared to what is heard, differences may be observed and changes made in how linguistic knowledge is represented. Meta-abilities may, therefore, be the cause of developmental change. This comparison, or awareness of a structure, may manifest

Table 24-3. Stages in the development of automaticity

Time I	*Time II*	*Time III*
Processing Strategies Set I	Processing Strategies Set II	Processing Strategies Set III
Intuitive Knowledge Rules Set I	Intuitive Knowledge Rules Set II	Intuitive Knowledge Rules Set III
	Conscious Knowledge Rules Set I	Conscious Knowledge Rules Set II
		Automatic Processing Rules Set I

itself in a variety of behaviors. One such behavior may be alternation of rules (Menyuk, 1964). Such alternation of rules has been observed in the development of all aspects of language. The child alternates between newly acquired rules with the use of older rules. For example, in early syntax development (1) articles are and are not used, and at a later age (2) rules for embedding relative clauses are and are not observed. Some examples of 1 and 2 appear below.

1. "I see girl" and "I see the girl."
2. "I know what is he doing" and "I know what he's doing."

Another manifestation of early awareness of categories and relations in the process of being learned are observed in the young child's introduction of differences that do not exist in the language, that is, creation of rules. Some examples of this are children's introduction of (3) phonemic differences to disambiguate words (Leopold, 1939). This indicates that the child is aware of the need to differentiate among words by marking phonological differences. Another example is (4) the child's use of modals in unique ways to convey differential intent (Ervin-Tripp, 1987). This provides some evidence that the child is aware of the possible use of modals to convey intent as well as aspect. Still another manifestation of overt comparison of linguistic categories and relations is the child's response to requests for clarification. Such responses indicate (5) an awareness that the message might have been misunderstood for varying linguistic structural (phonetic, phonological, lexical, semantactic) or pragmatic reasons. Further, in order to clarify, the child (6) manipulates these categories by offering a variety of corrections (Stokes, 1976). Along with the ability to modify utterances when requests for clarification are made is (7) the very young child's ability to self-correct (Muma, 1986).

A final and very familiar manifestation of awareness of linguistic categories and relations is (8) the child's ability to judge and correct anomalous and nongrammatical sentences. This ability does not suddenly appear at age 8 but rather appears early on with linguistic material that the child is in the process of acquiring. Two-year-olds reject sentences such as "The apple ate the boy" and correct them by modifying meaning (Gleitman, Gleitman & Shipley, 1972). Three- and four-year-olds reject sentences with missing determiners, nouns, verbs, and modals (Menyuk, 1963), and spontaneously add them. Ten-year-olds think sentences such as "Do you want the tiger to chase you or the lion" are funny (Flood & Menyuk, 1983).

The argument being presented is that awareness of linguistic categories and relations is not the end result of linguistic knowledge but rather a part of the acquisition of such knowledge. A further argument being made is that it is just this aspect of language knowledge that the language-disordered child has great difficulty with but, obviously, eventually achieves. It is obvious, by virtue of the fact that these children do progress in language development. The data obtained in the study of development of metalinguistic abilities described above clearly indicates that SLI children do make progress in these abilities. Awareness of linguistic categories and relations are needed to firmly establish linguistic representations and to retrieve them automatically. The language-disordered child intuitively acquires knowledge of language and then has a great deal of difficulty in achieving conscious awareness of that knowledge. Since this is the case, the further development of firm establishment of linguistic representations and automatic retrieval is delayed and, in this way, language development is delayed.

There are further facts that such an explanation might account for. In the beginning of this chapter, two other explanations for language delay were presented. The first of these were that these children suffer a reduced rate of processing speech information. For a long time it has been known that automaticity of processing information speeds up that processing (Flavell, 1985). The second explanation provided was that these children have a memorial problem. They cannot keep appropriate chunks in mind for appropriate encoding and, therefore, also exhibit retrieval problems. Speeding up rate of processing permits the processor to operate on more of the material. Thus, difficulties in metalinguistic abilities could theoretically subsume the other two explanations of language delay: reduced rate of processing and immediate memory problems.

FURTHER QUESTIONS

The above discussion presents a possible explanation for the delays in language development that have been observed in language-disordered children. I have argued that the delays are primarily caused by these children's particular difficulties in bringing to awareness what they know about language. To support this argument, data obtained in a number of studies of both normal and delayed language development have been cited. It has been found that normally developing children exhibit awareness of the categories and relations in language from the beginning of their development. As they mature linguistically, they are able to bring more mature aspects of language to awareness. After awareness of structures, automaticity in the processing of these structures occurs. Automaticity increases the rate at which structures can be processed, and the amount of information about structures that can be processed. In this way automaticity leads to further development. Given these data, I have argued that awareness is part of the acquisition of knowledge of language. Awareness of a structure is an indication of firm establishment of that structure. Further, such firm establishment is needed as a basis for comparison of what is known with what is still to be acquired and for automatic processing of structures. In these two ways, awareness of structure is needed for developmental change.

Studies of SLI children have found that they have difficulty in bringing to awareness categories and relations in all aspects of language. Limited developmental data are available but there are indications that these difficulties occur at the earliest stages of these children's language development and continue as their language develops. Not only is the development of these abilities remarkably slow in these children but, also, they plateau in these abilities, just as they plateau in language development. I have argued that these findings support the notion that delay is caused by metaprocessing difficulties since awareness of structures precedes and is necessary for comparison of what is known to what is still to be learned and for automatic use of structures. Automaticity is needed for rapid processing of the linguistic signal and an increase in the amount of the signal that can be processed.

The explanation for language delay presented above is quite speculative. However, there are at least three kinds of questions that might be asked about this possible explanation. The first set of questions are developmental ones. The course of language development in language-disordered children could be studied by comparing what they know about language during an age period and what aspects of language they are aware of during that same period. In this way, the posited relation between knowledge and awareness could be systematically examined. It would not matter that there is variation in the degrees and kinds of language knowledge among language-disordered children. The question being asked is not what the child knows about language but, rather, what the child is aware of in language in relation to what is known.

The second set of questions is concerned with intervention. The first question might be, how can these children be helped to become aware of the categories and relations in language that they are beginning to use? There are strategies that normally developing children use to help them encode and then retrieve linguistic information. For example, there are a number of features that can be used to store lexical items in memory. It may be the case that SLI children (and other children who suffer language delay) use a very small set of features for encoding. Use of a larger set can be taught. Deliberate and then automatic use of this wide range of features can be taught to speed up retrieval. The second question might be, Can one change these children's rate of language development by teaching them to be consciously aware of what they know about language?

This third set of questions is concerned with the academic problems the language-disordered child might encounter because of an inability to metaprocess language. This last set of questions is the one that is being seriously addressed at present. For example, the relation between language awareness in these children and their ability to learn to read is being examined in a number of studies (e.g., Kahmi & Catts, 1986; Kahmi, Catts, Mauer, Apel, & Gentry, 1988; Liebergott et al., 1988). Additional understanding might be obtained in other areas of research if the language-disordered child's awareness of rules was directly assessed. It seems to me that a very good candidate for this kind of approach might be studies of the learning-disabled child's knowledge of pragmatic rules—knowledge of, for example, speech acts and figurative language. Automatic use of such knowledge seems to be highly dependent on an initial awareness of the rules.

REFERENCES

Bailystok, E. (1986). Factors in growth of linguistic awareness. *Child Development, 57*, 498–510.

Bricker, W., & Bricker, D. (1974). An early language training strategy. In R. Schiefelbusch & L. Lloyd (Eds.), *Language perspectives: Acquisition, retardation and intervention* (pp. 431–486). Baltimore: University Park Press.

Curtiss, S. (1981). Dissociation between language and cognition. *Journal of Autism and Developmental Disorders, 11*, 15–30.

Ervin-Tripp, S. (1987). *Speech acts and syntactic development: Independent or linked.* Paper presented at the Annual Boston University Conference on Language Development, October, Boston.

Flavell, J. (1985). *Cognitive development.* Englewood Cliffs, NJ: Prentice-Hall.

Flood, J., & Menyuk, P. (1983). The development of metalinguistic awareness and its relation to reading. *Journal of Applied Developmental Psychology, 4*, 65–80.

Gleitman, L., Gleitman, H., & Shipley, E. (1972). The emergence of the child as grammarian. *Cognition, 1*, 137–164.

Kahmi, A., & Catts, H. (1986). Toward an understanding of developmental language and reading disorders, *Journal of Speech and Hearing Disorders, 51*, 337–347.

Kahmi, A., Catts, H., Mauer, D., Apel, K., & Gentry, B. (1988). Phonological or spatial processing abilities in language and reading. *Journal of Speech and Hearing Disorders, 53*, 316–327.

Kahmi, A., Lee, R., & Nelson, L. (1985). Word, syllable and sound awareness in language disordered children. *Journal of Speech and Hearing Disorders, 50*, 207–212.

Karmiloff-Smith, A. (1986). From meta-processes to conscious access: Evidence from children's metalinguistic and repair data. *Cognition, 23*, 95–147.

Leonard, L. (1972). What is deviant language? *Journal of Speech and Hearing Disorders, 37*, 427–446.

Leopold, W. (1939). *Speech development of a bilingual child: A linguist's record: Vol. 1.* Evanston, IL: Northwestern University Press.

Liebergott, J., Menyuk, P., Chesnick, M., & Korngold, B. (1988). *Language processing abilities and reading achievement in children.* Mini-seminar presented at the Annual Convention of the American Speech, Language and Hearing Association, November, Boston.

Menyuk, P. (1963). A preliminary evaluation of grammatical capacity in children. *Journal of Verbal Learning and Verbal Behavior, 2*, 429–439.

Menyuk, P. (1964). Alternation of rules in children's grammar. *Journal of Verbal Learning and Verbal Behavior, 3,* 480–488.

Menyuk, P. (1978). Linguistic problems in children with developmental dysphasia. In M. Wyke (Ed.) *Developmental dysphasia* (pp. 135–158). London: Academic.

Menyuk, P. (1983). Language development and reading. In T. Gallagher and C. Prutting (Eds.), *Pragmatic assessment and intervention issues in language* (pp. 151–170). Austin, TX: PRO-ED.

Menyuk, P. (1988). *Language development: Knowledge and use.* Glenview, IL: Scott, Foresman/Little Brown College division.

Miller, J. (1987). Language and communicative characteristics of children with Down syndrome. In S. Puschel, C. Tingey, J. Rynless, A. Crocker, & D. Crutchen (Eds.) *New perspectives on Down syndrome* (pp. 233–262). Baltimore: Brooks.

Muma, J. (1986). *Language acquisition: A functionalist perspective.* Austin, TX: PRO-ED.

Stokes, W. (1976). *Children's replies to requests for clarification: An opportunity for hypothesis testing.* Paper presented at the Annual Boston University Conference on Language Development, October, Boston.

Tallal, P., & Stark, R. (1980). Speech perception of language delayed children. In G. Yenikomshian, J. Kavanaugh, & C. Ferguson (Eds.), *Child phonology: Vol. 2.* (pp. 155–171). New York: Academic.

CHAPTER 25

Back to the Future: Research on Developmental Disorders of Language

PAULA TALLAL

In thinking about looking forward into the future and imagining what the next 10 years will bring in furthering our understanding of developmental language disorders, it is important to first look back to the past. In science, as in so many other areas, the accomplishments, as well as the failures, of the past greatly influence the directions for the future. So in looking into the future decade, we must do so by looking through the past decade.

In science, "facts" as well as cherished "myths" come to hold an esteemed place in our minds. Once established, it often takes more data to alter them than were originally required for their establishment. That is, once specific concepts enter our thinking about a particular topic, they take on a life of their own in guiding future theoretical constructs, which are the basis for future research. It may be for this reason that research often appears to be cyclical, with certain themes, techniques, or ideas dominating for a period of time and then residing.

Two important examples from the past come to mind. For a period of time you couldn't open a journal pertaining to the neural basis of speech and language without finding numerous papers reporting results of experiments using the dichotic listening technique (Kimura, 1967). There were literally hundreds or perhaps even thousands of papers published during the past decade reporting the results of dichotic listening studies. The enormous appeal of the dichotic listening paradigm was that it allowed us to investigate questions pertaining to hemispheric specialization in healthy subjects, using a noninvasive procedure. Previously, such questions could be addressed only by studying patients with brain lesions or by applying invasive procedures such as the Wada Test (Wada & Rasmussen, 1960). But with the development of the dichotic listening test, for the first time we could address questions pertaining to the normal distribution of function in the two cerebral hemispheres of normal individuals, using noninvasive, behavioral techniques. This was indeed an exciting breakthrough, and it is not surprising that studies of cerebral laterization and hemispheric specialization, specifically for auditory events including speech and language, dominated the research literature for almost a decade. To a great extent, as a result of research using this procedure, "hemispheric specialization" became a topic of household conversation. Hemispheric dominance was discussed at cocktail parties as well as in the popular press. It became "scientific folklore" that humans have a left, dominant hemisphere for speech and language, and a right, nondominant hemisphere that is more responsible for nonverbal events. I am not suggesting that this dichotomy had not already been well established in the scientific literature over a hundred years previously, based on case histories of patients with unilateral brain injury. However, once issues pertaining to cerebral laterization of function were able to be explored in normal subjects using noninvasive, behavioral procedures, research into hemispheric specialization absolutely exploded. Thus, the development of a model to explain how information is processed from the periphery through the cerebral hemispheres, and perhaps even more importantly, the development of a simple paradigm for testing this model in normal subjects, had a major impact on the direction of research for years to come.

A second example of how research trends develop and are maintained pertains to the role of visual perceptual deficits in children with developmental reading disorders. Based on the observation that developmentally dyslexic children have difficulty with reversible letters (such as *b* and *d*) and reversible words (such as *was* and *saw*), the hypothesis was developed that dyslexics "saw backwards." Indeed, to this day, the popular press perpetuates the notion that developmental dyslexia results from visual perceptual deficits that result in letter reversals. More than a decade of research focused on investigating the visual perceptual abilities of children with developmental reading impairments (Doehring, 1973). Although this research has taught us a great deal about patterns of strengths and weaknesses of dyslexic children, it has failed to support a hypothesis that dyslexic children "see backwards" or "read backwards." For example, research has shown that difficulties with visually reversible letters such as *b, d, g, p,* are likely attributable to phonological confusibility, as the sounds represented by these letters differ by only distinctive feature and also are characterized by an acoustic spectra incorporating rapidly changing formant transitions (Moscicki & Tallal, 1981; Tallal, 1984). The work of Isabelle Liberman and Donald Shankweiler and their colleagues has provided considerable data that now supports a model of reading disorders that is based on deficits in phonological analysis (Liberman & Shankweiler, 1979). The work in my laboratory has suggested that deficits in phonological analysis, themselves, may result from a more basic deficit in integrating acoustic information in the nervous system quickly in time (Tallal & Stark, 1981). Interestingly, more recent studies on dyslexia using eye movement techniques, electrophysiological techniques, and behavioral psychophysical techniques have indicated that the visual perceptual impairments that do occur in some dyslexics result from more general temporal integration deficits (Lovegrove, Martin & Slaghuis, 1986; Stark & Tallal, 1988; K. Gross-Glen, personal communication).

However, despite research advances in our understanding of the neural basis of developmental reading disorders, old "myths" die hard, even in science. A good example appeared on the front page of a prominent newspaper. In an article reporting the remarkable discoveries made by Galaburda and Kemper (1979) of specific and replicable neuroanatomical differences in the postmortem brains of dyslexic individuals, despite accurate reporting of the highly technical anatomical findings, the article began by describing dyslexia as a disorder in which children "read backwards"! Thus, research of the future must deal with the promises as well as the challenges created by research of the past.

As we approach the 1990s we can conclude that dyslexia does *not* result in most cases from a primary visual-processing deficit. Similarly, cerebral dominance for processing auditory information can no longer be conceived of as a simple left/right, verbal/nonverbal dichotomy. Left-brain damage, but not right-brain damage, has now been found to disrupt not only speech perception, but also the perception of *nonverbal*, rapidly changing stimuli (Tallal & Newcombe, 1978). Similarly, not all speech perception is disrupted by left-hemisphere damage. Rather, patients with left-hemisphere damage have particular difficulty in discriminating and producing speech sounds that are characterized by brief, rapidly changing temporal cues. (Tallal & Newcombe, 1978; Blumstein, Cooper, Zurif & Caramazza, 1977). Normal adult listeners show a right-ear advantage (left hemisphere specialization) not only for speech stimuli, but also for nonverbal stimuli incorporating rapid frequency modulations (Cutting, 1974). Similarly, not all speech stimuli show a right-ear advantage. Speech stimuli that are characterized by slowly changing or steady-state acoustics spectra are *not* processed preferentially by the left hemisphere (Cutting, 1974; Dorman, Cutting, & Raphael, 1975). Using the dichotic listening paradigm,

Schwartz and I showed that the degree of right ear advantage (left-hemisphere specialization) for speech discrimination could be significantly manipulated by altering the rate of change of the formant transitions within speech stimuli. In this study we demonstrated that normal adult listeners correctly reported significantly more speech stimuli (*ba, da, ga, pa, ta, ka*) presented to their right ear when these stimuli incorporated rapidly changing (40 msec) formant transitions. However, when the *duration* of the formant transitions within the same speech stimuli were computer extended to 80 msec, the advantage for the right ear was significantly reduced (Schwartz & Tallal, 1980).

Thus, we can enter the last decade of the 20th century with an altered understanding of hemispheric specialization for acoustic events, which is not based on a verbal/nonverbal dichotomy. We approach speech research in the 1990s with a new perspective, that the left hemisphere may be particularly specialized for temporal integration of rapidly changing sensory information, of which speech is a good example. This is not to suggest, of course, that the left hemisphere does not preferentially process language specific functions such as semantic representation (Neville, 1985). Rather, it suggests that the basic processes that underlie speech, and subsequently language perception and production, may not be specifically linguistic in nature.

In reviewing the state-of-the-art of research in language disorders, I would conclude that during the last decade, research has been primarily product or function oriented. That is, in the broad sense, language has been conceived of as incorporating receptive and expressive functions. These language functions have been further subdivided into phonology, morphology, syntax, semantics, and pragmatics. Each of these functions has been investigated separately. Furthermore, patients with language disorders have been characterized in terms of their patterns of ability and disability as they relate to these functions. For example Broca's aphasics have been characterized primarily as having difficulty with the expressive functions of speech and language, whereas Werniche's aphasics have more difficulty with receptive functions. Standardized language tests for children also allow for assessing receptive and expressive language functions, which can be further broken down into the individual component parts of language.

I anticipate that in the coming decade there will be a major shift in both clinical and theoretical thinking, away from function-based models and toward process-based models for language. Aphasiologists will focus more on the *processes* that are disrupted by differential brain damage and on how these disrupted processes manifest themselves in the language system of individual patients. Specifically, the effects of discreet brain damage on attention, perception, motor, memory, and conceptual processes, and how these interact with speech and language processes, will be the focus of research in the coming decade. I believe this to be the case for several reasons. First, the combination of research in speech and language disorders over the past several decades has resulted in the breakdown of previously held dichotomies and classifications such as the verbal/nonverbal dichotomy for hemispheric specialization and the expressive/receptive dichotomy for Broca's and Werniche's aphasias.

In the area of developmental language disorders, similar changes in perspective are emerging. For example, Susan Curtiss and I have come to some surprising conclusions based on findings from our longitudinal study evaluating the outcomes of early language impairments in children (Tallal, Curtiss, & Kaplan, 1988). In this study, 100 well defined children with specific developmental language impairment and 60 control children matched for age, I.Q., and SES were followed from ages 4 to 8 years. During this study children were assessed using receptive language measures, elicitation measures, and a free speech language sample. Based on standardized tests children were classified at the age of 4 years as having primarily an expressive language deficit or both receptive and expressive language problems. What we found as the result of detailed linguistic analyses was that although these children had serious developmental language delay, their problems could not be classified along specifically linguistic lines. Rather, we found that individual children performed the same linguistic function differently, depending on *different task processing demands.*

Children who had been classified as having primarily an expressive language deficit had a particularly hard time accessing their linguistic knowledge in a free speech setting. In such a setting the "expressively" impaired child may produce a language sample that suggests that he or she has not yet acquired specific linguistic rules (such as past tense or plurals). Quite surprisingly, however, the *same* child may demonstrate quite adequate mastery of the *same* linguistic rules under different task-processing constraints. For example, these children may respond quite normally to plurals or past tense in an expressive task where they are asked to complete a carrier phrase in an elicitation-type procedure or to point to an appropriate picture in a comprehension-type task. Conversely, children who had been diagnosed as having receptive language deficits demonstrated most difficulty in accessing their linguistic knowledge in tasks that were highly constrained by the experimenter, such as tasks that required the child to pay attention to a specific command or carrier phrase, hold information in memory, choose between competing alternatives, and formulate appropriate responses. However, the same "receptively" impaired children demonstrated adequate knowledge of the same linguistic structures that they had previously failed on comprehension and elicitation tasks when they were allowed to demonstrate their linguistic abilities in a free speech setting.

Importantly, results showed that whether the task required comprehension or expression of linguistic structure per se was *not* the determining variable. Rather, performance appeared to hinge on *nonlinguistic* task constraints. Based on these dramatic results, it seems appropriate that we change our interpretation of the nature of the deficit that we see in children with language impairments from a function-based concept to a process-based concept. That is, we see little evidence of specific linguistic deficits in these children. Rather, these children seem to be differentially characterized by the manner in which they are able to access, or fail to access, their linguistic knowledge under different *processing* constraints. This suggests that the deficit underlying developmental language disorders may be process, rather than function specific. "Receptive" language difficulty may result from an inability to focus attention on relevant aspects of the signal or to utilize sequential memory strategies appropriately in organizing incoming information, for example, rather than from difficulty in comprehending linguistic intent, per se. The *product* of such deficits may be a failure to comprehend linguistic intent. But the *process* that is at the root of the impairment may not, in itself, by language specific.

In the coming decade I would expect to see research in language disorders focusing on identifying the pattern of neural processes that characterizes different individuals, groups, or subgroups of patients who have been identified by common linguistic profiles. It should be the goal of such research to link specific neural substrates to specific neural processes, which in turn would be linked to specific linguistic functions. In order to accomplish this important goal as it pertains to the study of language disorders, advances in neuroscience, cognitive science, and speech and language sciences will need to be integrated.

There have been two recent advances toward such an integration that have enormous implications for research on speech and language disorders in the coming decade. The recent development of noninvasive brain imaging procedures has opened a remarkable window into the living human brain. Computed tomography (CT) scanning, magnetic resonance imaging (MRI), and positron emission tomography (PET) have revolutionized our ability to study the anatomy, morphology, and metabolic activity of the living human brain. The application of these technologies to patients with developmental communication disorders has provided, for the first time, an opportunity to evaluate their brain structure. Future advances in MRI and PET neurotransmitter labeling should open up even broader horizons for integrating hypotheses pertaining to brain structure and function, specifically as it applies to higher cortical function in humans.

In my laboratory, we have begun to apply several of these new technologies to individuals with developmental language and reading disorders. Jernigan, Hesselink, and I (1987, 1989) have recently reported the results of MRI studies in children with developmental language disorders. We found little evidence of frank brain damage, or even differences, in the posterior left hemisphere, as might have been hypothesized based on previous behavioral research. However, we did find significantly aberrant cortical asymmetries as well as subcortical differences, particularly in the area of the caudate nucleus, between language-impaired and normal children. Whereas only one language-impaired child showed frank lesions in the caudate region (Tallal, Jernigan, Trauner and Hesselink, submitted), the language-impaired children as a group showed significantly reduced volume in the size of the caudate area as compared to normal (Jernigan, Tallal & Hesselink, 1987; Jernigan, Hesselink & Tallal, submitted). Aram, Rose, Rekate, & Whitaker (1983) have also recently reported finding that children with caudate lesions show persistent deficits in speech and reading, whereas children with left hemisphere lesions do not. These results suggest that in the coming decade, research will focus more on understanding the pathways between subcortical and cortical systems and the neurotransmitters within these systems, which are important for processes that subserve language.

Research has also recently exploded in the area of cognitive science with the development of computational computer models that simulate higher cortical functions. These models provide important information that demonstrates top-down and bottom-up parallel processes for speech production, perception, reading, and other important cortical functions. Although the original computational models focused primarily on the reading process, more recent models for speech recognition and pronunciation have been developed (see McClelland & Rumelhart, 1987, for review). These models may prove to be exceptionally useful in conjunction with studies of developmental speech, language, and reading disorders. Having established a pattern of results from an impaired subject population, computer models can be used to simulate data to approximate that of the impaired subjects. Depending on the specificity and sophistication of the model, considerable information can be obtained by changing variables (which represent specific neural processes) in such a way as to simulate actual task performance of impaired subjects. Such an approach was used successfully by Christopher Chase in his recently completed doctoral dissertation (Chase, 1988) to study letter recognition processes in developmental dyslexia. The development of parallel distributed processing computational models has provided a new avenue of research, which, if correctly applied, will enhance our ability to conceptualize and model important higher cortical functions in humans.

My vision of the coming decade of research on language disorders is that it will be characterized as the decade of integration. We are in a unique position to integrate information from the neurosciences coming from the study of neuroanatomy, neurochemistry, and neurophysiology. Information being obtained by cognitive scientists through computational modeling of specific neural processes can also now be linked with information obtained from the clinical sciences pertaining to higher cortical function and dysfunction in humans. If we are to eventually understand brain/ behavior relationships underlying language disorders, such multidisciplinary scientific integration will be necessary. Cognitive scientists who are developing computational models have shown us the importance of parallel distributed processes. They've also shown us the equal importance of bottom-up and top-down analysis. Perhaps future research in our field can use such models as an analogy for progress. Neuroscientists can provide the key to the basic bottom-up processes. Cognitive and clinical scientists have a view from the top, that is the higher cortical functions in humans. It is my hope that the coming decade will hold the key to their integration through parallel, multidisciplinary interaction and collaboration.

REFERENCES

Aram, D. M., Rose, D. F., Rekate, H. L., & Whitaker, H. A. (1983). Acquired capsular/striatal aphasia in childhood. *Archives of Neurology, 40.*

Blumstein, S. E., Cooper, W. E., Zurif, E., & Caramazza, A. (1977). The perception and production of voice onset time in aphasia. *Neuropsychologia, 15,* 371–383.

Chase, C. H. (1988). Toward a distributed interactive model of developmental dyslexia. Unpublished doctoral dissertation, University of California, San Diego.

Cutting, J. E. (1974). Different speech-processing mechanisms can be reflected in the results of discrimination and dichotic listening tasks. *Brain and Language, 1,* 363–373.

Doehring, D. (1973). *Patterns of impairment in specific reading disability.* Montreal: McGill University Press.

Dorman, M. F., Cutting, J. E., & Raphael, J. (1975). Perception of temporal order in vowel sequences with and without formant transitions. *Journal of Experimental Psychology; Human Perception and Performance, 104,* 121–129.

Galaburda, A. M., & Kemper, T. L. (1979). Cytoarchitectonic abnormalities in developmental dyslexia. A case study. *Annals of Neurology, 6,* 94–100.

Jernigan, T., Hesselink, J., & Tallal, P. Cerebral morphology on MRI in language/ learning impaired children. Submitted to *Annals of Neurology,* 1989.

Jernigan, T. L., Tallal, P., & Hesselink, J. (1987). Cerebral morphology on magnetic resonance imaging in developmental dysphasia. *Society for Neuroscience Abstracts, 13*(1), 651.

Kimura, D. (1967). Functional asymmetry of the brain in dichotic listening. *Cortex, 3,* 163–178.

Liberman, I. Y., & Shankweiler, D. (1979). Speech, the alphabet, and teaching to read. In L. B. Resnick & P. A. Weaver (Eds.), *Theory and practice in early reading. Vol. 2.* Hillsdale, NJ: Lawrence Erlbaum.

Lovegrove, W., Martin, F., & Slaghuis, W. (1986). A theoretical and experimental case for a visual deficit in specific reading disability. *Cognitive Neuropsychology, 3,* 225–267.

McClelland, J. L., & Rumelhart, D. E. (1987). *Explorations in parallel distributed processing.* Cambridge, MA: MIT Press.

Moscicki, E., & Tallal, P. (1981). A phonological exploration of oral reading errors. *Applied Psycholinguistics, 2,* 353–367.

Neville, H. J. (1985). Effects of early sensory and language experience on the development of the human brain. In J. Mehler & R. Fox (Eds.), *Neonate Cognition: Beyond the blooming buzzing confusion* (pp. 349–363). Hillsdale, NJ: Lawrence Erlbaum.

Schwartz, J., & Tallal, P. (1980). Rate of acoustic change may underlie hemispheric specialization for speech perception. *Science, 207,* 1380–1381.

Stark, R. E., & Tallal, P. (1988). *Language, speech and reading disorders in children: Neuropsychological studies.* Austin, TX: PRO-ED.

Tallal, P., & Newcombe, F. (1978). Impairment of auditory perception and language comprehension in dysphasia. *Brain and Language, 5,* 13–24.

Tallal, P., & Stark, R. E. (1981). Speech acoustic-cue discrimination abilities of normally developing and language-impaired children. *Journal of the Acoustical Society of America, 69,* 568–574.

Tallal, P. (1984). Temporal or phonetic processing deficit in dyslexia? That is the question. *Applied Psycholinguistics, 5,* 167–169.

Tallal, P., Curtiss, S., & Kaplan, R. (1988). The San Diego longitudinal study: Evaluating the outcomes of preschool impairment in language development. In S. Gerber & G. Moncher (Eds.), *International perspectives on communication disorders* (pp. 86–126). Washington, DC: Galludet University Press.

Tallal, P., Jernigan, T., Trauner, D., & Hesselink, J. Developmental bilateral damage to the head of the caudate nuclei. Submitted to *Annals of Neurology,* 1989.

Wada, J., & Rasmussen, T. (1960). Intercarotid injection of sodium amytal for lateralzation of cerebral speech dominance. *Journal of Neurosurgery, 17,* 266–82.

Index